HORMONAL CORRELATES OF BEHAVIOR

Volume 2: An Organismic View

HORMONAL CORRELATES OF BEHAVIOR

Volume 1: A Lifespan View

Volume 2: An Organismic View

HORMONAL CORRELATES OF BEHAVIOR

Volume 2: An Organismic View

Edited by

**Basil E. Eleftheriou and
Richard L. Sprott**

The Jackson Laboratory
Bar Harbor, Maine

PLENUM PRESS • NEW YORK AND LONDON

Library of Congress Cataloging in Publication Data

Main entry under title:

Hormonal correlates of behavior.

Includes bibliographies and indexes.
CONTENTS: v. 1. A lifespan view.–v. 2. An organismic view.
1. Hormones. 2. Human behavior. 3. Animals, Habits and behavior of. I.
Eleftheriou, Basil E. II. Sprott, Richard L. [DNLM: 1. Behavior–Drug effects.
2. Hormones–Pharmacodynamics. WK102 E38h]
QP571.H65   599'.05   75-5938
ISBN 0-306-37504-4 (v. 1)
ISBN 0-306-37505-2 (v. 2)

© 1975 Plenum Press, New York
A Division of Plenum Publishing Corporation
227 West 17th Street, New York, N.Y. 10011

United Kingdom edition published by Plenum Press, London
A Division of Plenum Publishing Company, Ltd.
4a Lower John Street, London W1R 3PD, England

Printed in the United States of America

PREFACE

Our aim in this volume, as in Volume I, Hormonal Correlates of
Behavior: A Life Span View, has been to provide a critical assessment of the state of behavioral endocrinology as well as the more
usual summary of extant data. Each contributor was asked to probe
the strengths and weaknesses of his area as candidly as possible.
As a result, we hope the reader will find this Volume useful as a
reference source and as an honest evaluation of our present knowledge of the interaction between hormones and behavior.

                                            R. L. Sprott
Bar Harbor, 1975   B. E. Eleftheriou

CONTRIBUTORS

Robert Ader, Ph.D., Department of Psychiatry, University of Rochester School of Medicine and Dentistry, Rochester, New York 14642.

F. R. Brush, Ph.D., Experimental Psychology Laboratory, Syracuse University, Syracuse, New York 13210.

Robert M. Benson, M.D., Pediatric Endocrine Clinic, Children's Medical and Surgical Center, The Johns Hopkins Hospital and University, Baltimore, Maryland 21205.

John J. Christian, Sc.D., Department of Biological Sciences, University of New York at Binghamton, Binghamton, New York 13901.

David A. Edwards, Ph.D., Department of Psychology, Emory University, Atlanta, Georgia 30304.

Carl Eisdorfer, Ph.D., M.D., Department of Psychiatry and Behavioral Sciences, School of Medicine, University of Washington, Seattle, Washington 98101.

Basil E. Eleftheriou, Ph.D., The Jackson Laboratory, Bar Harbor, Maine 04609.

Merrill F. Elias, Ph.D., Department of Psychology and All-University Gerontology Center, Syracuse University, Syracuse, New York 13210.

Penelope K. Elias, Ph.D., All-University Gerontology Center, Syracuse University, Syracuse, New York 13210.

J. C. Froehlich, Ph.D., Experimental Psychology Laboratory, Syracuse University, Syracuse, New York 13210.

Roger A. Hoffman, Ph.D., Department of Biology, Colgate University, Hamilton, New York 13346.

Arthur Kling, M.D., Department of Psychiatry, Rutgers Medical School, Piscataway, New Jersey 08854.

James A. Lloyd, Sc.D., Program in Reproductive Biology and Endocrinology, The University of Texas Medical School at Houston, Houston,
Texas 77025.

Albert H. Meier, Ph.D., Department of Zoology and Physiology, Louisiana State University, Baton Rouge, Louisiana 70803.

Claude J. Migeon, M.D., Department of Pediatrics, Johns Hopkins
University, School of Medicine, Baltimore, Maryland 21205.

Howard Moltz, Ph.D., Committee on Biopsychology, Department of Behavioral Sciences, University of Chicago, Chicago, Illinois
60607.

John Money, Ph.D., Department of Psychiatry and Behavioral Sciences
and Department of Pediatrics, Johns Hopkins University School
of Medicine and Hospital, Baltimore, Maryland 21205.

Jack Panksepp, Ph.D., Department of Psychology, Bowling Green State
University, Bowling Green, Ohio 43403.

Murray Raskind, M.D., Department of Psychiatry and Behavioral Sciences, School of Medicine, University of Washington, Seattle,
Washington 98101.

Frank A. Rowe, Ph.D., Department of Psychology, Illinois Institute
of Technology, Chicago, Illinois 60607.

Michael H. Sheard, M.D., Department of Psychiatry, Yale University
School of Medicine, New Haven, Connecticut 06508.

Burton M. Slotnick, Ph.D., The American University, Washington,
D.C. 20000.

Richard L. Sprott, Ph.D., The Jackson Laboratory, Bar Harbor, Maine
04609.

Karen L. Stavnes, Ph.D., Department of Psychiatry and Behavioral
Sciences, University of Oklahoma Health Sciences Center, 800
N. E. 13th Street, Oklahoma City, Oklahoma 73190.

John G. Vandenbergh, Ph.D., Division of Research, North Carolina
Department of Mental Health, Raleigh, North Carolina 27602.

CONTENTS

VOLUME I

VOLUME II

CONTENTS

INTRODUCTION

Richard L. Sprott and Basil E. Eleftheriou

The myriad interactions between an organism and its environment, which contribute to its behavior, are the subject of this volume. It is both a fascinating and a frustrating subject. Any discussion of hormones and behavior can be made so complex as to be virtually unintelligible since the possible interactions between hormonal systems, feed back mechanisms, environmental conditions, and behavioral consequences are almost limitless. Too often, however, the temptation is to over simplify, with the underlying assumption that better science ensues, or at least that a naive reader can pick his way from tree to tree best by ignoring the forest. We hope we have chosen a middle ground. The contributors to this volume have presented their understanding of what is known in their respective areas. They have also attempted to point out the problems within given areas, and suggest the approaches needed to resolve these problems.

Eleftheriou's presentation emphasizes the great need for well controlled genetic experiments in all areas of hormones and behavior as a means of understanding the genetic control and influences upon the various behaviors involved. Until a few years ago, most of us had to resort to basic comparative data among and within various species to help us understand genetic variability and control. In recent years, however, the availability of new genetic strains, such as the recombinant inbred strains, opened new frontiers into the area of understanding genetic control of complex behaviors involved in hormones and their effects. Thus, the availability of genetic models which can be used to study physiologic, endocrine, and behavioral mechanisms facilitate an experimental approach to understanding complex interrelationships in hormones and behavior. The availability of strains where linkages of genes controlling various phenomena, such as Phr for pheromones, Bfo for bell-flash ovulation, Spl for serotonin, and Hnl for hypothalamic norepinephrine levels, gives us the first opportunity to attempt experimentation which will ultimately lead into the understanding of the complex relationships of genetic control of hormones and behavior. Such knowledge becomes invaluable as a tool for future research.

441

Dr. Meier makes a clear case for the importance of biological rhythms in the organization of an organism's behavior. He presents a comprehensive view of the relationship between the neuroendocrine system and cellular rhythms which accounts for circadian, estrous, lunar, and annual cycles of behavior. Dr. Meier's categorization of the roles of hormones as rhythm entrainers, modifiers and inducers provides some order in an otherwise hopeless welter of interactions. Thus, the entrainers, mainly catecholamines and adrenal corticosteroids, acting separately and synergistically appear to be the principal hormonal agents of entrainment. The modifiers, thyroid hormones and pineal gland products, influence the amplitude of the rhythms, the relations of individual rhythms to each other, and the sensitivity of the entraining system to the environment. The inducers act synergistically with the entraining hormones, stimulating those processes that are inducible at the time of day when the inducers are present. In short, the entrainers set rhythms of metabolic and behavioral responses to the inducers. The temporal relation of the daily rhythms of entrainers and inducers may be modified from day to day and produce the infradian cycles. Dr. Meier's approach is a novel one, but one which integrates the available knowledge in a comprehensible and realistic manner.

Possibly, one of the most significant advances in the area of endocrinology in recent years is the availability of a new and highly accurate technique for measuring levels of circulating hormones through radioimmunoassays. This permits us to measure, with a high degree of accuracy, hormones which had hitherto been assayed by rather crude techniques. Of the same magnitude of importance, is the recent recognition of the substances known as pheromones. Within the last 10 years, data has rapidly accumulated which indicates that pheromones play a significant and, often times, primary role in such diverse hormonal-behavioral relationships as acceleration of puberty, ovulation, pregnancy, learning, estrus activity, aggression, and perhaps other behaviors involving various systemic hormones. Vandenburgh's presentation emphasizes the importance of these substances in the daily life of the organism. In this instance, it should be emphasized that pheromologists owe considerable appreciation to the economic entomologist whose early work on insect pheromones gave considerable impetus to the field of mammalian pheromonology. Unfortunately, the remarkable success in identified insect pheromones and their utility to solve practical problems has not been shared in similar fashion in mammalian pheromones. Thus, biochemical identification and synthesis of mammalian pheromones, remains essentially untouched and open to expansive research. Additionally, we should stress the need for more detailed and expansive research in the specific area of behavioral alterations induced by pheromones or pheromonal communication. Here, the surface has not even been broached.

Slotnick gives us a masterful and successful presentation of the integrated neural and hormonal basis of maternal behavior. Although the available hormonal data far surpasses the information on neural basis of this behavior, an understanding of the integrative approach to the function and causative mechanisms involved in this rather complex behavior is presented. Thus, we see that lesions confined to the limbic system, particularly the cingulate cortex, hippocampus, septal area, and the related mammillary nuclei of the hypothalamus, cause severe disturbances in maternal behavior. Although, in view of such available data, the temptation is to ascribe such disturbances in the central nervous system that interfere with proper neuroendocrine reflexes, a role as the ultimate causes of deficits in maternal behavior. However, it appears that the disturbances caused by lesions in these brain regions may indeed have nothing to do with the concomitant disturbances in hormonal balance, but may affect maternal behavior of the postpartum animal without interfering with hormonal factors underlying the initiation or maintenance of maternal care. Indeed, it appears that deficits due to limbic lesions appear to stem from a disruption of sequential activities involved in maternal behavior. These lesions may alter the animal's perception of otherwise appropriate stimuli, or may disrupt pathways essential for integration of sequentially organised behaviors. Finally, it appears that the available studies have emphasized that brain lesions interfere with maternal care, but they have provided little information as to where in the nervous system hormones or experiential factors act to stimulate the onset of maternal behavior. According to Slotnick, it seems reasonable to assume that a neural substrate exists which is responsive to appropriate environmental and hormonal stimulation and, in turn, mediate the display of nesting, retrieving, nursing, and other activities involved in maternal behavior. As with all other areas where we have interaction of hormones, the central nervous system, and behavior, this area also needs further experimentation to help us understand the intricate relationships involved.

As Dr. Panksepp points out, the hope of finding a solution to serious human problems, such as obesity, by understanding and controlling the interaction between hormones and feeding behavior has made his area one of the most exciting in recent years. However, while his frank evaluation of the area acknowledges the great potential which exists, he clearly tells us how much we still don't know. While we are still not certain as to how hunger and feeding are regulated, the weight of the evidence points to a satiety factor produced in or monitored by the hypothatamus. Although the nature of this factor is the subject of considerable controversy, Panksepp's argument for a lipostat is quite persuasive. The most important contribution of this chapter, however, may well be his careful description of the actions of hormones as they modulate energy use and storage.

The pineal gland typifies the nature of the problems involved
in assessing interrelationships of organs secreting hormonal or
neurohumoral substances and the role of the substances upon various
types of behavior. It is ensconced in the deepest recesses of the
brain and although embryologically it is derived from the brain,
indications are that its neural input is supplied solely by the postsynaptic fibers from the superior cervical ganglia, as is the case
in the rat. From anatomical data derived from comparative studies
dealing with a number of different species, there are certainly variations on this anatomical relationship. Confounding the anatomical
situation is the nature of the relationship of neurotransmitters
that may be involved in stimulation, suppression, or modification
of this gland. Generally, the function of the pineal gland has remained enigmatic, due in large part to the fact that its removal
does not give rise to any consistent untoward effect and to the fact
that any presumed secretion is released in such minute amounts that
it cannot be easily detected in the circulatory system. Indeed,
as Hoffman points out a current controversy exists as to whether
the pineal secretes its products into the systemic circulation, or
into the cerebrospinal fluid of the third ventricle. However, it
appears that the pineal exerts a diversity of effects influencing,
directly or indirectly, such varied functions as the alpha rhythm
in electroencephalographic tracings, reproductive mechanisms, pho-
toataxis in pigment migration, spontaneous activity, wheel-running
activity, ethanol preference, exploratory activity, feeding and
drinking behavior, the pituitary gland in general, and a number of
other functions too numerous to mention here. The nature of the
control, the mediation and its causative mechanisms once again e-
ludes us at this time. However, we can tentatively ascribe to the
pineal a central role as a neurohumoral transducer by which environmental information of daily and seasonal time, superimposed upon
circadian rhythms, is directly or indirectly received and transmitted to the appropriate centroneural areas.

The chapters by Brush and Froehlich, Sprott and Stavnes can
be taken as a unit. Together, they cover the hormonal interactions
involved in an organism's attempt to adapt to its environment. All
three chapters clearly point out that in the area of learned behaviors, hormones have a role, but we know very little more than
this. Since research in this area is rarely conducted by endocrinologists and behaviorists working together, the literature is full
of over simplification and over optimism. The temptation is obvious:
problems of motivation, emotion, and learning are important and
solutions have enormous potential for improving the human condition.

As Dr.'s Brush and Froehlich point out, the major role of hormones in the control of adaptive behaviors is their modulation of
motivation. The role of hormones as modifiers of learning processes
is more difficult to assess. Sprott suggests that there is no con-

vincing evidence that hormones (other than neurotransmitters) have
demonstrable effects upon learning processes apart from their effects on motivation and activity. Hormones may effect the learning
process indirectly (e.g. steroids and thyroxin) by modifying the
action of neurotransmitters. On the other hand, the evidence that
neurotransmitters are directly involved in learning processes is
much more convincing. Dr. Stavnes provides a particularly lucid
description of the role of these biogenic amines in the modification of activity and avoidance learning behaviors. As the authors
of all three chapters point out, there are still many problems to
solve in this challenging area, not the least of which is the almost complete reliance upon avoidance studies for testing hormone-
learning hypothesis.

CHAPTER 12

HORMONES AND BEHAVIOR: A GENETIC APPROACH

Basil E. Eleftheriou, Ph.D.

The Jackson Laboratory
Bar Harbor, Maine   04609

CONTENTS

INTRODUCTION

"A hormone is a physiologic organic chemical agent liberated by living cells of a restricted area of the organism which diffuses, or is transported to a distant site in the same organism where it brings about an adjustment that tends to integrate the component parts and actions of the organism."

For many of us, the above definition of a hormone is reminiscent of our basic course in endocrinology. With such a definition, many an endocrinology teacher has attempted to encompass, in a short and concise description, the nature of a hormone: its specificity, its function, its integrative influences, its mode of transportation, its ultimate fate. If in a philosophical mood, most of us would argue - in the analogous pattern of the philosophers of the Middle Ages and their pins and angels: What is more crucial to the organism, a hormone, an enzyme, or a vitamin?

Time and space do not permit us the luxury of arguments ex cathedra or quid pro quo regarding hormones or their significance in the daily life of an organism. Most of us would accept the significant role these chemical substances play in living organisms. Indeed, since the dawn of history, many scientists have repeatedly attempted to understand functional systems, causative mechanisms, and chemical mediators of the living system. Possibly, with Hippocrates and his theory of the balance of humors, the basis was formed for a chemical (hormonal) concept of medical theory and treatment. Thus, the ancients, some Chinese but mostly Greeks observed that castrating bulls pacified them; administering burnt sponge reduced many symptoms of thyroid dysfunction; administering testicular tissue for sexual debility and impotence reduced the associated malfunction; fractionating human urine resulted in partially purified steroids for alleviating sexual problems associated with impotence (Needham & Gwei-Djeu, 1968). The accompanying behavioral observations probably formed the beginning of a concept of hormonal basis of behavior and the historical birth of psychoendocrinology. However, not until Berthold's (1849) classic experiments on castration and testicular transplants in fowl, which were accompanied by observations on behavioral alteration, did we receive the benefit of an experimental verification of some of the ancient concepts of the role of hormones and behavior.

Historically, Claude Bernard's observations on carbohydrate metabolism and behavior, and Canon's (1915, 1927) theory of fright, fight, or flight further emphasized the role of hormones in behavior. However, it was the publication of Hormones and Behavior by Dr. Frank Beach (1948) which resulted in the recent extensive interest in the areas of hormones and behavior. The hormonal determinants of behavior are manifold, and the role of hormones in behavior is well established. After all, the objective of this entire treatise was to summarize just this role. Thus, I shall not attempt to elaborate on various hormones and their respective influences on various behaviors in different species of animals. Rather, the objective of this chapter is to focus the attention on the availability and use of genetically defined species and, specifically, the mouse, for deriving optimum benefit when experimenting in the general area of hormones and behavior where genetic basis of such interaction is needed.

Early in the development of this field of hormones and behavior,
the comparative approach received considerable attention. Physiolog-
ically and metabolically, hormones were found to act identically in a
great number of species. The expression of a particular behavior e-
licited by each hormone, singly or in combination with other hormones,
however, could vary significantly. This particular finding attracteu
and still attracts the fascination of a great number of distinguished
comparative scientists dealing in this area. The generation of the
comparative data on hormones and behavior is now in geometric relationship to the number of investigators participating. Even within
a given species, however, this extensive accumulation of data has
not helped in elaborating causative or controlling mechanisms. In
reality, oftentimes we have been losing the "forest for the trees,"
and, thus, our ultimate objective within this area of hormones and
behavior.

THE GENETIC APPROACH

An alternative to the comparative approach is the use of strains
of a given species whose background is known. This approach offers
a unique insight into the genetic controlling mechanisms of hormones
and subsequent behavior, as well as the genetic control of behaviors
which may, in turn, influence hormonal levels. Unfortunately, the
availability of such strains is limited to a few species. Among
these, the one species where such availability is high and where
genes have been mapped is the house mouse, Mus musculus. In this
chapter, a brief discussion will be presented on the availability
of strains of mice that can be used for behavior-endocrine-genetic
experiments. In short, because of the obvious advantages of mouse
populations, the discussion will concentrate on three available
genetic systems of breeding: (a) inbred lines; (b) recombinant-
inbred lines; and (c) congenic lines. With these three basic genetic
procedures, an experimenter wishing to avail himself of these genetic
tools can enhance and further his research objectives dealing with
behavior and hormones.

Inbred Strains

The experimental approach of using various strains in comparative studies is used widely in the area of behavior and hormones.
Usually, the subjects can come from strains chosen with respect to
the same trait used in the comparison study. More frequently, the
strains were developed for quite different traits, oftentimes not
related to hormones and behavior. Inbred strains are maintained
not by selection, but by adherence to a particular mating system.
Comparisons between non-inbred stocks are also useful in hormones
and behavior. For example, the laboratory albino rat is significant-

ly different from those caught in the wild. Nevertheless, the
genetic homogeneity achieved by inbreeding provides a research
tool for which there is no substitute.

Inbreeding is the mating of animals more closely related than
the average, and its quantitative expression is in relative terms
which have reference only to a specified foundation stock in genetic equilibrium. All of the individuals of a given species are related to some extent, but usually only the closer degrees of relationship bear significance for the problem of inbreeding. Inbreeding is a relative concept, and its intensity varies over a wide
range because of the different types of inbreeding regimens that
are used. However, the brother-sister and parent-offspring matings
represent the most intense form possible with animals incapable of
self-fertilization, such as the mouse. Breeding to other families
within a strain, represents outbreeding with relation to the family group, but inbreeding (if families are related) with respect to
the species as a whole. The primary goal of inbreeding is to enhance the probability that offspring will inherit the same genes
from both parents. Thus, it leads to a decline in heterozygosis
and the fixation of genotypes. The rate of fixation is a function
of inbreeding intensity, and Wright's (1923) coefficient of inbreeding is designed to express the expected decrease of heterozygosis in relation to the original foundation stock. In contrast,
there is no way of expressing the degree of heterozygosis of a
random-bred stock in terms of the number of loci involved, although
knowledge of the origin and phenotypic variability of a group may
enable the experimenter to judge it as relatively great or small.
For clarification and theoretical treatment of the various inbreeding regimens, the reader is referred to any basic text in genetics.

Intense inbreeding over a long period of time leads to the
production of very homozygous stocks. Whether such stocks or
strains ever attain a completely isogenic state is quite unknown.
Usually, inbreeding is accompanied by a decline in vigor and reproductive capacity, although some strains are fertile and active after 50 or more generations of brother-sister matings. It is possible that the necessity of selecting for viability results in the
maintenance of some heterozygosity, but it must be relatively small
and can usually be neglected. The experimenter who uses these
strains, however, cannot assume that the removal of genotypic variants necessarily eliminates phenotypic variants. There is ample
evidence that homozygous individuals are less well buffered against
minor environmental agents and inbred animals may be no more uniform
in response than random-bred subjects (McLaren & Michie, 1956). The
use of Fl hybrids between any given inbred strains retains the advantages of genetic uniformity, while adding the advantages of superior developmental and physiological homeostasis. Most of the
evidence to support this view is derived from physiological and mor-

phological studies (Lerner, 1954). Unfortunately, however, there
are a few complications in applying the concept of developmental
homeostasis to behavioral characters, that can also be indirectly
associated to behaviors affecting hormones (Mordkoff & Fuller,
1959). An increase in behavioral variability which may, in turn,
effect hormones may actually facilitate aspects of physiological
homeostasis. An organism must develop in only one of a number of
possible patterns, and it can behave successfully in a multitude
of ways while affecting differentially the same hormones. Thus,
by necessity, this phenomenon of differential effects upon the
same hormones by different behaviors must be explained on the basis
of thresholds and related phenomenan. This complicates the genetic
approach to behavior and hormones considerably.

A hybrid between two inbred strains may actually be more variable than either parent if the hybrid genotype happens to fall in
a critical range for determination of a given trait. For example,
almost all C57BL/6J mice are resistant to audiogenic seizures,
and almost all DBA/2J mice are susceptible. Their F_1 hybrid is
intermediate, hence much more variable from individual to individual (Fuller & Thompson, 1960). However, in spite of this reser-
vation, F_1 hybrids are highly recommended for general experimental
purposes. In one instance, Meier (1964) has found less variability among F_1 hybrids than their respective inbred parents. Once
homozygosity has been reached, inbred lines retain their genetic
characters for long periods of time in the absence of outcrossing.
Over many generations, mutations will undoubtedly occur, and the
characteristics of the strain can change. However, general experience in biological research suggests that the drift is usually
small and unimportant over a given experimenter's lifetime. There
are some instances, however, wherein an occassional investigator
has described a cryptic mutation which altered the behavior of
mice of a line separated from the main one for 30 generations
(Denenberg, 1959).

It is imperative that the cautious investigator dealing in
genetic research with hormones and behavior should take steps to
prevent subline differentiation where possible. However, in reality, this is inevitable when stocks are separated over a period of
generations or by geographic necessity. A case in point is the
recently found differences in open-field behavior, corticosterone,
and hypothalamic norepinephrine levels in the subline C57BL/6J and
C57BL/6By which have been separated from each other for some time
(Eleftheriou, unpublished). To prevent such variability and a subline differentiation, comparisons with other workers will be facilitated if a breeding stock is regularly replaced from a mammalian
genetics center. Workers using the same source will have genetically nearly identical subjects. On a small scale, a controlled mating
system may be used to prevent diversification within a single colony.

Generally, however, the experimenter using inbred strains from a
genetic center should also be aware of the major effects upon mice
of different strains due to transportation, season of the year,
and general handling and housing within a given laboratory. Thus,
extreme caution should be applied to obtain results which approximate given environmental conditions. Different laboratory conditions may affect behavioral responses and, consequently, hormonal
levels due to hitherto unknown factors in a given experimental
laboratory (Sprott & Eleftheriou, 1974; Eleftheriou et al., 1975).

Genetic uniformity among animals within inbred strains implies
that differences in a given phenotype of individual mice of the
same strain are almost exclusively non-genetic in origin, except
for the necessary sex and occassional mutation dimorphism. Differences between strains which exceed the varibility observed within
them indicate phenotypic differences attributable to a difference
in heredity. Therefore, the amount of genetic determination can
be estimated statistically by comparing phenotypic variants between
and within inbred strains. This knowledge has been applied extensively in the area of behavior genetics, to a limited extent in
the area of genetics and hormones, but it has almost never been
applied to the area of behavior and hormones. Unfortunately, however, even comparative studies of given inbred strains that are
not followed by further crossbreeding or backcrossing of a given
trait provide, at best, the limited information that variation in
a particular trait characteristic is affected by genotype. In
short, it is not sufficient to study given traits in a number of
inbred strains.   Rather, for a true genetic approach one must
pursue the problem further by attempting to isolate the genetic
determinants of the particular trait. In order to accomplish this,
crossing and backcrossing of various strains, that usually exhibit
the extremes of a given trait, is necessary. This procedure of
crossing and backcrossing is time-consuming and the average investigator may find it not only experimentally unfeasible, but tedious
and expensive. As a consequence, many investigators have avoided
the pursuit of characterizing genetic controlling mechanisms of
particular traits which to them were of great interest.

In short, the detection of differences between pure breeding
stocks is only the first step of a genetic analysis. Segregation
and linkage analyses are additional necessary steps. Particular
investigators doing genetic research have found the majority of
the more interesting strain differences are usually controlled by
more than one pair of alleles, or are influenced by uncontrollable
environmental variation, or both. This situation usually prevents
Mendelian analysis of given traits. Even in instances where Mendelian
segregation ratios have been observed, linkage tests are usually laborious and uncertain. A given investigator who has ample animal
housing facilities, finances, and considerable time on his hands

can pursue the genetic characterization of a particular trait of his interest in order to obtain linkage. Unfortunately, however, usually only geneticists exhibit the patience required for this time-consuming approach. The average investigator interested in the area of hormones and behavior would rather have a tool which will offer him an answer in a rather short period of time since his major interest is not genetics.

Recombinant Inbred Strains: A New
Approach in Genetic Analysis

In recent years, the number of potential useful single-gene markers has increased as a result of the discovery of isozyme and immunological polymorphisms (Roderick et al., 1971; Snell & Cherry, 1971). These developments have increased the number of loci that can be followed in a linkage test, thus enhancing the probability of linkage detection (Hutton & Coleman, 1969). Unfortunately, however, typing individuals with respect to these loci is generally more laborious than typing for visible markers. Such typing is frequently destructive, precluding additional observations on the test animal. Recently, Bailey (1971) has developed a method of segregation and linkage analysis, the recombinant inbred strains (RI), that capitalizes very effectively on the existence of these cryptic genetic markers. This method offers a simple and unique approach to the detection of strain differences regarding segregation and linkage analysis. The method is generally applicable to otherwise difficult traits. The RI method's utility relies upon the fact that polymorphic variation is very extensive in cross fertilizing species (Lewontin & Hubby, 1966; Harris, 1966), a fact that is reflected in multiple genetic differences between inbred strains. Mammals have sufficient DNA to code for thousands of genes, and a significant proportion of loci exhibits polymorphic variation. Thus, unrelated strains differ by hundreds, possibly thousands, of genetic loci. The usual test for segregation and linkage analyses are limited since they only have a few loci that can be followed in a single segregant individual. The recombinant-inbred method developed by Bailey (1971) circumvents this difficulty by developing a number of inbred lines from the F_2 generation produced from the cross of two unrelated but highly inbred strains (Fig. 1). The recombinant inbred strains comprise a genetically fixed population of segregants at hundreds of loci that has continuity in space and time. Thus, this method, developed by Bailey, differs in principle from traditional approaches to linkage studies in that data gathered at different times and at different places are cumulative. Furthermore, this approach offers a workable procedure for extending segregation and linkage analysis to complex characters.

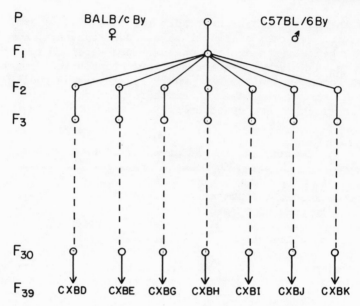

Fig. 1. Derivation of the recombinant-inbred strains from the inbred progenitor strains BALB/cBy and C57BL/6By. In the generations following the F_1, each RI strain was independently developed and maintained by a brother-sister mating regimen.

        The method is remarkably and uniquely simple. The RI strains were derived from the cross of two unrelated, but highly inbred progenitor strains, and then maintained independently from the F_2 generation under strict regimens of brother-sister inbreeding. This procedure genetically fixes the chance recombination of genes as full homozygosity is approached in the generations following the F_2 generation. The resulting battery of strains can be looked upon in one sense as a replicable recombinant population. The utility of such strains for analyzing gene systems is described elsewhere (Bailey, 1971). Of the several original RI strains developed, seven are now in existence (CXBD, CXBE, CXBG, CXBH, CXBI, CXBJ, and CXBK). These were derived from a cross of strains, BALB/cBy (C) by C57BL/6By (B6), followed by over 40 generations of full-sib matings. The letters D through K were arbitrarily chosen to denote the different strains, while the letters C and B denote the original progenitor strains which were crossed. Additionally, two reciprocal F_1 hybrids (B6CF$_1$ and CB6F$_1$) are also available. The rationale for the development of this genetic procedure is that linked genes will tend to become fixed in the same combinations (progenitor) as they entered the cross. Unlinked genes are randomly assorted in the F_2 generation and are, therefore, equally likely to be fixed in progenitor or recombinant

phases. Such a group of inbred strains may be thought of as a
fossilized segregating population.

In the actual use of these RI strains for segregation analysis,
it is expected that for a given trait which is controlled by a single pair of segregating genes, two classes of RI strains will be
apparent in equal frequency, the two classes resembling the two
progenitor strains. Generally, if the trait is controlled by more
than one pair of genes, intermediate or more extreme classes are
expected. In cases of epistasis, types to be expected may be
beyond and/or below the progenitor strains. If many segregating
loci influence the given trait, with small additive effects, a
continuous distribution of RI phenotypes is expected. Environmental factors and incomplete penetrance can be reduced to insig-
nificance by measuring numerous individuals from each strain.
Whereas the number of subjects required for a strain will depend
on the heritability of a given trait, the number of RI strains
required depends on the genetic complexity of that trait. If the
goal is to distinguish between one- and two-locus models with the
several types of epistasis possible, as many as 20 RI strains are
usually desirable. Those traits which are controlled by more than
two segregating loci are probably beyond the practical limits of
complete analysis, although it may be possible to detect a major
locus even when numerous minor loci are segregating. Detection
of a major locus in such cases will usually depend on the close
linkage of the major locus to a suitable marker.

The most important use of the RI strains is in the linkage
analyses per se. Once fixation is attained, no genetic changes
occur save mutation. Consequently, each RI strain needs to be
typed only once for a given character. Typing of the group RI
strains for a single locus defines a strain distribution pattern
(SDP) for that locus. This SDP can be compared with the SDP of any
other segregating locus, whenever the latter information becomes
available. If the respective SDP's reveal a significant excess
of progenitor types, linkage may not be possible. The SDP of a
particular locus identifies a chromosome region in which the locus resides. Once the RI strains have been characterized for numerous segregating loci scattered throughout the genome, newly discovered segregating loci can be mapped simply by typing each RI
strain. Although matching SDP's indicate possible identity or
close linkage of two loci, it should be kept in mind that two
SDP's may match merely by chance $[p = (\frac{1}{2})^k$, where k is the number
of RI strains$]$. As the linkage map becomes more complete, the
procedure would establish ultimately the correct order of the
genes, with the exception of closely linked factors.

In addition to detecting linkage, it is desirable to determine
the linear order of the genes on a given chromosome. The facility

with which multiple markers can be followed using RI strains lends
itself to chromosome mapping. The study of such genes confined to
a short segment of a chromosome is called fine structure analysis.
The RI strains lend themselves quite easily to fine structure analysis inasmuch as discrete products of recombination events can be
recovered an analyzed. Rather than deliberately attempting to un-
cover rare recombinants in specified regions, RI strains offer the
opportunity for analysis of recombination events where they occur.

The power of the RI strains for fine structure analysis can
be computed (Taylor, 1971). RI strains derived by brother-sister
mating have a mean of 0.04 of crossovers per centiMorgan (cM) per
line. In this respect, among 25 RI strains, one crossover would
be expected to have occurred on an average in some line for each
cM of chromosome (Taylor, 1971). Expressing this another way, a
chromosome 100 cM in length would be partitioned into approximately
100 parts. If inbreeding were delayed a number of generations beyond the F_2 generation, the opportunity of crossing over is increased, making the derived RI strains less valuable for linkage
detection, but more valuable for fine structure analysis. For
each generation of random mating prior to inbreeding, the probability of crossing over increases by 0.005 per cM per line. Thus, 8
generations of random mating prior to inbreeding doubles the utility
of these lines for fine structure analysis. This type of approach
might be impractical unless an F_2 derived, large, random mating
population, having been in existence for some time were available.
It is important that population size remain large during the period
of random mating, in order to minimize genetic drift and the attending complications (Taylor, 1971).

Congenic Lines

In the ultimate analysis, the RI strains have been enhanced
in their utility by the availability of additional lines of mice.
This battery of mice is called congenic lines, and they are not to
be confused with the RI strains. The congenic lines were developed
independently from the initial cross of C57BL/6By to BALB/cBy by a
regimen of skin-graft testing and backcrosses to B6 for at lease 12
generations. This procedure resulted in congenic B6 lines, each of
which differ from B6 itself by only an introduced chromosomal segment including a C-strain allele at a distinctive histocompatibility
(H) locus. Each of these congenic lines has been tested against
RI strains by means of skin-grafts to find which of the RI strains
carry the C-strain allele and which the B6 -allele at a particular
H locus, thereby establishing their strain distribution patterns
(SDP). A brief outline of the regimen followed for the development of the congenic lines is presented in Fig. 2.

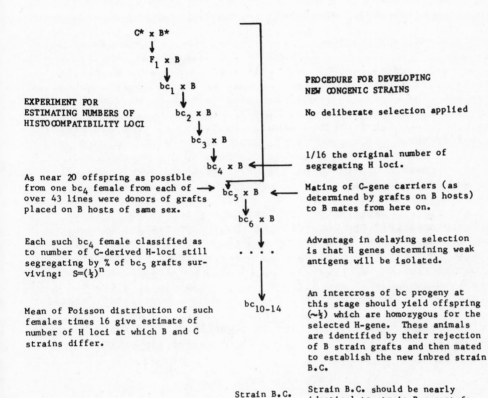

EXPERIMENT FOR
ESTIMATING NUMBERS OF
HISTOCOMPATIBILITY LOCI

PROCEDURE FOR DEVELOPING
NEW CONGENIC STRAINS

No deliberate selection applied

As near 20 offspring as possible
from one bc_4 female from each of
over 43 lines were donors of grafts
placed on B hosts of same sex.

1/16 the original number of
segregating H loci.

Mating of C-gene carriers (as
determined by grafts on B hosts)
to B mates from here on.

Each such bc_4 female classified as
to number of C-derived H-loci still
segregating by % of bc_5 grafts surviving: $S=(\frac{1}{2})^n$

Advantage in delaying selection
is that H genes determining weak
antigens will be isolated.

Mean of Poisson distribution of such
females times 16 give estimate of
number of H loci at which B and C
strains differ.

An intercross of bc progeny at
this stage should yield offspring
($\sim\frac{1}{4}$) which are homozygous for the
selected H-gene. These animals
are identified by their rejection
of B strain grafts and then mated
to establish the new inbred strain
B.C.

Strain B.C.

Strain B.C. should be nearly
identical to strain B except for
the selected difference at a
single H locus.

*C-BALB/c mouse strain)
 B=C57BL/6 mouse strain) Any two inbred strains may be employed
 bc=backcross progeny
 n=number of H-loci

Fig. 2. Bailey's method for the development of new congenic lines
and for estimating numbers of histocompatibility (H) loci. Repro-
duced by personal consent of Dr. D. W. Bailey.

Fig. 2 summarizes briefly Bailey's (1971) development of the congenic lines which he has used recently to good advantage in analyzing the complex murine histocompatibility system. In short, it should be emphasized that both the congenic lines and the RI strains are used for functional genetic analysis in order to establish linkage with the least amount of effort.

In actual application of this system, when a given trait is analyzed, the SDP of the RI strains is considered and examined with SDP of other traits already available through research of other investigators. When an SDP matches that of the locus represented by an existing congenic lines, the latter line is then tested for that particular trait. In order for linkage to be detected, the congenic line which is tested usually must resemble the BALB/cBy progenitor strain in regard to the trait of concern. This is necessary because of the nature of the development of the congenic lines. When such correlation of a given trait between a congenic line and BALB/c occurs, it is concluded that a locus, at which differences in that trait are determined, is linked or is pleiotropic with the histocompatibility locus carried by the congenic line. If the histocompatibility locus, carried by the particular congenic line, has been mapped on a chromosome then the subsequent trait which an investigator examines is also determined. By comparing the position of the F_1 hybrids, one is also able to determine whether there is dominance for the high or the low aspects of a trait. Additionally, if the reciprocal F_1 hybrids do not exhibit any significant differences between each other, maternal effects are also eliminated. Conversely, if there is significant difference between the two reciprocal F_1's, maternal effects can be suspected.

APPLICATION OF THE METHOD

The RI method of genetic analysis combined with a congenic line approach possesses a unique advantage in that one can determine quickly the probable location of a new gene by matching its pattern of distribution with those of other genes among a set of inbred strains that already have been developed. This is a great advantage over conventional approaches but derived from the replacement of the individual by the RI line as a unit of segregation. By the use of the RI method, one is able to identify genetic determinants in a short time, since the RI lines are already available and, in most instances, do not necessitate further crosses of various types as, for example, is the case with conventional Mendelian analysis. Additionally, the RI method has the advantage over conventional approaches in that (a) tissue from different individuals within an RI line may be pooled without introducing genetic heterogeneity; (b) once the RI strains are established, the time dealy required for production of the segregating generations can be avoided; (c) the

Table 1. SUMMARY OF THE VARIOUS LOCI IDENTIFIED THROUGH THE USE OF THE RI STRAINS AND CONGENIC LINES BY ELEFTHERIOU AND CO-WORKERS (1972-1974).

Symbol	Explanation	Chromosome (Linkage Group)	Possible Action or Influence	Reference
Aal	Active avoidance learning performance	9(II)	Active avoidance performance in shuttle box	Oliverio & Eleftheriou, 1973
Bfo	Bell-flash ovulation	4(VIII)	Ovulatory response in females following exposure to intermittent ringing of bell or flashing of high intensity light	Eleftheriou & Kristal, 1974
Cpl-1 Cpl-2	Corticosterone plasma levels	- -[†]	Circulating plasma levels	Eleftheriou & Bailey, 1972
Cpz	Chlorpromazine	9(II)	Modification of avoidance behavior by chlorpromazine	Castellano et al., 1974
Eam	Ethanol activity modifier	4(VIII)	Modification of toggle box activity by ethanol	Oliverio & Eleftheriou, 1975
Exa	Exploratory activity	4(VIII)	Exploratory activity in toggle box	Oliverio et al., 1973
Hnl	Hypothalamic norepinephrine activity levels	unknown[*]	Activity levels of hypothalamic norepinephrine	Eleftheriou, 1974
Phr	Male pheromone	- -[†]	Pheromonal facilitation of ovulation in PMS-primed females	Eleftheriou, 1972
Sco	Scopolamine	17(IX)	Scopolamine effects on exploratory activity	Oliverio et al., 1973
Wra	Wheel-running activity		Influences activity level in wheel	Eleftheriou, 1975

(*) The locus exerting an influence on hypothalamic norepinephrine activity levels is linked to the histocompatibility gene, H-23, whose linkage group is as yet unknown.

(†) In these two instances, no linkage was obtained.

recessive characteristics of both progenitor strains are expressed
in RI strains; (d) genetic differences tend to be maximized due to
the elimination of heterozygotes; (e) genetic associations, due to
either pleiotropy or linkage may be detected between traits expressed in utero, adult characteristics - male limited traits and
female limited traits - and traits that require killing individuals
at different stages or require different pretreatments, and (f) the
F_1 hybrid of the progenitor lines accepts tissue or organ grafts
from any of the RI strains.

Thus, using this approach of recombinant-inbred strains and
congenic lines, Eleftheriou and co-workers have identified and, in
some instances have found the linkage of genes that control various
behavioral and hormonal determinants (Table 1). It should be emphasized that all this work by Eleftheriou and co-workers was conducted within the short period of approximately three years. Using
conventional techniques, the same amount of work would, in all
probability, have absorbed many times that amount of time. Thus, the
utility of the RI strains is typified in the economy of time, which
is of prime interest to the investigator dealing with a hybrid
science such as gentics, behavior and endocrinology.

Table 1 presents genetic analyses dealing with various loci
that exert a controlling influence upon a number of behaviors, drug
and hormonal changes. Additionally, a number of other genetic studies were conducted that led to clarification of some of the biochemical aspects of morphine-binding protein in the brain and analgesia
(Shuster et al., 1975; Barran et al., 1975), effects of halothane
anesthesia on learning (Elias & Eleftheriou, 1975), and several
others which are not necessary to mention here.

In reality, the reader may question the wisdom of continuing
such investigations when, in essence, the relationship between
genetics, behavior, hormone or drug has not been clarified, nor
have the causative mechanisms underlying this relationship been
amplified. In answer to this, one may underscore the significance
of this research and the embryonic stage that it presently occupies.
It is now time to apply this available knowledge. The proposed
uses of the available information could be amplified quite extensively. However, because of the brevity of space, I should like
to only concentrate on one example. This deals with the relationship of the locus dealing with active avoidance learning (Aal),
hypothalamic norepinephrine (Hnl), and serotonin (Spl).

For some time now, there has existed an impressive body of
evidence indicating that disturbances in serotonin metabolism in
the brain can lead to profound changes in behavior of human beings
and laboratory animals. Similarly catecholamines, and serotonin,
have been extensively implicated, in various significant altera-

tions of behavior (Woolley, 1962; Woolley & Shaw, 1954a, 1954b).
The impetus for controlled direct determinations of these amines
in the brain, and their relationship to learning behavior was initiated by the early work of Woolley and van der Hoeven (1963) who
reported that high amounts of cerebral serotonin decreased maze-
learning ability of adult mice, whereas a decline in both serotonin
and catecholamines improved it. However, subsequent research into
the role of these amines in learning behavior, using methods of
direct determination as well as indirect methods of estimation
through the use of various pharmacologic inhibitors, blocking
agents, or competitors have both confirmed and negated some of the
original assumptions. We now possess evidence that rats depleted
of brain norepinephrine display facilitation of acquisition of a
shuttle-box response (Cooper et al., 1973), or exhibit a decrement
in motor activity and shuttle-box avoidance responding (Hanson,
1967; Rech et al., 1966, 1968). This abvious contradiction has
been clarified, at least partially, by the recent work of Ahlenius
and Engel (1971) who reported that norepinephrine plays a significant role in the effective performance of conditioned avoidance
behavior, but that dopamine must be present in order to maintain
this function. Furthermore, the same investigators (Ahlenius &
Engel, 1972) in a later study, as well as Nakamura and Thoenen
(1972), reported indications of hyperirritability with significant
reduction in brain norephinephrine. Based on these findings, one
must postulate that the obvious contradictions, in the various
studies previously cited, may well be due to differential levels
of inhibition of norepinephrine. Thus, it must follow that a
critical level of these amines is necessary for exhibiting various
degrees of enchancement or decrement of avoidance behaviors. Alternatively, we must consider the probability that different concentrations of the inhibitors used in these studies result in
significant changes in the equilibrium constants and homeostatic
mechanisms maintained in free, bound, and turnover rates for each
amine or for a combination of brain amines.

Of some significance is the finding that conditioned reactions,
especially the negatively reinforced conditioned avoidance responses
that are significantly altered by changes in brain amine levels,
can be reversibly reinstated, but there exists a species and strain
specificity regarding the degree of reinstatement (Orshinger, 1961;
Herz, 1960; Oakley, 1963; Seiden & Hanson, 1964; Seiden & Carlsson,
1963, 1964). Thus, it must be assumed that strong genetic determinants play a dominant role in the mediation and response of each
species of animal. Similar results have been obtained with specific
experiments dealing with memory and recall associated with avoidance
behaviors (Murphy & Henry, 1972; McFarlain & Bloom, 1972). These
results, however, are not surprising inasmuch as recent data reported by Eleftheriou (1971) indicate significant differences in
norepinephrine disappearance rates in a number of mouse strains.

An additional point that deserves emphasis is the experimental approach used by the various investigators who have dealt with the subject. For a number of years, results from experiments dealing with localization of electrolytic lesions or electrical stimulation of specific brain regions underscored the importance of the regional approach to neural phenomena associated with behavior, physiology, or endocrinology. Unfortunately, either due to lack of advanced technology or due to personal bias of a particular investigator, most of these studies ignored the importance of analyzing amine changes in various regions of the brain. Instead, the entire brain was usually considered as a single entity, and regional brain determinants of behavior and neurochemistry were ignored. Only recently have attempts been made to explore the significance of the relationship of behavior and amine concentrations in various brain regions rather than in the entire brain. Thus, Wimer et al (1973) report significant differential activity in serotonin and norepinephrine associated with mouse strain (C57BL/6J vs. DBA/2J) and brain region analyzed (amygdala, frontal cortex, hypothalamus, and hippocampus). Similarly, experiments with rats indicate differential changes in regional brain norepinephrine resulting in specific behavior associated with particular brain region (Anlezark et al., 1973). Thus, it now becomes imperative that genetic studies of a highly sophisticated nature be undertaken to analyze and elucidate the mechanisms involved in these relationships.

One manner in which such genetic studies can be conducted is by analyses which determine whether the single locus active avoidance effect (Aal) and the single locus controlling either serotonin (Spl) or hypothalamic norepinephrine (Hnl) are the same or are indeed quite different. In short, the relationship between active avoidance learning and brain serotonin and norepinephrine which has been postulated for some time can be clarified in a short period of time, at least in the mouse, using the available information derived from the recombinant-inbred strains. Additionally, I should emphasize that the same type of approach can be implemented to clarify relationships between other loci as, for example, wheel-running activity (Wra) and corticosterone (Cpl-1 or Cpl-2) and norepinephrine levels (Hnl). Thus, confirmation of the possible genetic control and linkage for any combination of these traits offers a new tool of enormous importance for the study of genetic, behavioral and endocrine relationships.

In conclusion, it is hoped that this short presentation has offered some awareness to those interested in pursuing the genetic approach to behavior and hormones to offer them unique ways in which they can pursue their respective interests in this general area. It is hoped that the reader may be stimulated to take up this approach.

REFERENCES

AHLENIUS, S., & ENGEL, J., 1971, Behavior and biochemical effects
    of L-DOPA after inhibition of dopamine-β-hydroxylase in reser-
    pine pretreated rats. Naunyn-Schmiedebergs Arch. Pharmakol.
    270:349.

AHLENIUS, S., & ENGEL, J., 1972, Effects of dopamine-β-hydroxylase
    inhibitor on timing behaviour. Psychopharmacologia 24:243.

ANLEZARK, G., CROW, T. J., & GREENWAY, A. P., 1973, Impaired learn-
    ing and decreased cortical norepinephrine after bilateral locus
    Coeruleus lesions. Science 181:682.

BAILEY, D. W., 1971, Recombinant-inbred strains: an aid to finding
    identity, linkage and function of histocompatibility and other
    genes. Transplantation 11:325.

BARAN, A., SHUSTER, L., ELEFTHERIOU, B. E., & BAILEY, D. W., 1975,
    Opiate receptors and analgesic response in mice: Basis for
    genetic difference. Brain Res. (in press).

BEACH, F. A., 1948, Hormones and Behavior, Harper (Hoeber), New York.

BERTHOLD, A. A., 1849, Transplantation der Hoden, Arch. Anat. Physiol.
    u. wiss. Med. 16:42.

CANNON, W. B., 1915, Bodily Changes in Pain, Hunger, Fear and Rage,
    Appleton, New York.

CANNON, W. B., 1927, The Janus-Lang theory of emotions: a critical
    examination and an alteration. Amer. J. Psychol. 39:106.

CASTELLANO, C., ELEFTHERIOU, B. E., BAILEY, D. W., & OLIVERIO, A.,
    1974, Chlorpromazine and avoidance behavior: A genetic analy-
    sis. Psychopharmacologia 34:309.

COOPER, B. R., BREESE, G. R., GRANT, L. D., & HOWARD, J. L., 1973,
    Effects of 6-hydroxydopamine treatments on active avoidance
    responding: evidence for involvement of brain dopamine. J.
    Pharmacol. & Exp. Ther. 185:358.

DENENBERG, V. H., 1959, Learning differences in two separated livers
    of mice. Science 130:451.

ELEFTHERIOU, B. E., 1971, Regional brain norepinephrine turnover
    rates in four strains of mice. Neuroendocrinology 7:329.

ELEFTHERIOU, B. E., 1973, A gene influencing hypothalamic norepinephrine levels in mice. <u>Brain Res</u>. (in press)

ELEFTHERIOU, B. E., & BAILEY, D. W., 1972a, Genetic analysis of
plasma corticosterone levels in two inbred strains of mice.
<u>J. Endocrinol</u>. 55:415.

ELEFTHERIOU, B. E., & BAILEY, D. W., 1972b, A gene controlling
plasma serotonin levels in mice. <u>J. Endocrinol</u>. 55:225.

ELEFTHERIOU, B. E., BAILEY, D. W., & ZARROW, M. X., 1972c, A gene
controlling male pheromonal facilitation of PMS-induced ovulation in mice. <u>J. Reprod. Fert</u>. 31:155.

ELEFTHERIOU, B. E., & KRISTAL, M. B., 1974, A gene controlling
bell- and photically-induced ovulation in mice. <u>J. Reprod.
Fert</u>. 38:41.

ELEFTHERIOU, B. E., ELIAS, M. F., CHERRY, C., & LUCAS, L. A.,
1975, Wheel running activity: A genetic investigation.
Physiol. & Behav. (in press).

FULLER, J. L., & THOMPSON, W. R., 1960, Behavior Genetics, Wiley,
New York.

HANSON, L. C. F., 1967, Biochemical and behavioral effects of tyrosine hydroxylase inhibition. <u>Psychopharmacologia</u> 11:8.

HARRIS, H., 1966, Enzyme polymorphisms in man. <u>Proc. Roy. Soc.
Lond</u>. 164:298.

HERZ, A., 1960, Drugs and the conditioned avoidance response. <u>Int.
Rev. Neurobiol</u>. 2:229.

HUTTON, J. J., & COLEMAN, D. L., 1969, Linkage analyses using biochemical variants in mice. II. Levulinante dehydratase and
autosomal glucose 6-phosphate dehydratase. <u>Biochem. Genet</u>.
3:517.

LERNER, I. M., 1954, Genetic Homeostatis, Wiley, New York.

LEWONTIN, R. C., & HUBBY, J. L., 1966, A molecular approach to the
study of genic heterozygosity in natural populations. II.
Amount of variation and degree of heterozygosity in natural
populations of <u>Droxophila pseudobscura</u>. <u>Genetics</u> 54:595.

MCFARLAIN, R. A., & BLOOM, J. M., 1972, The effects of PCPA on brain
serotonin, food intake, and U-Maze behavior. <u>Psychopharmacolo-
gia</u> (Berl.) 27:85.

MCLAREN, A., & MICHIE, O., 1956, Variability of response in experi-
    mental animals. A comparison of the reactions of inbred F1
    hybrid, and random bred mice to a narcotic drug. J. Gent.
    54:440.

MEIER, G., 1964, Differences in maze performances as a function of
    age and strain of house mice. J. Comp. Physiol. Psychol. 58:
    418.

MORDKOFF, A. M., & FULLER, J. L., 1959, Heritability of activity
    within inbred and crossbred mice: A study in behavior genetics.
    J. Hered. 50:6.

MURPHY, D. L., & HENRY, G. M., 1972, Catecholamines and memory:
    enhanced verbal learning during L-DOPA administration. Psy-
    chopharmacologia (Berl.) 27:319.

NAKAMURA, K., & THOENEN, H., 1972, Increased irritability: a
    permanent behavior change induced in rats by intraventricular
    administration of 6-hydroxydopamine. Psychopharmacologia
    24:359.

NEEDHAM, J., & GWEI-DJEN, L., 1968, Sex hormones in the Middle Ages.
    Endeavour, 27:130.

OAKLEY, S. R., 1963, The effect of tranquilizers on positively and
    negatively motivated behavior rats. Psychopharmacologia (Berl.)
    4:326.

OLIVERIO, A., ELEFTHERIOU, B. E., & BAILEY, D. W., 1973a, Explora-
    tory activity: genetic analysis of its modification by
    scopolamine and amphetamine. Physiol. & Behav. 10:893.

OLIVERIO, A., ELEFTHERIOU, B. E., & BAILEY, D. W., 1973b, A gene
    influencing active avoidance performance in mice. Physiol.
    Behav. 11:497.

OLIVERIO, A., CASTELLANO, C., & ELEFTHERIOU, B. E., 1975, Morphine
    sensitivity and tolerance: A genetic investigation in the
    mouse. Psychopharmacologia (in press).

OLIVERIO, A., & ELEFTHERIOU, B. E., 1975, Motor activity and alcohol:
    Genetic analysis in the mouse. Pharm. Biochem. & Behav. (in
    press).

ORSHINGER, O. A., 1961, The effects of monoamine oxidase inhibitors
    on the deconditioning action of reserpine in rats. Psycho-
    pharmacologic (Berl.) 2:326.

RECH, R. H., BORYS, H. K., & MOORE, K. E., 1966, Alterations in behavior and brain catecholamine levels in rats treated with α-
methyltyrosine. J. Pharmacol. Exp. Ther. 153:412.

RECH, R. H., CARR, L. A., MOORE, K. E., 1968, Behavioral effects of
α-methyltyrosine after prior depletion of brain catecholamines.
J. Pharmacol. Exp. Ther. 160:326.

RODERICK, T. H., RUDDLE, F. H., CHAPMAN, V. M., & SHOWS, T. B.,
1971, Biochemical polymorphisms in feral and inbred mice.
Biochem. Genet. 5:457.

SEIDEN, L. S., & CARLSSON, A., 1963, Temporary and partial antagonism
by L-DOPA of reserpine-induced suppression of a conditioned
avoidance response. Psychopharmacologia (Berl.) 4:418.

SEIDEN, L. S., & CARLSSON, A., 1964, Brain and heart catecholamine
levels after L-DOPA administration in reserpine treated mice:
correlations with a conditioned avoidance response. Psychopharmacologia (Berl.) 5:178.

SEIDEN, L. S., & HANSON, L. C. F., 1964, Reversal of the reserpine-
induced suppression of the conditioned avoidance response in
the rat by L-DOPA. Psychopharmacologia (Berl.) 6:239.

SNELL, G. D., & CHERRY, M., 1972, Loci determining cell surface
alloantigens. In RNA viruses and host genome in oncogenesis,
p. 221-228. P. Emmelot & P. Bentvelzen (eds.). North-Holland
Publishing Co., Amsterdam.

SPROTT, R. L., & ELEFTHERIOU, B. E., 1974, Open-field behavior in
aging inbred mice. Gerontologia 20:155.

SHUSTER, L., WEBSTER, G. W. YU, G., & ELEFTHERIOU, B. E., 1975, A
genetic analysis of the response to morphine in mice: Analgesia
and running. Psychopharmacologia (in press).

WIMER, R. E., NORMAN, R. L., & ELEFTHERIOU, B. E., 1973, Serotonin
levels in hippocampus: striking variations associated with
mouse strain and treatment. Brain Res. (in press).

WOOLLEY, D. W., 1962, The Biochemical Basis of Psychoses. Wiley,
New York.

WOOLLEY, D. W., & SHAW, E., 1954a, A biochemical and pharmacological
suggestion about certain mental disorders. Proc. Nat. Acad.
Sci. U.S. 40:228.

WOOLLEY, D. W., & SHAW, E., 1954b, The role of catecholamine in mental disorders. Brit. Med. J. 1954-II:122.

WOOLLEY, D. W., & VAN DER HOEVEN, T., 1963, Alteration in learning ability caused by changes in cerebral serotonin and catecholamines. Science 139:610.

WRIGHT, S., 1923, Mendelian analysis of pure breeds of livestock. I. The measurement of inbreeding and relationship. J. Hered. 14: 339.

CHAPTER 13

CHRONOENDOCRINOLOGY OF VERTEBRATES

Albert H. Meier, Ph.D.

Department of Zoology and Physiology
Louisiana State University
Baton Rouge, Louisiana   70803

CONTENTS

INTRODUCTION

Research in biological rhythms has grown rapidly since 1960.
However, the study of biological clocks is a relatively old area
of research having begun almost 250 years ago. Bünning (1967)
has attributed the first demonstration of an endogenous time sense
within living systems to de Mairan, an astronomer, in 1729. De
Mairan discovered that the daily alternation of the opening and
folding of the leaves of a plant persisted underground in the absence of external photoperiodic cues.

The subsequent history of research in biological rhythms is
an interesting lesson in itself. Insufficient credit has been
given to the thin line of naturalists who continued to study biological clocks often in the face of ridicule or studied indiffer-

ence. Although widely discussed in Europe, no one bothered to duplicate de Mairan's simple experiment for 30 years. Significant
new research was reported in 1832 by De Candolle who also studied
leaf movements, cited by Bünning (1967). He found that the daily
rhythm persisted in continuous light with a period of 22.5 to 23.0
hours. In addition, he discovered that the phase of the leaf rhythm
could be reversed by inverting the daily schedule of light and dark.
Thus, the daily cycle of illumination did not directly cause the
rhythm but it did entrain or synchronize the phase of the rhythm.

Sustained work with animals began during the late 1920's.
Most of these early studies were performed with invertebrates and
involved rhythms of behavior such as locomotor activity and orientation. It gradually became evident that many daily cycles that
were thought to result from reactions to environmental changes
were actually endogenous rhythms that persist under constant conditions of temperature and light. The periods of the free-running
rhythms were found to approximate 24 hours (<u>circa dies</u>), but to differ sufficiently so that, the phases of the rhythms tend to drift
with no obvious environmental entrainment. Temperature has little
influence on the periods of the rhythms, although it may sometimes
act as an entrainer. The principal environmental time setter
(entrainer or synchronizer) is the daily photoperiod.

The presence of endogenous daily rhythms of organismal behavior
indicate that there must also be rhythms of neural and metabolic
activites supporting them. One of the first studies of a physiological rhythm in vertebrates was made by Forsgren (1928, 1935) who
reported a daily rhythm of liver glycogen content in mice. During
the past 40 years, innumerable reports have documented the existence
of daily rhythms of oxygen consumption, of daily variations in blood
and urinary concentrations of metabolites and electrolytes, and of
other manifestations that the internal environment is not constant,
but rather periodic.

Although much of the substantive work, at the cellular level,
has been done with organisms such as unicellular algae, it is now
evident that endogenous daily, or circadian, rhythms are present in
individual cells as well as in multicellular organisms. That is,
the individual cell measures out the basic unit of biological time,
the circadian rhythm. Because the cellular clocks are imprecise and
the periods of the rhythms tend to vary from 24 hours and from each
other, they must be synchronized in order to produce organismal
rhythms. The neuroendocrine system is peculiarly well suited to
monitor the environmental cues and to transmit that information to
the cells so that the individual rhythms may be organized for the
production of meaningful physiological and behavioral integration
of the organism within itself and in relation to its environment.
The hormones that seem most likely to be involved would be those

produced by nervous tissues, or those dependent on neurohormones. These hormones include catecholamines and the hormones of the pituitary and the pineal glands.

The importance of biological rhythms was not immediately recognized by the majority of vertebrate physiologists and endocrinologists. They labored under a dogmatic view that physiological mechanisms were simply homeostatic systems in which the principal function was to maintain a constant internal condition despite a changing external environment. The presence of daily variations seemed merely to indicate that the internal mechanisms lagged somewhat in reacting to the environmental cycles.

Although endocrinologists were slow to discover the significance of rhythms, they have since responded with an avalanche of research reports. Already, it is impossible to provide a complete review of research in hormone rhythms in an article of this scope. In addition, only tentative conclusions can be drawn at this stage of exponential growth of knowledge with the hope that they may serve as guidelines for further research and with the expectation that some of them will be proven incorrect within an embarrasingly short time. Although this review is restricted to vertebrate studies, it should be remembered that much of this research was inspired by studies that were first performed with plants and invertebrate animals.

DAILY RHYTHMS OF ADRENAL CORTICOIDS

General Characteristics

The corticosteroid hormones are among the most important hormones in the vertebrates. They are best known for their roles in mineral and carbohydrate metabolism. But their activities are extremely diverse. Because the corticoids are recognized as potent and basic hormones, it is not surprising that a considerable amount of research has been accomplished with respect to their daily rhythms. This research has centered on the glucocorticosteroids such as cortisol and corticosterone which respond to stimulation by adrenocorticotropic hormone (ACTH) elaborated by the adenohypophysis.

A daily rhythm in the concentration of corticosteroids was first reported by Pincus (1943) who found a daily rhythm of urinary excretion of corticoid metabolites in young men. These studies were continued and expanded by Halberg and his coworkers (1959), and by numerous other investigators who reported daily rhythms of plasma corticoid concentrations in vertebrate species ranging from fish (Boehlke et al., 1966; Garcia & Meier, 1973) to fowl

(Boissin & Assenmacher, 1971; Dusseau & Meier, 1971; Joseph & Meier, 1973) and from mice (Halberg et al., 1959) to man (Bartter et al., 1962).

In many of the animals investigated, the phase of the corticoid rhythm is apparently controlled by the daily schedule of light and dark. For example, a change in the schedule of the daily photoperiod is followed by an appropriate shift in the phase of the corticoid rhythm. In some instances, the hormonal shift is immediate and in others it occurs gradually over a period of days.

In a detailed study of the Japanese quail, Coturnix coturnix, a shift in the light-dark schedule resulted in almost immediate adjustments in the concentration rhythm of plasma corticosterone (Boissin & Assenmacher, 1971). The corticoid rhythm could be entrained to a 35-hour day (26L:9D) as well as to a 13-hour day (6L:7D). Variations in plasma concentrations of corticoids and ACTH in rats and humans can also be entrained by an ultradian (< 20 hours) or an infradian (> 28 hours) light cycle (Orth et al., 1967). These findings seem to stretch the definition of a circadian rhythm.

In the human, the cycles of sleep and wakefulness and of activity and rest do not have fixed relations to the daily alternation of light and dark. The cycle of sleep and wakefulness has often been postulated to synchronize the corticoid rhythm. These conclusions were largely drawn from studies of night workers. Adrenal responses to reversals in the sleep-wakefulness pattern varied considerably from one study to another. Rephasing of the plasma rhythm of corticoids required 4 to 8 days (Perkoff et al., 1959) or longer than two weeks (Weitzmann et al., 1968). On the other hand, Migeon and coworkers (1956) reported that partial reversal of the activity cycle had no modifying effect on the rhythm of plasma corticoids. Unfortunately, it was often not possible to control the light-dark conditions in these studies. In continuous light or continuous dark, a sleep-wakefulness cycle does entrain a corticoid rhythm that is similar in phase with one entrained by an illumination cycle when the onset of light is equated with the onset of wakefulness (Krieger et al., 1969).

It now seems clear that the light-dark cycle is a principal entrainer for corticoid rhythms in humans as well as in other animals even when the activity cycle does not coincide with it. Neither continuous activity for 48 hours (Halberg et al., 1961) nor complete bed rest for 36 hours (Reinberg et al., 1970), or even as long as 54 days (Vernikos-Danellis et al., 1972), had any appreciable effect on the expected normal pattern of corticoid concentrations (See Fig. 1).

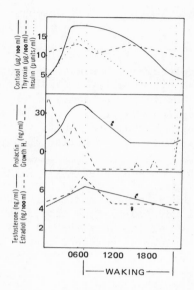

Fig. 1. Daily patterns of plasma hormone concentrations in humans. A composite of the literature.

Orth and his coworkers (Orth et al., 1967; Orth & Island, 1969) performed a series of studies in which they varied the cycle of sleep and wakefulness with respect to the schedule of light and dark. In one study, darkness was prolonged for 4 hours after awakening. After an adaptation period of 2 weeks, they found that the peak phase of the 17-hydroxycorticosteroid rhythm coincided with the onset of light indicating that the cycle of illumination rather than that of activity set the rhythm. However, in other studies in which the relations of the sleep-wakefulness and illumination cycles were varied, there were sometimes two peaks in the daily corticoid rhythm, one apparently set by the illumination cycle and the other set by the sleep-wakefulness cycle. In these instances, one peak occurred at the onset of light and the other occurred at the onset of the activity period.

In addition to the normal peak occurring early during the photoperiod, a second daily peak of urinary excretion of ketosteroids was found in men during the evening shortly before a daily exercise period (De Lacerda & Steben, 1974). The second peak developed after one week of exercise and disappeared within a few days after the exercise regimen was halted. It appears that the second peak reflects an anticipatory or preparatory response of the adrenal for locomotor activity. Although rhythms of urinary ketosteroids have been interpreted to reflect rhythms of adrenal activity, a portion of the urinary ketosteroids are derivatives of the testes. Consequently, it might be useful to repeat this interesting experiment using assays that are more specific for adrenal corticoids.

Because varying the phase of corticoid rhythm with respect to other hormonal rhythms may have important consequences on metabolism and behavior (discussion in subsequent sections), the production of secondary corticoid peaks bears further investigation. Auxilliary peaks in humans may be produced by the sleep-wakefulness cycle if it does not coincide with the effective daily photoperiod, and perhaps by daily periods of exercise (DeLacerda & Steben, 1974) or social contact (Mills, 1966). In addition, Krieger and coworkers (1971) found 2 minor peaks that coincided with the times of feeding (noon and evening). Although these peaks persisted for 2 days after feeding was stopped and replaced with continuous intravenous glucose administration, the findings that circadian rhythms may persist for 2 days in adrenal tissue cultures (Andrews & Folk, 1964) would indicate that feeding may still have accounted for these minor peaks.

The limitation of water availability to one hour during the day also modifies the plasma corticosterone rhythm in rats (Coover et al., 1971; Johnson & Levine, 1973). The principal peak occurred shortly before the time of watering regardless of its relation to the photoperiod and the time of the normal peak. This anticipatory peak resembles the one observed in the urinary excretion of ketosteroids in subjects undergoing a daily exercise regimen (DeLacerda & Steben, 1974) in that both alterations require more than a week to develop. It also follows that stresses that cause the release of corticosteroids would influence the pattern of hormonal relations and cause changes in physiological conditions if repeated often enough (Meier et al., 1973). Abnormalities in the daily rhythm of plasma cortisol have been reported in patients with psychic depression (Fullerton et al., 1968; Jacobsson et al., 1969). If the abnormal rhythm has a causative influence on the behavior, it might be worthwhile to treat the rhythm. In turn, the treatment might involve simple behavioral adjustments.

According to a strict interpretation, a daily rhythm must persist for at least 2 complete cycles in conditions of constant light intensity in order to be considered an endogenous daily, or circadian, rhythm. In this sense, the adrenal cycle of mice is circadian in that it persists under conditions of continuous dark (Halberg et al., 1953). In rats maintained in continuous light, some (Dunn et al., 1972) have reported that the rhythm of plasma corticosterone concentration persists whereas others (Cheifetz et al., 1968) have reported that the rhythm is eliminated. A loss of the daily rhythm in concentration of plasma corticosterone was also reported for the common pigeon after 15 days in continuous light (Joseph & Meier, 1973). Conroy & Mills (1970) cited a study in which the plasma cortisol rhythm was found to disappear in a man during the time that he spent 4 months underground with no external cues.

Pathways for Photoperiodic Entrainment

Photoperiodic entrainment of any rhythm implies the existence

of photoreceptors. Critchlow and coworkers (1963) tested whether
the eyes are necessary for photoperiodic entrainment of the rhythm
of plasma corticosterone in rats. They found that the corticoid
rhythm became free-running following optic enucleation in rats
maintained on a daily schedule of light and dark. However, destruction of the rod layer of the rat retina by prolonged exposure
to continuous light did not prevent subsequent entrainment by a
daily photoperiod (Dunn et al., 1972). Other cell types may have
been involved because the blinded rats could still respond to light-
dark patterns. Blinding by interruption of the optic nerve modifies or abolishes the rhythms of ACTH and of the plasma corticoids
in rats and mice (Saba et al., 1965; Haus et al., 1964, 1967;
Halberg, 1969). Haus and coworkers (1964) observed that the hormone rhythm persisted in blinded mice but the phase of the rhythm
was the inverse of that found in normal animals. Curiously, in-
version of the rhythm of plasma corticoids has also been noted in
dogs following ablation of the olfactory bulbs (Arcangeli et al.,
1973). After 2 months, the phase of the rhythm returned to normal.
Blindness may be accompanied by differences in the plasma cortisol
rhythm in humans (von Hollwich, 1969; Bodenheimer et al., 1973).
Because the daily rhythm in humans may also be influenced by the
activity schedule, it is difficult at this time to decide what role
the photoperiodic regimen may have in entraining adrenal corticoid
rhythms in the blind.

The available data seem to indicate that some cells in the eye
of mammals are sensitive to photoperiodic cues and that this information is passed along the optic nerve. However, there appear to be
other sensors located elsewhere. In the absence of the eye, these
sensors and pathways may still exert an entraining effect on the
rhythm of the corticosteroids although the phase angle of the rhythm
with respect to the photoperiod may differ from that found in normal
animals. The multiplicity of photosensors that are involved in the
entrainment of daily rhythms is well established and a role for
special external photoreceptors as parts of entraining mechanisms is
the exception rather than the rule among the vertebrates as well as
the invertebrates (review, Menaker, 1972).

Pathological conditions have sometimes proved beneficial in
understanding normal regulatory mechanisms in humans. Plasma corticoid rhythms were lost in patients with pretectal and temporal lobe
diseases (Krieger, 1961; Oppenheimer et al., 1961; Alvisi & Ferrara,
1969) and in patients with lesions of the fornix (Ganong, 1969).
Mason (1958) also reported that section of the fornix as well as
damage to the hippocampus in monkeys caused a loss in the normal
daily variations in plasma corticoids. Krieger & Krieger (1966)
studied 48 patients with focal diseases of the central nervous system and found that plasma corticoid rhythms were disturbed but that
there was no loss of consciousness nor of the normal sleep pattern.

Abnormalities of the daily pattern of plasma cortisol levels have been reported in some cases of pituitary tumors with suprasellar extension (Hokfelt & Luft, 1959; Osterman et al., 1973). In most instances, however, it is not possible to discern whether the areas involved are integral parts of the neural mechanism controlling the corticoid rhythms or whether they have one of a multitude of indirect or permissive influences.

In rodents, there is considerable justification for the view that the daily rhythm reported in concentration of plasma corticosterone (Guilleman et al., 1959; Halberg et al., 1959a; McCarthy et al., 1960; Glenister & Yates, 1961) depends on a daily rhythm of release from the adrenal cortex (Halberg et al., 1959b; Retiene et al., 1968) that in turn is driven by a daily release of pituitary ACTH (Cheifetz et al., 1968; Retiene et al., 1968) resulting from the stimulation of a daily rhythm of hypothalamic corticotropin releasing factor (CRF) Ungar, 1964; Cheifetz et al., 1969; Hiroshige & Sakakura, 1971; David-Nelson & Brodish, 1969; Seiden & Brodish, 1972). Although a rhythm of hypothalamic CRF is present in adrenalectomized as well as hypophysectomized rats, the phases of the peak values are shifted several hours earlier than in the normal animal (Hiroshige & Sakakura, 1971; Takebe et al., 1972). Isolation of the medial basal hypothalamus (Halasz et al., 1967; Palka et al., 1969) and lesions in the suprachiasmatic nucleus (Halasz, 1969) and median eminence (Saba et al., 1969) abolishes the normal daily rhythm in rats. In addition, cortisol is secreted episodically in humans with quiescent periods between secretory intervals (Weitzmann et al., 1966; Hellman et al., 1970), and the correspondence between the times of peaks of plasma corticoid levels and those of ACTH levels is good (Berson & Yalow, 1968). A daily rhythm of CRF was also reported for the common pigeon and its phase appears to precede by 4-6 hours the phase of the rhythm of plasma corticosterone (Sato & George, 1973).

Although the evidence appears to build a strong case for a pituitary role in regulating a daily rhythm of plasma adrenal corticosteroids, the proofs are correlative. Because the rhythms of CRF, ACTH, and adrenal and plasma corticosteroids are in synchrony, the evidence suggests the possibility but does not necessarily prove that one rhythm depends on another.

A direct test for pituitary involvement was made on a teleost fish, Fundulus grandis (Srivastava & Meier, 1972). The regulation of adrenal cortical activity is essentially the same in fish and other ectothermic vertebrates as in the endothermic vertebrates. However adrenal cortical tissue in fish is capable of producing reduced amounts of hormones sometimes for several weeks following hypophysectomy. Pituitary ACTH is necessary for the long-term maintenance of adrenal function. Following hypophysectomy, a clear daily variation in plasma cortisol concentration was still present

in <u>Fundulus grandis</u> after 15 days. Although the levels were lower
than those in the intact fish, the pattern appeared to be identical.
In addition, inverting the photoperiod caused the phases of the
rhythms to invert in the hypophysectomized as well as in the intact
fish (Fig. 2).

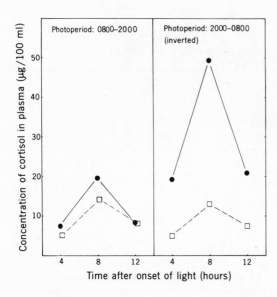

Fig. 2. Daily variation in
concentration of cortisol in
plasma of intact (circles)
and hypophysectomized
(squares) <u>F. gradis</u> at two
12-hour daily photoperiods
(light from 0800 to 2000,
and from 2000 to 0800).
From Srivastava & Meier,
Science <u>177</u>, 185-187 (1972).
Copyright 1972 by the American Association for the Advancement of Science.

Similar studies were performed with the laboratory rat (Allen
<u>et al</u>., 1972) and the Japanese quail, <u>Coturnix coturnix</u> (Boissin
<u>et al</u>., 1971). However, in these studies the adrenal cortex was
supported in the hypophysectomized animals by heterotopic pituitary
transplants under the kidney capsule. The daily rhythm of plasma
corticosterone persisted in hypophysectomized rats, and the pattern
was similar to that in the normal rats. Because pituitary transplants were present, the authors concluded that hypothalamic CRF
may have been released periodically into the blood and subsequently
induced a daily rhythm of release of ACTH from the transplants. This
possibility needs to be reexamined in view of the study with hypophysectomized fish. Although Boissin and coworkers (1971) were unable to demonstrate a statistically significant rhythm of plasma
corticosterone with a limited number of quail, the daily pattern of
the corticosterone concentrations appear similar to that found in
normal birds.

There is evidence that the adrenal stress response and the daily
rhythm of plasma corticoids involve separate mechanisms. The stress
response depends on the release of pituitary ACTH in all vertebrates
tested, including fish (Donaldson & McBride, 1967). The pituitary,
however, is not necessary for the entrainment of a daily rhythm of

plasma cortisol in a fish (Srivastava & Meier, 1972). In addition,
lesions in the medial basal hypothalamus in rats affect the daily
rhythm of the adrenal corticoids but they do not prevent the stress
response (Osterman et al., 1973). Another difference is that
stress is followed by an increase in plasma corticoid levels within a few minutes, generally reaching maximum levels in 15-30 minutes
and subsiding to former levels in less than 2 hours (Ader et al.,
1967) whereas the interval between the release of CRF or ACTH and
the increase of plasma corticoid levels may be 2 hours or more
(see Hiroshige et al., 1973; Sato & George, 1973). In addition,
Hiroshige and coworkers (1973) discovered that a sharp peak of hypothalamic CRF occurred at 0800 (photoperiod:0600-1800) in normal
female rats and at 1200 in ovariectomized rats but the phases of
the plasma corticosterone rhythms were the same in both groups with
peaks at 1600.

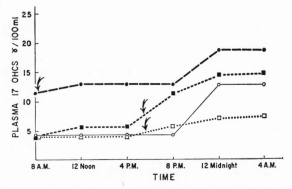

Fig. 3. Effect of atropine administered in different dosages and at
different time of day on circadian pattern of plasma 17-OHCS in a
cat (No. 224). Arrows indicate time of administration of drug. Key:
O———O, control day: □———□, atropine, 1.2 mg subcutaneously (0.4
mg/kg) at 6 p.m.; ■———■, atropine 0.6 mg subcutaneously (0.2 mg/kg)
at 6 p.m.; ●———●, atropine, 1.2 mg subcutaneously at 8 a.m. From
Krieger & Krieger, Science 155:1422 (1967). Copyright 1967 by the
American Association for the Advancement of Science.

Cholinergic mechanisms appear to be involved in the regulation
of the corticoid rhythm. Injections of atropine, an anticholinergic
agent, blocked the expected daily rise in plasma corticosterone in
rats when injections were made 4 hours earlier (Krieger & Krieger,
1967). Atropine was ineffective at other time (Fig. 3). Although
atropine blocked the daily rise of plasma concentrations, it did
not block the adrenal response to ACTH, the pituitary-adrenal response to vasopressin, or the hypothalamic-pituitary-adrenal response to insulin-induced hypoglycemia or bacteria-induced stress.
Further, the plasma corticoid rise produced by intrahypothalamic im-

plants of cholinergic agents was blocked with prior atropine administration but not by prior administration of dexamethasone which has a strong negative feedback on ACTH production. These findings also indicate a degree of separation of the systems controlling the stress response and the daily rhythm of plasma corticoids. Because many of the antihistamine drugs have atropine-like activities, it might be worthwhile to determine whether they alter the daily rhythm of corticosteroids in humans.

Pentobarbital, a depressant of the central nervous system, similarly blocked the expected daily rise of plasma corticosterone levels in rats (Krieger & Krieger, 1967). This drug is recognized for its ability to block ovulation in rodent estrous cycles and avian egg-laying cycles. Morphine has also been reported to alter the daily rhythm of plasma corticosterone concentrations in rats (McDonald et al., 1959).

Catecholaminergic mechanisms have been investigated in rats with regard to a possible role in regulating corticoid rhythms. Injections of 2 drugs (k-methyl-p-tyrosine or 6-hydroxydopamine) that reduce brain catecholamine concentrations caused an increase in plasma concentrations of corticosterone 4 to 11 hours later, and L-dopa, a precursor for norepinephrine, partially prevented the effect (Scapagnini et al., 1970; Van Loon et al., 1971; Jori et al., 1973). On the other hand, Ulrich & Yuwiler (1973) were unable to abolish the daily rhythm of serum corticosterone in rats by injections of 6-hydroxydopamine although it reduced total brain norepineprine and dopamine by 29% and 53%, respectively.

Although not usually considered, sex differences in the rhythms of plasma corticoids and hypothalamic CRF have been reported. In a teleost fish, Fundulus grandis, during the reproductive season there was a bimodal pattern of plasma cortisol concentrations in males and a unimodal pattern in females (Garcia & Meier, 1973). In the laboratory rat, the sex differences are even more curious (Hiroshige et al., 1973). Although the plasma rhythms of corticosterone were similar in males and females with peaks at the onset of dark, the phases of the rhythms of hypothalamic content of CRF differed markedly. The peak occurred at 1800 in males and at 0800 in females (photoperiod:0600-1800). Ovarian hormones were responsible, apparently, for only a part of the differences. This finding provides additional reason to question the concept that CRF rhythms drive plasma corticoid rhythms by way of ACTH rhythms.

Ontogeny of Corticoid Rhythms

The ontogeny of hormone rhythms has received little attention and the studies are almost entirely restricted to the adrenal corticoids in rats. There is general agreement that the mature adult rhythm in rats forms at some time between 21 and 30 days of age (Allen & Kendall, 1967; Ader, 1969; Ramaley, 1973). Ramaley (1973) reported that daily rhythms were present at day 18 (females) and 19 (males), but that the phases of the rhythms differed from the adult pattern that was developed by day 26. By way of contrast, the corticosterone response to either stress began on day 15 (Allen & Kendall, 1967) and a rhythm of hypothalamic CRF content was fully developed during the third week (Hiroshige & Sato, 1970). The adult rhythm of the adrenal corticoids in humans is established between one and 3 years of age (Franks, 1967).

If postnatal rats are handled often, the maturation of the rhythms of both plasma corticosterone and of locomotor activity can be advanced to as early as day 16 (Ader, 1969). On the other hand, large doses of cortisol on days 2 to 4 virtually suppressed the rhythm of plasma corticosterone at day 30 and severely reduced growth rates (Krieger, 1972). These results suggest the possibility that early experiences may have lasting influences on the animal by affecting hormone rhythms.

Functions of Corticoid Rhythms

Studies concering the regulation of adrenal corticoid rhythms received considerable incentive from the discoveries that the corticoid rhythms have important roles in physiology and behavior. Pincus (1943) was first to associate daily rhythms of glucocorticoids with another rhythm. Pincus found a daily rhythm of blood eosinophil concentrations and demonstrated that this rhythm depends on a daily rhythm of adrenal corticoids. Halberg and coworkers (1953, 1959a) carried out further studies with mice which demonstrated that the daily rhythms of blood eosinophils and lymphocytes depended on the corticoid rhythm.

Because many of the early studies of vertebrate rhythms involved the monitoring of locomotor activity, the studies by Halberg and his coworkers (Halberg, 1959, 1962; Halberg et al., 1959b) which associated the rhythms of the adrenal cortex with daily rhythms of locomotor activity provided convincing information that the endocrine system has a central role in regulating organismal rhythms. At the time Halberg initiated his studies, knowledge of the adrenal cortical response to stress had conditioned many to assume that increased concentrations of plasma corticoids should be expected as the consequences of increased tensions of living and that a daily rhythm of corticoid levels would result from a daily rhythm of locomotor activity. Halberg and coworkers, however, demonstrated that the daily rise in concentrations of plasma corticoids preceded by several hours the onset of daily activity in both the nocturnally active mouse as well as in the diurnally ac-

tive mouse as well as in the diurnally active human. They concluded that the daily increase in plasma corticoids was preparatory for daily activity rather than a consequence of the activity
(Fig. 4). A role for adrenal corticoids in regulating avian migratory activity is discussed later.

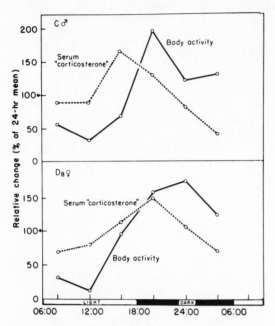

Fig. 4. Daily changes in
gross body activity of two
populations of mice in relation to corresponding
changes in serum cortico-
sterone. The latter rhythm
leads the former. From
Halberg et al., Endocrin-
ology 64, 228-230, (1959).

Several studies support a role for a daily rhythm of adrenal
corticoids in affecting the nervous system. The peak of the daily
rhythm of general activity of the EEG in humans is preceded by 1-2
hours by the peak of the daily rhythm of plasma corticoids (Frank,
1961; Frank et al., 1966). Several hours also elapse from the
time of cortisol injection to the peak of brain sensitivity measured by electroshock seizure thresholds and to the time of intra-extra-
cellular electrolyte and amino acid fluxes in rat brain (Woodbury
et al., 1957). Thus an interval of time may be involved between an
increase in plasma corticoid concentrations and the neural responses.
Whether this lag is sufficient to account for the apparent unrelated-
ness of the daily rhythms of the corticoid hormones and the rhythm
of locomotor activity in the meadow vole (Seabloom, 1965) and the
common pigeon (Joseph & Meier, 1973) is unclear. In the diurnally
active pigeon, the daily rise of plasma corticosterone occurs early
during the dark hours of 12 and 16-hour daily photoperiods. In
evaluating possible entrainers or synchronizers of daily rhythms,
such as the corticoid hormones, it should be recognized that an
entrained event may occur up to 24 hours after the entraining stimulus. A synergistic role of prolactin and corticosterone in regulating locomotor activity in a migratory sparrow is discussed in
the section titled ANNUAL CYCLES.

The peak of the plasma cortisol rhythm in humans was reported to lead the peak of the intraocular pressure in glaucomatous eyes by about 4 hours, and disruption of the corticoid rhythm disrupted the rhythm of intraocular pressure (Boyd & McLeod, 1964). Adrenalectomy also abolished the daily rhythm of paradoxical sleep in rats (Johnson & Sawyer, 1971). Metyrapone, an inhibitor of corticosterone and cortisol synthesis, obliterated the daily rhythm of learning ability in rats (Stroebel, 1967).

Responses to drugs administered at different time of day has attracted considerable interest. Reinberg and his associates (Reinberg et al., 1965, 1969) studied the cutaneous response to intradermal injections of histamine in humans. They found a peak near midnight and a trough in the morning. Response rhythms with similar phases were also observed in allergic subjects given scratch tests with penicillin and house dust. The phases of these rhythms were approximately the reciprocal of normal rhythms of plasma corticoids which tend to reduce allergic reactions. On this basis the authors concluded that allergic response rhythms are caused by the plasma corticoid rhythms.

Daily rhythms of activity of several liver microsomal enzymes have been positively correlated with the rhythm of the plasma corticoids (Radzialowski & Bousquet, 1967, 1968; Jori et al., 1971). Hickman and coworkers, (1972) reported that the daily rhythm of cholesterolgenesis in rat liver was removed by adrenalectomy. In addition, Rapoport and coworkers (1966) found a relation between the daily variations of mouse liver tryptophan pyrrolase (TP) activity and those of plasma corticosterone. They also reported that adrenalectomy abolished the pronounced enzyme rhythm. On the other hand, adrenalectomy did not remove the rhythm of rat liver tyrosine k-ketogulutarate transaminase (TKT) Wurtman & Axelrod, 1967). Both TP and TKT activities can be induced by glucocorticoids.

The rhythm of mitosis has been investigated with respect to the adrenal cortex in several vertebrates. Taken as a whole, the rhythm of mitosis may be damped considerably by hypophysectomy but it is not lost completely in most instances. Bullough & Lawrence (1964) concluded that both adrenalin and the glucocorticoids are responsible for setting the rhythms of mitosis in mice. They believe that adrenalin decreases mitosis by enhancing the effect of epidermal chalone and that the corticoids prolong the action of adrenalin. Their studies with parabiotic twins indicated that the synchronizing factor for the rhythm of mitosis is carried by the blood. Kiely & Domm, (1973) reported a rhythm of DNA synthesis in the rat incisor, as measured by the uptake of tritiated thymidine. A rhythm persisted in hypophysectomized animals although the phase was altered. They also found that cortisone has a strong stimulatory effect on DNA synthesis at certain times of day but not at

others. Kiely suggested that the corticoid hormones act synergistically with the catecholamines in normal animals in regulating the
rhythm of mitotic rates.

Summary and Conclusions

The daily cycle of illumination is the principal environmental
entrainer of the daily rhythms of plasma corticoids. Other environmental cues repeated daily may modify the hormonal rhythms. The eye
is an important photosensor in photoperiodic entrainment of the corticoid rhythms in mammals, but it is less important in the other vertebrate classes. Although considerable correlative evidence suggests
that photoperiodic entrainment is mediated by the hypothalamic-pituitary-adrenal pathway, other research indicates that the plasma corticoid rhythms do not depend on the cyclic release of pituitary ACTH.

The daily rhythms in plasma concentrations of the adrenal corticoids are important entrainers of many behavioral and metabolic
rhythms. However some rhythms persist in adrenalectomized animals
and in animals lacking daily rhythms of corticosteroids. The catecholamines appear to be responsible for maintaining some of those
rhythms that are not dependent on the corticoid rhythms.

RHYTHMS OF THYROID HORMONES

Relatively little research has been performed on the daily
rhythms of hormones associated with the thyroid gland as compared
with those of the other major endocrine glands. One possible reason
is that the thyroid is poorly understood despite the many years of
diligent research. It appears to be involved in general metabolism
and in the maturation of the nervous system and in some aspects of
behavior. Although it is well known for a role in oxygen consumption and temperature regulation in endothermic vertebrates, this
function is of little or no importance in many of the ectothermic
vertebrates which are probably closer to the organismal mold in
which the thyroid evolved. Thus there is reason to believe that
the basic functions of this gland are still to be delineated.

Daily rhythms of pituitary content or plasma concentrations
of thyroid-stimulating hormone (TSH) have been reported in rats
(Bakke et al., 1965; Singh et al., 1967; Retiene et al., 1968)
and humans (Blum et al., 1968; Vanhaelst et al., 1972). Daily
rhythms in plasma concentrations of thyroid hormones, measured as
protein-bound iodine, were reported in rabbits (Laird & Fox, 1970)
and humans (Auerbach, 1963).

Both thyroxin and triiodothyronine concentrations in the plasma
were found to vary during the day in the ambulatory human (Vernikos -

Danellis et al., 1972). However, the hormone levels varied errat-
ically during bedrest, and the authors concluded that the daily
rhythms of the thyroid hormones may be posture dependent. This explanation may also be valid for the absence of TSH rhythms in several subjects examined by Webster and coworkers (1972) inasmuch as
some of them were patients.

A daily rhythm in the plasma concentration of any hormone may
reflect variations not only in secretion rates but also in disappearance. Walfish and associates (1961) reported a daily rhythm in the
disappearance of radioiodine - labelled thyroxine from human blood
with the maximum occurring during the day. A daily rhythm of thyroxin disappearance was also found in calves with the maximum rate
observed during the day when they were awake and feeding (Nathanielsz,
1969). Inverting the feeding schedule caused the phase of the hormone disappearance rhythm also to be inverted. The magnitude of the
role that the hormone disappearance rhythm has in producing the plasma
concentration rhythm has not been ascertained. Conceivably, the
rhythm of disappearance could even provide the driving force for
rhythms of hormone secretion by way of feedback activities. However, a rhythm of pituitary TSH content persisted in mice treated
with propylthiouracil, a substance that blocks the secretion of
thyroid hormones (Bakke & Lawrence, 1965). The phase of the TSH
rhythm in the treated rats differed from that in the normal rats.

The functions of thyroid hormones with respect to rhythms fall
into 2 possible categories: a) thyroid hormone rhythms drive other
rhythms, and b) thyroid hormones permit the expression of other
rhythms. Thyroidectomy, which may be expected to have an affect on
either role, has produced equivocal results. The daily rhythms of
oxygen consumption and body temperature were greatly damped, if not
abolished, in rats following thyroidectomy (Popovic, 1956). On the
other hand, thyroidectomy did not appear to interfere with the
rhythm of locomotor activity in axolotl larvae maintained on a photoperiodic regimen or in continuous light (Kalmus, 1940). Natural
and artificially-induced hypothyroidism in humans is associated with
a different pattern and a lower amplitude in the rhythms of plasma
corticoid concentrations and urinary excretion of the corticoids
(Fig. 5) than those present in euthyroid subjects (Martin et al.,
1963).

There is evidence in a fish, Fundulus chrysotus, that thyroxin
may drive other rhythms (Meier, 1970). Thyroxin injections entrained
a rhythm of sensitivity to prolactin activity so that there was a
fixed phase angle between the time of thyroxin injection and the peak
of sensitivity. However these results may also be interpreted in a
manner that assigns a permissive role only to high levels of thyroxin.
The entrainment itself could have resulted from the daily disturbances
of the injections.

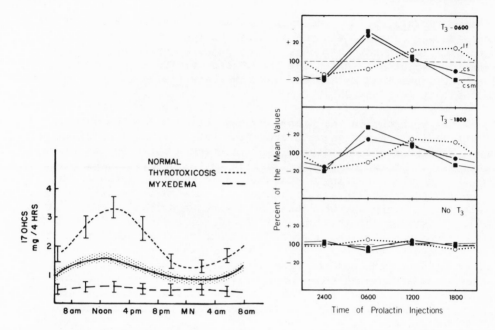

Fig. 5. (Left) Mean variation in urinary 17-OHCS excretion in 25
normal subjects, 13 patients with thyrotoxicosis and 8 patients with
myxedema. The shaded area represents the standard error of the mean
for the control subjects and the vertical bars represent the standard
error of the mean for the patients with thyroid dysfunction. From
Marin et al., J. Clin. Endocrinol. Metab. 23, 243-260 (1963).

Fig. 6. (Right) Triiodothyronine and circadian crop sac and fattening responses to prolactin. c s = crop sac weight; c s m = dry crop-
cas mucosal weight, l f = liver fat (% dry weight). From Meier et
al., J. Interdiscipl. Cycle Res. 2, 161-171 (1971).

        Contrary to the results in fish, thyroxin and triiodothyronine
injections did not entrain rhythms of sensitivity to prolactin in
common pigeons, Columa livia (John et al., 1972). The hormones
appear to have permissive roles. In pigeons maintained in continuous
light, the phases of free-running rhythms of crop sac sensitivity to
prolactin were in synchrony in groups treated with thyroid hormones
either at 0600 or at 1800. The rhythms of both groups, however,
were out of synchrony with an untreated group. The changes in the
phases of the free-running rhythms of the hormone-treated groups
may have resulted from a change in the period inasmuch as Wahlström
(1965) has shown that thyroxin increased and thiourea decreased
the period of a free-running rhythm of self-selected activity in
canaries. After 2 weeks in continuous light, the sensitivity rhythm
dampened out in the untreated pigeons but persisted in the birds
treated with thyroid hormones (Fig. 6).

At this stage of research, the evidence seems to favor a permissive role for thyroid hormones. Such a role could involve the sensitivity of the phase-setting mechanism to environmental cues as well as the integrity of endogenous free-running rhythms. Because thyroxin decreases the activities of hormones involved in the inactivation of catecholamines (D'Torio & Leduc, 1960; Levine et al., 1962) and because thyrotoxicosis and sympathetic nervous system overactivity are similar (Harrison, 1964; Waldstein, 1966), catecholamine activities are apparently potentiated by thyroxin. A permissive role for thyroid hormones, then, could signify a role for catecholaminergic mechanisms in the entrainment and maintenance of circadian rhythms.

DAILY RHYTHMS OF GROWTH HORMONE

Most of the studies of growth hormone rhythms have been performed with humans in which there is a distinct rhythm in subjects kept on a normal daily regimen (Hunter et al., 1966; Quabbe et al., 1966; Takahashi et al., 1968; Weitzmann et al., 1968; Honda et al., 1969; Sassin et al., 1969; Nakagawa, 1971; Molnar et al., 1972). Although various events, such as exercise (Roth et al., 1963), may influence the concentrations of plasma growth hormone, the most characteristic and prominent daily increase occurs during the early period of sleep and is associated with slow wave sleep (stages 3 and 4) (Sassin et al., 1969) (Fig. 7). Deprivation of sleep prevented the normal occurrence of plasma increase in growth hormone and reversal of the sleep-wakefulness schedule caused a prompt adjustment of the growth hormone rhythm (Weitzmann et al., 1968; Sassin et al., 1969).

The drug diazepam, while suppressing phenomena related to stage 4 was also reported to suppress the release of growth hormone during sleep (Stokes et al., 1972). However, Rubin and co-workers (1973), were unable to duplicate the suppression of growth hormone release using a similar drug, flurazepam, although it did abolish slow wave (stage 4) sleep. Thus it is presently unresolved whether slow wave sleep is necessary for the sleep-stimulation of growth hormone release or whether slow wave sleep and growth hormone release coincide as a result of common elements in the regulatory mechanisms.

A daily rhythm in concentration of plasma growth hormone has also been reported in swine (Topel et al., 1973). The lowest levels occurred during the afternoon hours. Higher concentrations occurred at night during sleep with the peak occurring shortly after dawn. On the other hand, no rhythms of growth hormone were found in lactating cows (Koprowski et al., 1972) or in rats (Muller et al., 1970). These findings, however, do not necessarily indicate that growth hormone concentrations are unaffected by sleep in those animals. Cows are known to sleep irregularly and laboratory rats may also be irregular at times under some laboratory conditions.

Unlike some of the other hormones, then, the daily rhythm of growth hormone is largely dependent on a behavioral rhythm that is easily modified, at least in humans. According to a strict usage of the term, its rhythm may not be circadian (endogenous under constant environmental conditions) and it may be controlled primarily by the sleep-wakefulness cycle. These possibilities deserve further experimentation.

Almost nothing is known regarding the utility of a daily rhythm of, or of timed release of, growth hormone. An interesting finding is that the mitotic rate in mouse liver can be increased by growth hormone injection at only one time of day and not at other times (Halberg & Howard, 1958). In view of the cumulative effects that prolactin has when injected daily at specific times (see section on prolacin), it would be interesting to learn whether growth depends on the release of growth hormone at a specific time during the circadian system. If it does, the manipulation of a sleep-wakefulness schedule with respect to a daily L:D cycle could have important consequences economically and medically.

DAILY RHYTHMS OF PROLACTIN

General Characteristics

Although prolactin is most famous for its mamotropic activities, its presence in the lower vertebrates offers clear testimony that these effects are recent, though not unwelcome, evolutionary contributions. Because prolactin has a multitude of metabolic and behavioral effects, Riddle (1963) concluded that prolactin is a generalized tropic hormone affecting many organs and systems. Unlike other hormones of the adenohypophysis which are under stimulatory control, prolactin is regulated in part by an inhibitory factor elaborated in the hypothalamus.

Daily rhythms of prolactin were first reported in 1964 in hamsters (Kent et al., 1964) and rats (Clark & Baker, 1964). In both species, greater amounts were observed in the pituitaries in the evening than in the morning. In rats maintained on 12-hour daily photoperiods (0600-1800), the peak of pituitary prolactin content occurred at 1600 (Clark & Baker, 1964). The fall in pituitary levels probably signifies the release of prolactin into the blood stream because the highest blood concentrations of prolactin in male rats on a 14L:10D regimen occurred during the dark (Dunn et al., 1972).

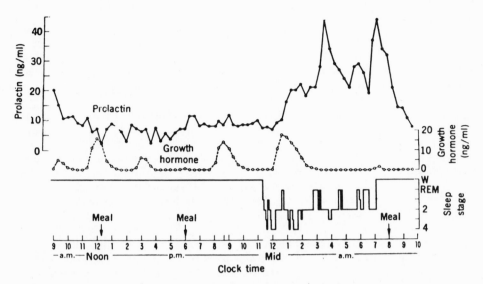

Fig. 7. Prolactin, growth hormone, and sleep stage in a male subject, age 23. The results of this 24-hour catheter study are representative of 24-hour pattern seen in six subjects; W, wake. From Sassin et al., Science 177, 1205-1207 (1972). Copyright 1972 by the American Association for the Advancement of Science.

In virgin heifers, plasma concentrations of prolactin were found to be low during the dark and high during the light except for a short interval about noon (Swanson & Hafs, 1971). The pattern of prolactin in lactating cows differed somewhat (Kropowski et al., 1972). Low levels were observed between 0400 and 1000 and highest levels were found during the afternoon.

In adult humans, highest concentrations of plasma prolactin have been found during the dark (sleep) (Nokin et al., 1972; Van Haelst et al., 1973). Although both growth hormone and prolactin are released at night in humans, the patterns do not match, suggesting different mechanisms of control (Sassin et al., 1972) (Fig. 7). The patterns of the daily rhythms of thyrotropin-releasing hormone (TRH) and prolactin also differ (Vanhaelst et al., 1973) indicating that although TRH can cause the release of prolactin (Jacobs et al., 1971), it probably does not control the daily rhythm.

A bimodal rhythm of plasma concentrations of prolactin has been reported in the goldfish, Carassius auratus (Leatherland & McKeown, 1973). On a 14-hour daily photoperiod (0600-1800), the peaks occurred at 0600-0900 and at 2100-2400 in fish maintained both in fresh water and 30% sea water (Fig. 8).

Most studies of prolactin rhythms as well as daily rhythms of
other hormones do not take into account the possibility of seasonal
changes. This neglect may be justifiable in some of the common experimental animals but it is no longer appropriate for animals which
undergo marked seasonal changes in metabolism and behavior. Seasonal
variations in the daily rhythm of pituitary prolactin content have
been reported in a migratory bird, the white-throated sparrow, Zonotrichia albicollis (Meier et al., 1969). During May when the birds
were metabolically and behaviorally ready for the vernal migration,
the daily rise occurred sharply at midday and declined during the
afternoon. The daily rise also occurred at midday during the inter-
migratory period in August but the levels did not decline until close
to dawn. Apparently, the time of prolactin synthesis remained constant at midday but the time of day when the hormone was released in
the blood varied seasonally.

Studies of possible environmental synchronizers of prolactin
rhythms are needed. Although it is possible to argue from several
sources that the prolactin rhythm is entrained by the daily photoperiod, direct experimentation seems to be lacking. There seems
to be no constant environmental behavioral cue that can be correlated
with the phase of the rhythm in the animals investigated. High levels may be found in either light or dark, or during activity or rest.
It has not been ascertained whether the rhythm persists under constant environmental conditions.

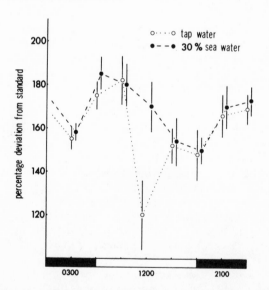

Fig. 8. Changes in the concentration of plasma prolactin in goldfish, Carassius auratus, during a 24-hour period. The fish were
acclimated to tap water or 30% artificial sea water. Modified from
Leatherland & McKeown (1973).

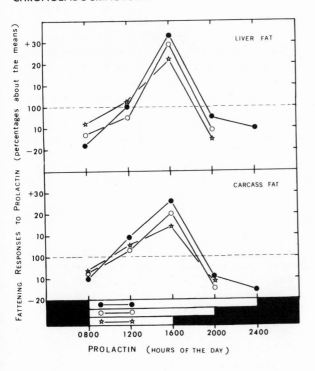

Fig. 9. Daily varia-
tions in fattening re-
sponses to prolactin.
From Joseph & Meier,
J. Exp. Zool. 178:
59-62 (1971).

Daily Rhythms of Responses to Prolactin

Possible function of daily rhythms of prolactin have been
studied in only several laboratories. Daily injections of prolactin have yielded results suggesting that the daily rhythms may
have important metabolic, reproductive, and behavioral roles. The
time of day when prolactin is given is critically important. Injections of prolactin at midday of 16-hour daily photoperiods e-
licited large gains in body fat stores in the migratory white-
throated sparrow (Zonotrichia albicollis) measured after a week of
treatment (Meier & Davis, 1967). However, injections given early in
the photoperiod caused losses in fat stores.

Since this initital discovery in a migratory sparrow, daily variations in fattening responses to prolactin have been found in teleost
fishes (Lee & Meier, 1967; Mehrle & Fleming, 1970; Joseph & Meier,
1971; de Vlaming & Sage, 1972), amphibians (Meier, 1969), reptiles
(Meier, 1969; Trobec, 1974), birds (John et al., 1972; MacGregor,
1974), and mammals (mice and hamsters) (Meier, 1972; Joseph & Meier,
1974). In all instances, prolactin had an inhibitory effect on fat
stores when given daily at certain times and a stimulatory effect
when administered at other times. Increases of 200 to 400% in fat

stores with appropriate increases in body weight have often been
reached in one week of treatment. Decreases of 50% in fat content
within a week were also common as a result of prolactin injections
at specific times of day. The animals that fattened in response to
prolactin also consumed more food than those that did not fatten.
However, prolactin did not appear to cause fattening by stimulating
food consumption. Fat stores were maintained in starved fish at
the expense of other tissues of the body indicating that increased
food consumption was a consequence of the hormonally induced fattening rather than a primary inducer (Meier, 1969). These findings
may have considerable import concerning the treatment of obesity if
they can be related to humans.

The effect of photoperiod on the rhythm of fattening response
to prolactin was examined in a brackish water killifish, Fundulus
grandis (Joseph & Meier, 1971). When daily injections were made
at 0, 4, 8, 12, or 16 hours after the onset of light, the greatest amount of fattening occurred in the 8-hour group regardless of
whether the daily photoperiod was 9, 12, or 16 hours. In addition,
the peak of fattening occurred 8 hours after the onset of light regardless of whether the daily photoperiod began at 0800 or at 1200.
Thus the phase of the response rhythm is set by the onset of light
in the killifish (Fig. 9).

Several other responses to prolactin have been studied with
respect to daily variations. A daily rhythm of sensitivity or
response was found in every instance. One of the more interesting
responses is that of the pigeon crop sac which served as the principal assay for prolactin for almost 40 years (Riddle et al., 1932).
In pigeons kept on a 12-hour daily photoperiod, injections of prolactin given early in the photoperiod had relatively little effect
compared to those given later in the day (Burns & Meier, 1971; Meier
et al., 1971) (Fig. 10A). The daily rhythm of crop sac sensitivity
was present whether the injections were given locally by intradermal
injections over the crop sac, or systemically.

Other daily variations in responses to prolactin include non-
lipid growth in fish (Lee & Meier, 1967), inhibition of amphibian
metamorphosis (Breaux & Meier, 1971), promotion of the red eft water
drive (Meier et al., 1971), locomotor activity (Fig. 11) and orientation in birds (Meier, 1969, Martin & Meier, 1974), and the antigonadal effect in birds (Meier, 1969b). The latter two responses
are discussed in the section on annual cycles.

Circadian rhythms of fattening responses to prolactin persisted
for at least 10 days in the killifish, Fundulus grandis, maintained
in continuous light (Meier et al., 1971). Both the rhythms of fattening responses and the rhythm of crop sac response persisted for
about 12 days in the common pigeon, Columba livia, maintained in
continuous light (John et al., 1972).

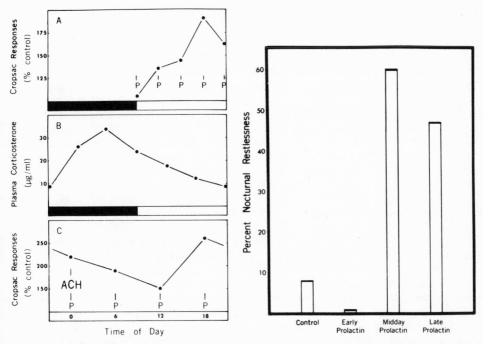

Fig. 10. (Left) Daily variations in the crop sac response to prolactin in Columba livia. In Experiment A, the responses to four
daily intramuscular injections of prolactin (P) given at one of
several times of day were tested in pigeons maintained on 12L:12D.
In Experiment B, the concentrations of plasma corticosterone were
measured at several times of day in pigeons maintained on 12L:12D.
In Experiment C, the crop sac responses to four daily intramuscular
injections of prolactin given at one of several times of day following
the injections of corticosterone were tested in pigeons maintained in
continuous light. From Meier & MacGregor, Am. Zoologist 12:257-271
(1972).

Fig. 11. (Right) Diurnal responses of nocturnal locomotor activity
to prolactin (2 μg/gm body weight) in the white-throated sparrow.
Zonotrichia albicollis, before the appearance of vernal Zugunruhe.
Caged birds were maintained outdoors in individual cages where the
locomotor activity was monitored using a microswitch assembly and
event recorder. Nocturnal restlessness were defined as continuous
activity for 2 hours or longer. Daily injections were made early,
at midday, and late during a natural photoperiod of about 13½ hours
early in April. From Meier, Gen. Comp. Endocrinol. Suppl. 2:55-62
(1969). Copyright by Academic Press.

The presence of daily variations in responses to prolactin
signify that another system with a circadian expression entrains
rhythms of metabolic and behavioral responses to prolactin and,

in turn, is entrained by the daily photoperiod. Such a system must be able to exert diverse influences throughout the body, a property that might be expected of several hormones. In addition, it should probably be under neural control in order to be responsive to environmental cues. With these considerations, there are relatively few known systems which could be involved. The hormonal components of several possible entraining systems have been investigated by placing animals in continuous light in order to remove photoperiodic entrainment of endogenous systems and by daily injections of hormones to simulate the endogenous daily increases in hormone concentrations. Although the thyroid may be involved in some lower vertebrates (see section on Thyroid), the adrenal cortex appears to have important roles in entraining daily responses to prolactin among representatives of all the major vertebrate classes. Daily injections of adrenal corticoids entrained daily rhythms of fattening responses to prolactin in 2 fish (Meier et al., 1971b; Meier, 1972), 2 reptiles (Meier et al., 1971b; Trobec, 1974), 3 birds (Meier & Martin, 1971; Meier et al., 1971b; Meier et al., 1971a), and 2 mammals (Meier, 1972; Joseph & Meier, 1974). That is, daily injections of adrenal corticoids and prolactin may cause losses or gains of fat stores in variable amounts depending on the temporal relations between the injections of the 2 hormones (Fig. 12). Injections of adrenal corticoids also entrained the following additional daily rhythms of responses to prolactin: locomotor activity and migratory orientation in the white-throated sparrow (Martin & Meier, 1974), reproductive photosensitivity and photorefractoriness in birds (Meier & Dusseau, 1973; Meier et al., 1971a), the red eft water drive (Meier et al., 1971c), and pigeon crop sac stimulation (Meier et al., 1971b, d). The significances of several of these temporal synergisms of adrenal corticoids and prolactin are discussed in later sections.

The studies of the pigeon are interesting in that they allow for a comparison of several rhythms of responses to prolactin in one animal. Systematic injections of corticosterone entrained the rhythm of crop sac response and the rhythms of fattening responses (Meier et al., 1971b, d). Both of the response rhythms free-run on continuous light for about 10 days but eventually disappear unless treated with thyroid hormones (John et al., 1972). In no instance did the daily peaks of fattening responses coincide with the daily peaks of crop sac responses. The phases of the response rhythms of obviously related parameters such as abdominal fat content, liver fat content, food consumption and intestinal lengths and weights did coincide. Because prolactin stimulates the crop sac to produce "milk" for the young, it is curious that as much prolactin was apparently produced and released in immature pigeons as in incubating adults (Schooley & Riddle, 1938). It has been suggested that the temporal relations of corticoid and prolactin rhythms may change during maturation so that prolactin may account for the high levels of fat in the young and for crop sac stimulation in incubating adults (Meier et al., 1971d).

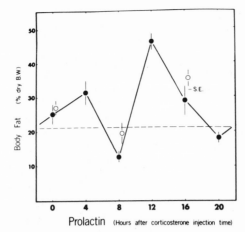

Fig. 12.   Temporal relations of corticosterone and prolactin controlling fat levels: Experiments 2 and 3.   In both experiments the light
was continuous; the injections of corticosterone were made on July 29
and 30, and August 3; the injections of prolactin were made daily,
August 1 to August 5.   In Experiment 2, photosensitive birds received
corticosterone injections at 0800; and prolactin at 0-, 8-, or 16-
hour intervals after the time of corticosterone injection.   The mean
levels of body fat are represented by open cicles.   In Experiment 3,
photorefractory birds received corticosterone injections at 0800-2000.
Prolactin injections were made at 0800, 1600, or 2400 in each corti-
costerone-treated group, so that there were 6 groups receiving prolactin at 4-hr intervals after corticosterone.   The mean levels of
body fat are represented by closed circles.   The dashed line represents the mean value of untreated birds.   From Meier & Martin, Gen.
Comp. Endocrinol. 17:311-318 (1971).   Copyright by Academic Press.

     The daily rhythms of plasma adrenal corticoids were investigated
in several vertebrate species in order to relate the endogenous
rhythms with the experimental results of injections.   By equating the
time of the daily rise of plasma corticoids with the time of daily
injections of the corticoids, it was found that the daily rise of
the endogenous hormone can account for the times of the daily fattening responses to prolactin in the white-throated sparrow (Dusseau
& Meier, 1971) and the killifish (Garcia & Meier, 1973), and for
the time of peak crop sac response in the pigeon (Joseph & Meier,
1973).   That is, the intervals between the injections of the adrenal
corticoids and the peak responses to prolactin in animals kept in
continuous light are the same as those intervals between the daily
rise of plasma corticoids and the peak responses to prolactin in
animals maintained on a daily photoperiodic regimen (Fig. 10).   Inasmuch as daily rhythms of plasma cortisol persisted in hypophysectomized fish (Srivastava & Meier, 1972), the observations that rhythms
of fattening responses to prolactin persisted in hypophysectomized
fish (Lee & Meier, 1967; de Vlaming & Sage, 1972) cannot be con-

sidered evidence against an important entraining role for corticoid rhythms.

Because disturbances or stresses of various sorts can cause the release of both corticoids and prolactin, it might be expected that prolonged disturbances of handling or control injections alone could affect the same parameters as those affected by the exogenous hormones. Studies in this regard were made on fish, lizards, birds, and mammals (Meier et al., 1973). Prolonged daily injections (10 days and more) of saline did elicit marked stimulatory or inhibitory effects on fat stores and the reproductive system depending on the time of day when the disturbances were made. This study did not determine how the daily rhythms of the hormones may have been modified. The results should serve as a warning to investigators who subject their animals to handling at the same time each day.

The effects of daily disturbances on fat stores and the reproductive system has other implications that may be of considerable economic and medical importance. It seems probable that the daily schedule of activities in humans, for example, may be responsible for some metabolic and reproductive problems. Consequently, conditions such as obesity might be alleviated by altering behavior patterns or by providing stimuli or drugs that could cause the release of corticoids or prolactin at specific times of day. Drinking water (inhibitory: Buckman & Peak, 1973) and mammary gland manipulation (stimulatory: Kolodny et al., 1972) or naps (stimulatory: Parker et al., 1973) are methods which may be used to control prolactin production during the day (or night) in (and by) both men and women.

DAILY RHYTHMS OF REPRODUCTIVE HORMONES

Long before the current concern with hormone rhythms in reproduction, Riley (1937) reported evidence of probable daily rhythms of the gonadotropic hormones in the house sparrow (Passer domesticus). Riley found that spermatogenesis was largely restricted to an interval of several hours late during the dark.

Studies of reproductive hormone rhythms in humans proliferated after techniques were developed to assay for reproductive hormones in the blood and it was no longer necessary to remove glands to obtain evidences of hormone activities. The highest concentrations of blood follicle-stimulating hormone (FSH) have been found during the early morning hours in the sighted (Faiman & Ryan, 1967; Saxena et al., 1968; Bodenheimer et al., 1973) as well as in the blind (Bodenheimer et al., 1973). Possible rhythms in blood concentrations of luteinizing hormone (LH) are not so evident as those for FSH concentrations (Boyar et al., 1972; Krieger et al., 1972; Nakin & Troen, 1972; Ruben et al., 1972). Like FSH, LH is released in apparently random pulses. Slightly greater amounts appear to be released during REM sleep (Ruben, 1972), an item of interest in that norepinephrine, a central neurotransmitter, has been implicated in both REM sleep (Jouvet, 1969) and in LH secretion (Wurtman, 1971). Daily rhythms of gonadotropic hormones have also been reported in Japanese quail (Tanaka et al., 1966; Bacon et al., 1969; Follett & Sharp, 1969).

Although a daily rhythm of plasma LH is not always apparent, the secretion of the hormones it stimulates, testosterone and estradiol, do exhibit prominent daily rhythms in human males (Dray et al., 1965; Resko & Eik-Nes, 1966; Faiman & Winter, 1971; Littmann & Gerdes, 1972; Bodenheimer et al., 1973) and females (Bodenheimer et al., 1973), respectively. The highest concentrations occur in the morning. Similar rhythms have been reported in the blind (Bodenheimer et al., 1973). As in the secretion of the gonadotropic hormones, testosterone secretion is pulsatile.

The amplitudes of the rhythms of the gonadotropic hormones are characteristically less than those of other hormones. However, small changes may be important inasmuch as the concentrations of FSH and LH are only slighly higher in adults than they are in prepubertal children (Odell & Moxer, 1971). In addition, daily rhythms of responses must be considered. Daily variations in ovarian and uterine responses to injections of human chorionic gonadotropin have been reported in mice (Bindon & La Mond, 1966) and daily rhythms of oviducal responses to mammalian gonadotropic hormones (FSH and LH) were reported in a sparrow (Meier, 1969). Thus reproductive functions may depend not only on rhythms of secretion but also on the phase relations of the secretion rhythms with respect to the rhythm of responses or sensitivity of the receptive tissues.

Because the concentrations of the gonadal hormones undergo daily variations it is not surprising to find daily rhythms in reproductive behavior. For example, the female medaka (Oryzias latipes), a cyprinodont teleost fish, lays a few eggs daily just before dawn (Robinson & Rugh, 1943; Egami, 1954). The time of egglaying is set by the photoperiod and becomes irregular in constant light. Similar results have been reported in 2 species of anabantoid fishes (Marshall, 1967). Spawning occurred during the last few hours of light. Inverting the photoperiod caused a rapid reversal in the time of spawning. Spawning became less frequent and irregular in continuous light. Sardines also spawn during a discreet period in the evening (Gamulin & Hure, 1956).

Many similar citiations of reproductive behavior at specific times of day could be made. Even the laboratory rat is sexually more active at one time of day (Lisk, 1969). Most copulatory activity occurred 3.5 to 5.5 hours after the onset of dark, at a time of low levels of plasma testosterone (Kinson & Liu, 1973). The daily

peak of testosterone was found late in the dark period. With the
information at hand, peaks of reproductive behavior do not coincide
with high levels of testosterone in either the human or rat.

Several advantages may be cited for the timing of reproductive
behavior at specific times of day. If the patterns of the male
and female are in phase, there is a more economical apportioning
of time. In some instances, the timing of mating may be more con-
ducive for a successful pregnancy. It might also serve as an iso-
lating mechanism to reduce interbreeding of closely related animals,
especially fish, residing in the same habitat and breeding at the
same time of year. Additional daily rhythms of reproductive hormones are cited and discussed in subseqent portions of this review.

DAILY RHYTHMS OF OTHER HORMONES

Pancreatic Hormones

Inasmuch as the hormones of the pancreas are not under direct
neural control, they are not likely to have central roles in temporal
organization. The daily rhythm of blood insulin in humans is similar
in phase to the rhythm of blood glucose and is probably largely responsive to it (Jolin & Montes, 1973). The plasma insulin rhythm
and the response rhythm of pancreatic cells to glucose were reported
to be in phase with the peak occurring late during a 12-hour daily
photoperiod (Gagliardino et al., 1972). Rhythms of blood insulin
and glucagon were observed in humans on a restricted caloric diet
of proteins with peaks at 1500 and 1800, respectively (daily photoperiod: 0730-2330).

The rhythms of the pancreatic hormones, then, appear to reflect
the rhythm of blood glucose. In addition, they may be influenced by
the rhythms of hormones such as the adrenal corticoids and growth
hormone that stimulate the secretion of insulin. The daily peaks
of blood insulin in the human and in the rat (Girard-Globa & Bourdel,
1973) occur about 6 to 9 hours after the peak in blood corticosteroids
and several hours after the onset of their respective activity periods.
It seems likely that the time of high levels of insulin may have important consequences on growth and fattening by acting synergistically
with the activities of other hormones.

Biogenic Amines

Biogenic amines are discussed elsewhere in this text and consequently they receive less attention here than they might otherwise merit in a discussion of daily rhythms of hormones. They are
also treated in this article with respect to their relations with

other rhythms. For example, norepinephrine is an important synaptic transmitter with important roles in the stimulation of pituitary and pineal hormones.

Peripheral rhythms of the catecholamines have been demonstrated in the human on the basis of their periodic release in the urine with a peak 4 hours after dawn (Reinberg et al., 1970). Jori and coworkers (1971) concluded on the basis of studies using inhibitors of catecholamine synthesis and by correlations with rhythms of corticoid hormones that the rhythms of several liver enzymes are entrained by catecholamine rhythms that are mediated by the adrenal cortex. Some rhythms of liver enxymes (tyrosine aminotransterase), however, appear to be directly controlled by a rhythm of catecholamine (Black et al., 1971).

Daily rhythms of brain serotonin and the catecholamines have been implicated in the control of the sleep-wakefulness cycle (Reis et al., 1968; Jouvet, 1969; Luce, 1970). The presence and the phases of the rhythms vary from one area of the brain to another. There is often a reciprocal relation between the phases of the rhythms of serotonin and norepinephrine.

The regulation of melatonin production in the pineal gland and the functions of this hormone are discussed elsewhere in this volume by Professor J. C. Hoffman. Consequently the discussion of the pineal gland is brief and limited to its role in reproduction and photoperiodism.

CYCLES IN REPRODUCTION

Estrous Cycle in Rodents

An enormous literature has accumulated dealing with the estrous cycle of rodents. This cycle serves to bring the animal to a peak of physiological and behavioral preparedness for mating and pregnancy every 4 or 5 days unless interrupted by a successful mating. For convenience, the cycle may be divided into estrus (the day of ovulation), followed by 2 or more days of diestrus and by proestrus.

Everett & Sawyer (1950) observed that ovulation occurs at a fixed time of day in the rat and is set by a neurogenic stimulus that occurs 9 to 11 hours earlier during the afternoon of proestrus. If a depressant of the central nervous system was given before this "critical period", ovulation could be prevented. This study has been duplicated by many other researchers and extended to other rodents, including the golden hamster, Mesocricetus auratus (review: Kent, 1968), with essentially similar results. The timing of the "critical period" and ovulation is set by the daily photoperiod (Critchlow,

1963; Everett, 1964). However, the circaquadridian estrous cycle persisted in hamsters maintained in continuous light for as long as 3 generations although ovulation occurred at random times during the day (Alleva et al., 1968).

Alleva and coworkers (1971) compared the free-running circaquadridian estrous cycle with the circadian rhythm of locomotor activity in the golden hamster maintained in continuous light. They observed that the period of the circadian rhythm was greater than 24 hours and that the circaquadridian cycle was about 4 times as long (> 96 hours). A spontaneous delay of a 4-day cycle to a 5-day cycle was not accompanied by a phase shift in the circadian rhythm of locomotor activity nor in the time of ovulation. The authors concluded that the same endogenous timer sets the circadian rhythm of locomotor activity as well as the daily events within the estrous cycle.

There is considerable agreement that LH has an important role in stimulating ovulation. The neurogenic stimulus that occurs during the "critical period" results in a surge of LH release from the pituitary and into the blood. Hypophysectomy performed before 1600 (photoperiod: 0500-1900) on proestrus prevented ovulation in 80% of cycling rats but 90% ovulated if hypophysectomy was performed at 1630 (Greig & Weisz, 1972). The increase in LH began around 1600 and peaked about 1700. Injections of sodium pentobarbitone between 1500 and 1600 on proestrous prevented both the LH surge and ovulation delaying them until the following day.

With the exception of proestrus, the plasma concentrations of LH were reported to be low throughout the estrous cycle in rats and exhibit no obvious daily rhythms. Apparently LH does account for the increasing amounts of estrogen secretion that begins on diestrus-2 and peaks on the morning of proestrus (Freeman et al., 1972). In turn, the increasing concentrations of estrogen prepare for the LH surge. In hamsters, luteinizing hormone releasing hormone (LH-RH) stimulated much greater release of LH during proestrus than during estrus and diestrus-1 (Arimura et al., 1972). Estrogen is believed to enhance the LH response to LH-RH (Arimura & Schally, 1971).

The plasma concentrations of FSH in the rat were found to rise on the afternoon of proestrus, remain high through the night, and return to base levels by noon of estrus (Taya & Igarashi, 1973). Thus the cyclic release of large quantities of FSH as well as of LH follow the cyclic increase of estrogen suggesting a positive feedback effect by estrogen. Comparable increases of the gonadotropic hormones prior to the increase in estrogen concentrations on diestrus have not been reported (see Fig. 13).

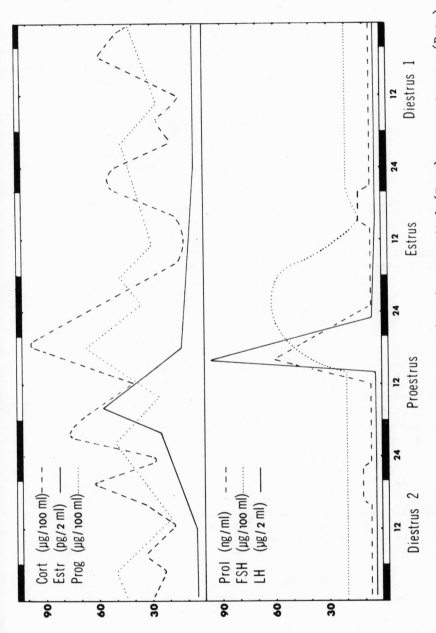

Fig. 13. Concentrations of corticosterone (Cort), extradiol (Estr), progesterone (Prog), prolactin (Prol), follicle-stimulating hormone (FSH), and luteining hormone (LH) in the rat estrous cycle. A composite from the literature.

Estrogen also primes the surge of prolactin that occurs on the afternoon of proestrus and terminates about midnight in the rat (Freeman et al., 1972). Treatment with anti-LH on the day before proestrus (diestrus-2) prevented the surge of prolactin and ovulation unless accompanied by diethylstilbesterol, an estrogenic compound.

In unmated rats, the prolactin surge terminates by midnight (Neill et al., 1971; Kalra et al., 1971). However, if mating occurs, plasma levels have be n reported to remain high until dawn of estrus (Butcher et al., 1972). Thereafter for the first 4 days of gestation, there was a bimodal daily (or semicircadian) rhythm of prolactin with peaks at the ends of the light and dark periods (Photoperiod: 0545-1815). Mating appears to have initiated the prolactin peak at the end of the dark period while permitting the continuation of the peak occurring at the end of the light period (Fig. 14).

This new peak of prolactin during gestation is of special interest in that daily injections of prolactin were found to prevent ovulation in the hamster provided the injections were made at 18 hours after the onset of a 12-hour daily photoperiod but not at 0, 6, or 12 hours after the onset of light (Joseph & Meier, 1974). In addition the cycle was arrested in hamsters maintained in continuous light by injections of prolactin given 12 hours after daily injections of corticosterone. Prolactin injections made at 0, 4, 8, 16, or 20 hours after the injections of corticosterone were ineffective. If this relation has a role in pregnancy, one would predict that the daily rise of plasma corticoids in the hamster during gestation should occur during the latter half of a 12-hour daily photoperiod. Unfortunately, this information appears to be lacking. Certain problems concerning the maintenance of pregnancy may result from an inadequacy of prolactin at specific times of day. On the other hand, some problems of fertility may be caused by large quantities of prolactin at those same times of day.

Because progesterone injections induce lordosis in female rats, it is not surprising that the greatest concentrations of plasma progesterone have been observed about the onset of darkness on proestrus (Mann & Barraclough, 1973) at a time when most matings usually occur. This peak is distinctive in that it was found only on the day of proestrus. The peak of a daily rhythm of progesterone was observed on each day of the cycle late during the dark. By obtaining samples of ovarian plasma at the same times that he obtained samples of peripheral plasma, Mann further concluded that the daily increase in plasma (peripheral) progesterone was produced by the adrenal and that the large increase on the evening of proestrus was largely produced by the ovary.

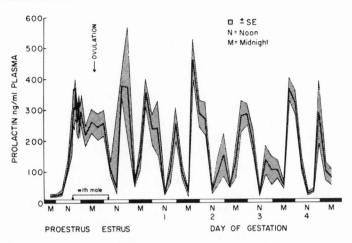

Fig. 14. Prolactin concentration in plasma of rats, 5 rats/group at 52 time periods and 4 rats/group at 5 time periods (3 AM, 2 PM, 2:30 PM, 6 PM or proestrus and 6 PM on day 2 of gestation) from 3 AM of proestrus to midnight of day 4 of gestation. Time intervals are 3 hr except from 2-7 PM of proestrus when the intervals are 30 min. Reference standard is NIAMD rat prolactin RP-1 (11 IU/mg by the mouse deciduoma assay). From Butcher et al., Endocrinology 90:1125-1127 (1972).

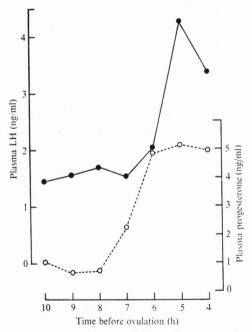

Fig. 15. Concentrations of luteinizing hormone (LH) (●————●) and progesterone (o————o) in plasma collected from hen A40 before ovulation. An increase in the level of progesterone preceded that of LH. From Furr et al., J. Endocrin. 57:159-169 (1973).

The pattern of plasma corticosterone concentrations during the
rat estrous cycle is also curious. The primary peak of the daily
rhythm of plasma corticosterone was observed near the end of a 14-
hour daily photoperiod (Raps et al., 1971). An additional prominent peak occurred late in the dark on proestrus. Secondary peaks
of low amplitude were also found to occur late in the dark on the
other days of the cycle (Fig. 13).

Slight modifications in the daily patterns of serotonin (Quay,
1963) and glycogen (Kachi et al., 1973) content in the pineal gland
during the estrous cycle have been reported in rodents. The daily
pattern of HIOMT activity (used as an index of melatonin synthesis)
also varies during the estrous cycle in rats (Wurtman et al., 1965).
These changes may be responses to other hormones, for example estrogen. Pinealectomy has no discernible effect on the estrous cycle
nor on the time of ovulation in hamsters maintained on normal stimulatory photoperiods (Morin, 1973).

The available information regarding the events of the estrous
cycle seem to favor the argument that the timing of ovulation is
controlled by the same circadian mechanisms that regulate the daily
rise of the plasma corticoids. This idea is based on the following
4 summations and one addition:

1. The LH surge as well as the increases in FSH, prolactin, and
progesterone occur at about the same time on proestrous as the daily
rise of plasma corticoids.

2. Continuous light sometimes obliterates the daily rhythm of
plasma corticoids and arrests the estrous cycle in rats.

3. The period of a free-running circadian rhythm of locomotor
activity (which has been correlated with a rhythm of adrenal corticoids) is one-fourth as long as circaquadridian estrous cycle of the
hamster.

4. Agents such as the barbiturates and atropine can block both
ovulation and the expected daily rise of plasma corticoids in some
rodents if injected before a critical period.

5. In addition, McCormack & Meyer (1962) were able to induce
ovulation and even pregnancy in immature rats as early as
day 22, an age when the daily rhythm of plasma corticoids first appears in rats (Ramaley, 1972).

The length of the cycle appears to depend in large measure on
the production of estrogen. When the concentration of estrogen is
sufficiently high, it triggers LH and prolactin surges on the following day.

Egg Laying Cycle in Birds

Egg laying in birds usually follows a pattern in which a sequence of eggs is layed, one each day. Most of the research concerning hormone mechanisms has been performed in domestic fowl, Gallus gallus domesticus, and in Japanese quail, Coturnix coturnix japonica. The mechanisms involved in timing ovulation in the hen (Fraps et al., 1947; Rothchild & Fraps, 1949; van Tienhoven et al., 1954; Fraps, 1955) appear similar to those described in a rodent (Everett & Sawyer, 1950). That is, LH appears to be the principal ovulation-inducing hormone, and depressants of the central nervous system can block ovulation when given before a critical period.

Opel (1966) has described a sequence of events in egg laying by Japanese quail maintained on a 14-hour daily photoperiod (0200-1600). Most (80%) eggs were layed during the last 7 hours of light and 13% were layed during the dark. The first egg of a sequence was layed 9 to 10.5 hours after the onset of the photoperiod and each successive egg was layed about 35 to 40 minutes later each day. The sequence was usually terminated when egg-laying would occur in the dark and a new sequence was initiated on the second day thereafter. Thus the interval between successive ovipositions (egg laying) in a sequence is about 24.6 hours. Because ovulation normally occurs about 35 to 40 minutes after oviposition and about 7 hours after LH injection, the neurogenic stimulus for the release of ovulation-inducing hormone would be expected to occur at about 3 hours after the onset of light on the first day of a sequence and about 7 hours after the onset of light on the last day. These findings are in substantial agreement with those provided by Wilson & Huang (1962) for the Japanese quail and they are basically similar to the pattern of egg laying reported for the domestic fowl (Fraps, 1954).

Several theories have been proposed to account for the occurrence of ovulation at a progressively later time each day during a sequence (Fraps, 1954, 1961; Bastian & Zarrow, 1955; Nalbandov, 1961). According to a hypothesis advanced by Fraps (1961) there is a daily rhythm in the threshold of a neural component concerned with LH release which is stimulated by a hormone secreted by the developing follicle. When high levels of the follicular hormone coincide with a low neural threshold a discharge of LH occurs. Because the follicular maturation cycle is longer than 24 hours, the production of the follicular hormone would follow a similar time course. Eventually the peak level of the follicular hormone would occur at a time when the neural mechanism is relatively refractory and the release of LH would not be stimulated until the second day when the neural mechanism is sensitive. The follicular hormone is probably progesterone (Fraps, 1961; Furr et al., 1973). (Fig. 15).

Considerable confusion has resulted from attempts to determine the precise time of release of LH. Furr and coworkers (1973) pro-

vided convincing arguments and evidences that the confusion resulted
from unreliable methodology for the assay of LH. Based on radioimmunoassay procedures, Furr reported that greater concentrations
of plasma LH occurred 4 to 7 hours before ovulation than at other
times of the cycle. This observation correlates well with the
finding that hens ovulated 6 to 7 hours after the intravenous injection of LH (Fraps et al., 1947). In addition, Furr reported
that the concentrations of plasma progesterone may account for the
increase in plasma LH as suggested by experiments in which progesterone injections induced ovulation apparently by causing the release of pituitary LH (Fraps, 1955; Ralph & Fraps, 1959).

The ovulatory cycle is endogenous, persisting under continuous
light with a periodicity somewhat greater than 25 hours in both
chickens (Fraps, 1959; van Tienhoven, 1961) and quail (Arrington
et al., 1962; Opel, 1966). The time of ovulation and egg-laying can
be set in continuous light by disturbances (van Tienhoven et al.,
1961; Arrington et al., 1962). Apparently the entraining mechanism
is responsive to disturbances as well as to cycles of illumination.
These results are consistent with the postulate that the same mechanism regulates both the daily rhythm of the adrenal corticoids and
the cycle of egg-laying.

Menstrual Cycle in Primates

The menstrual cycle of primates resembles in many ways the
estrous cycle of rodents. In the human, the average cycle length
is 29.5 days (about the same as a synodical month). Progressive
changes in hormone concentrations occur during the cycle, and
these changes are also associated with changes in behavior. Although the roles of the gonadotropic hormones in preparing for an
precipitating ovulation have been delineated and the feedback influences of the ovarian hormones have been utilized to arrest the
cycle and to prevent ovulation, much remains to be accomplished
concerning the role of hormones in the probably underlying circadian
organization. This topic has recently been reviewed in depth (Ferin
et al., 1974), and only a few studies are cited here that seem to be
of special interest.

In a study involving one woman volunteer who remained in a
cave isolated for 88 days from timing cues of the external world,
it was determined that the existence of a menstrual cycle was not
dependent on obvious cues (Reinberg et al., 1966). The circadian
rhythm of her activities averaged a little more (24.6 hour day)
than a day while in the cave, and her menstrual cycle averaged
25.7 days compared to her normal 29-day menstrual cycle.

An interesting study was reported by Dewan (1965) concerning
a woman who had a 16-year history of irregular menstrual cycles.

Reasoning that light may stimulate the production of the gonadotropic hormones, Dewan arranged to have indirect lighting in her room during the 14-15th to the 16-17th nights after the onset of her previous menstruation. For 3 cycles in succession, her menstrual cycle became regular at 29 days.

The efficaceous results of supplying light at night during midcycle when ovulation usually occurs compels a comment concerning a conceivable evolutionary significance. Before humans began to use fire and to live in shelters, adventuring at night by subdominant males may have been more practical and more often successful during full moon than at other times during the lunar cycle when darkness posed threats of physical hazards almost as serious as those posed by the group leader during the day. Appropriately, menstruation and the accompaning times of depression would then occur at new moon when the adventurous males would more likely remain close to their own nests. Studies of primitive cultures or of individuals willing to live in a primitive manner for long periods are indicated in order to determine whether the menstrual cycle can still be syncronized to a synodical month.

Lunar Cycle in Fish

The revolutions of the moon about the earth cause the moon's position with respect to the sun to vary continually. In consequence, the revolutions of the earth cause the sun to rise every 24 hours and the moon to rise every 24.8 hours. The difference between the solar and lunar day produces a cycle of changing relations that is completed every 29.5 days. The most notable changes during the cycle are those resulting from the reflected light of the moon and those (tides) resuting from its gravitational force. Both aspects have important influences in some invertebrate animals and also in a few vertebrates investigated.

The semilunar spawning activity of the California grunion, Leuresthes tenuis, is a well known phenomenon in which mechanisms sensitive to tidal fluctuations or other lunar influences are implicit (Thompson, 1919; Walker, 1952). Spawning occurs during the high nocturnal tides in spring and summer for several nights following the peak tides of the month that coincide with full and new moon. The eggs are laid in the sand along the high water mark and develop so that the agitation of high water 2 weeks later causes the larvae to hatch and to be swept out to sea. Similar reports for a number of teleosts have been reviewed by Schwassmann (1971).

Although Bünning (1967) has suggested that lunar cycles may occur as a result of a beat phenomenon in which cycles of unequal lengths (such as solar and lunar days) produce secondary cycles of relations between the 2 primary cycles, little experimental work

has been done to expose the vertebrate systems that may be involved.
Recently a study was reported that may have implications regarding
lunar cycles (Meier et al., 1973). In addition to the photoperiodic
cues of a daily schedule of light and dark, a series of vertebrates
including 2 species of fishes, one reptile, a bird, and a mammal
were provided another daily cue in the form of a disturbance. For
example, the fish were disturbed by netting them once daily (raising
them briefly above the water and replacing them immediately). Investigation of the animals used in this experiment as well as subsequent studies indicated that disturbances repeated daily for 2-3
weeks can produce substantial increases or decreases in body weight,
fat stores, and weights of reproductive organs and tissues depending on the temporal relations of the disturbances with respect to
the photoperiod. Fish are particularly sensitive to disturbances,
responding even to fine streams of bubbles applied for a few hours
daily in 50-gallon aquaria. Depending on the species and the parameter measured, there may be one or 2 times of day when the disturbances is stimulatory. A hypothetical extension of these results is
that a changing pattern of photoperiodic and mechanical cues (such
as those produced by tidal fluctuations) could impose lunar cycles
in metabolism and reproduction.

     The illumination and other more subtle changes produced by the
moon may also influence the behavior and physiological conditions
of some vertebrates. House sparrows (Passer domesticus), may be entrained by a dim light having an intensity of one-half that produced at full moon (Menaker & Eskin, 1967). Gwinner (1971) and
others have demonstrated that locomotor activity in birds is influenced by stages of the moon. The guppy, Lebistes reticulatus,
has a lunar rhythm of sensitivity to light of different colors being
most sensitive to yellow light at full moon and to violet and red
light at new moon. Apparently no research has yet been performed
to determine the manner of neuroendocrine involvement in these
activities. The above studies suggest, however, that photoperiodic
mechanisms may well be involved. In addition, the evidence seems
to favor the hypothesis that circadian mechanisms are modified and
utilized for the production of tidal and lunar cycles.

                              PHOTOPERIODISM

                           Bünning's Hypothesis

     The importance of day length in regulating changes in physio-
logical events during the annual cycle was first demonstrated in
the flowering of plants (Garner & Allard, 1920). Photoperiodic
mechanisms were subsequently discovered in insect diapause (Marco-
vitch, 1924) and avian reproduction and migration (Rowan, 1926).
Rowan demonstrated that events occurring normally in the spring in

the slate-colored junco, Junco hyemalis, (gonadal growth, premigratory fattening, and migratory behavior) could be induced during the winter in Edmonton, Canada, by artificially increasing the daily photoperiod by several hours. A role of the annual cycle of day lengths in setting annual cycles of reproduction has now been documented in many vertebrate species of the temperature zones from fish to mammals (reviews: Harrington, 1959; Atz & Pickford, 1964; Mayhew, 1964; Farner, 1964; Aschoff, 1955; Ortavant et al., 1964).

Our understanding of the underlying mechanisms in photoperiodism stem from the important theory advanced by Bünning (1936) who proposed that endogenous daily rhythms are involved in all photoperiodic phenomena. Summaries of the evidences and explanations of the theory are available (Bünning, 1960, 1967; Hamner & Takimoto, 1964; Pittendrigh, 1966). With respect to reproduction, light is thought to act in 2 capacities, as an entrainer of a daily rhythm of photosensitivity and as an inducer of gonadal stimulation. Entrainment of the photo-inducible phase(s) is set in some animals primarily by the onset of the daily photoperiod so that the photoinducible phase(s) occurs later in the day. If light is present during the photoinducible phase, it may induce changes in physiological conditions such as gonadal growth. This understanding of photoperiodism is probably too simple to cover every photoperiodic phenomenon, but it has served well as a working hypothesis.

The presence of 2 systems in photoperiodic stimulation of the vertebrate reproductive system was demonstrated in 2 passerine birds (Jenner & Engles, 1952). By placing the birds on nonstimulatory 6-hour daily photoperiods and interrupting the dark hours by 2-hour intervals of light at various times after the onset of the 6-hour photoperiods, Jenner & Engles determined that light interruptions were stimulatory for the reproductive system when given 16 to 18 hours after the onset of the 6-hour photoperiod. Using variations of the "interrupted night" experiment and designing his experiments patterned after studies made in plants, Hamner (1963, 1964, 1965) demonstrated that circadian systems are involved in the photoperiodic effect in the house finch, Carpodacus mexicanus. In one experiment, Hamner placed his birds on a 72-hour 'day' (6L:66D) and gave them an additional hour of light at 24, 36, 48, or 60 hours after the onset of the 6-hour photoperiod. Gonadal growth resulted only in the groups that received light at 36 or 60 hours after the 6-hour light phase. Apparently, the 6-hour duration of light sets a photoinducible phase that is circadian and is present 36 hours and 60 hours later in the absence of other interruptions by light. Other studies have demonstrated a similar role of circadian systems in fish (Baggerman, 1971), birds (Farner, 1965; Menaker, 1965; Wolfson, 1965; Follett & Sharp, 1969), and a mammal (golden hamster) (Elliott, Stetson, & Menaker, 1972) (see Figs. 16 & 17).

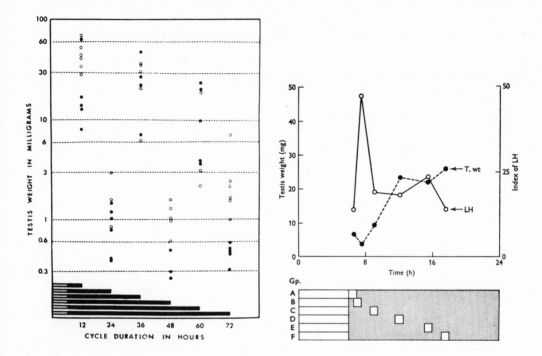

Fig. 16. (Left)   Data on the weights of the testes from birds in experiment 1 (solid circles) and experiment 2 (open circles).   Solid black bars represent different durations of darkness; open boxes represent standard light period of 6 hours.

Fig. 17. (Right)   The effect of asymmetric skeleton photoperiods on testicular development and plasma LH levels in Chloris.   A high peak of LH occurs in the group exposed to a light pulse 7·5 h from 'dawn', but this is not accompanied by testicular development.   From Lofts et al., (1970).   Cambridge University Press.

The presence of 2 responding systems in photoperiodism has also been demonstrated in the house sparrow, Passer domesticus (Menaker & Eskin, 1967). The birds were maintained on a 14-hour daily photoperiod in which the intensity of light was too low to stimulate gonadal growth but sufficient to entrain a daily rhythm of locomotor activity. A 1.5 hour interruption of bright light provided late during the dim light phase promoted testicular growth whereas a similar interruption of light given early during the dim light phase did not. The dim light phase entrained a photoinducible phase later in the day when 1.5 hours of bright light, but not dim light, could induce reproductive development.

Pineal Hypothesis

The most widely known hypothesis concerning neuroendocrine mechanisms in the photoperiodic control of reproduction involves the pineal body. Because the pineal is discussed separately in this volume by Professor J. C. Hoffman, only a brief outline of the role of the pineal in reproduction will be presented here. In the lower vertebrates, the pineal is primarily a photosensory structure although it can also produce melatonin in fish (Quay, 1965; Oksche & Kirschstein, 1967; Oguri et al., 1968; Fenwick, 1970). In mammals and birds, the pineal is glandular and produces melatonin (reviews: Kitay & Altschule, 1954; Wurtman et al., 1968).

Whereas the adrenal cortex has attracted considerable research in rhythms because of its recognized importance and significance in vertebrate function, the pineal has attracted similar attention, it seems, for the opposite reasons. Most of the research has been directed toward an understanding of the antigonadal activities of melatonin especially in the white rat and the golden hamster. The most impressive results by far have been those in the golden hamster (Hoffman & Reiter, 1966; Reiter et al., 1966). Pinealectomy can prevent the normal regression of the gonads in hamsters placed on a short photoperiod. Experiments with rodents indicate that the presence of light is transmitted by way of the eyes and neurons of the sympathetic nervous system to the pineal gland where it exerts an inhibitory effect on the production of melatonin (review: Wurtman et al., 1968; also see Hoffman, this volume). Melatonin, along with its precursor serotonin, when injected into the third ventricle of the brain can reduce the release of LH and FSH and increase the release of prolactin (Kamberi et al., 1970, 1971).

In the nonmammalian vertebrates, the pineal has at most a subsidiary role in photoperiodic control of the reproductive system. There is no convincing evidence that pinealectomy interferes significantly with photoperiodic stimulation. However, because the pineal is generally thought to exert only a negative role as a

result of melatonin production in the dark these experiments are
not necessarily conclusive. The crucial experiment, therefore, is
one that tests whether reproductive development can occur in pinealectomized animals on a short photoperiod that is nonstimulatory in
normal animals. When this procedure was administered in the white-
crowned sparrow (Oksche et al., 1972), only a minimal increase in
paired testes size (8 mg in pinealectomized vs. 2 mg in normal birds)
occurred in the pinealectomized birds when compared to the increase
(about 500 mg) that occurs in that bird on a long photoperiod for
the same length of time.

Inasmuch as the hamster is a hibernator, it may be of interest
to consider the antigonadal effect in terms of hibernation. Because atrophy of the gonads is one prerequisite for hibernation in
all species (Kayser, 1957, 1961; Popovic, 1960; Denyes & Baumber,
1964; Hoffman, 1964) the complete block of gonadal hormone production that may otherwise occur to some extent on short photoperiods
or continuous darkness could be an important role of the pineal antigonadal effect.

It seems clear that the pineal does not have a primary role in
photoperiodism in many of the vertebrates. The absence of an inhibitory effect alone does not appear to satisfy the requirements
for photostimulation. The presence of light over a longer period
of the day must also promote a stimulatory effect in addition to a
possible secondary role in reducing an inhibitory effect. The
pineal apparently has no more than a minor role in either the entrainment of photoinducible phases or in the photoinduction of
gonadal growth, requirements for photoperiodic mechanisms as illustrated by ahemeral light experiments in representative species from
fish to mammals, including the golden hamster (Elliott et al.,
1972).

                            Adrenal Hypothesis

Another hypothesis for the photoperiodic mechanism has been
advanced on the basis of studies of the white-throated sparrow,
Zonotrichia albicollis, and the house sparrow, Passer domesticus
(Meier & Dusseau, 1973). This hypothesis implicates the adrenal
cortex as a part of a mechanism that entrains intervals of photosensitivity. In one experiment with photosensitive white-throated
sparrows maintained on a nonstimulatory 6-hour daily photoperiod,
injections of corticosterone were made daily at 18, 12, or 6 hours
before the onset of light. After 11 days of injections, the testes
and ovaries were stimulated in the group that received corticosterone at 18 hours before dawn but not in the 12- or 6-hour groups nor
in the saline injected controls. Because photostimulation also includes the induction of vernal premigratory fattening and nocturnal

migratory restlessness in the white-throated sparrow, it is of
further interest that these events may also be induced by daily
injections of corticosterone given at 18 hours before a daily
photoperiod of 6 hours (Meier & Martin, 1971).

In another experiment with the house sparrow, the presence of
2 photoinducible phases for gonadotropic activities has been demonstrated (Meier & Dusseau, 1973). The reproductive systems were
fully matured in male and female sparrows maintained on a long
daily photoperiod (16L:8D). Handling alone (birds taken from the
cages and immediately replaced) was carried out daily for 6 days
at one of 4 different times (0, 8, 16, or 20 hours after the onset of light). Among the males, the paired testes weights were
reduced by 50% in those groups that were handled at either 0 or
at 16 hours after the onset of light. In addition, testosterone
activity as measured by bill color was much reduced in the 16-hour
group. On the other hand, no reduction in testicular weights nor
reduction in testosterone activity resulted in the groups that
were handled at midday or at midnight. The reactions of the female reproductive system were comparable. Meier postulated that
handling caused the release of corticosterone that, in turn, entrained the photoinducible phases for LH and FSH at 4 to 8 and
20 to 24 hours, respectively, after the handling. When handling
was performed at the onset of a 16-hour photoperiod, the photoinducible phase for FSH occurred during the dark with a loss of
testes weight but a retention of testosterone production. When
handling was performed at the offset of light, the photoinducible
phase for LH occurred during the dark causing a loss in testicular
weight and a loss of testosterone production. The photoinducible
phases for both FSH and LH occurred during the photoperiod when
handling was carried out at midday or midnight (Fig. 18).

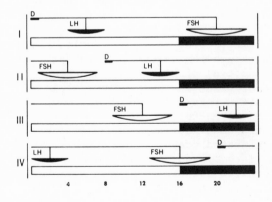

Fig. 18. A model of the entraining effect of disturbance (d) by handling on the
photoinducible phases for LH
and FSH in photosensitive
house sparrows maintained on
a 16-h photoperiod. Disturbances at the onset (I) and
the offset (III) of light reduces the gonadal weights.
Only the disturbance at the
offset of light reduces sterio-
dogenesis. Disturbances at
midday (II) and at midnight
(IV) have no effect. From
Meier & Dusseau, Biol. Reproduction 8:400-410 (1973).
Copyright by Academic Press.

The presence of 2 separate photoinducible phases for LH and
FSH has also been suggested for the house sparrow (Murton et al.,
1970a) as well as for the greenfinch, Chloris chloris (Murton et
al., 1969; 1970b). Light interruptions at 7 to 9 hours after the
onset of 6-hour daily photoperiods stimulated increases in plasma
LH and evidences of testosterone production whereas light interruptions at 16 to 18 hours after "dawn" caused testicular growth
which the authors attributed to FSH release inasmuch as LH has little or no effect on gonad weights in the absence of FSH (Lofts &
Murton, 1968) (Fig. 17).

Photic Pathways

Confusion concerning the pathways of photic effects on photoperiodic mechanisms stem in part from a lack of discernment that
light may affect several systems by way of separate pathways.
There are at least 3 systems responsive to light that may be expected to exert either major or minor influences on reproduction.
One system (the entraining pathway) is involved in the entrainment of most daily rhythms in an organism, including the rhythm
of photosensitivity of a second system (the inducing pathway).
The inducing system responds to the presence of light by stimulating the production and release of the gonadotropic hormones.
A third system (the pineal pathway) transmits impulses to the pineal. The entraining (e.p.) and inducing (i.p.) pathways are parts
of the systems predicted by Bünnings' (1960) hypothesis. Their
presence has been demonstrated by the ahemeral light experiments
discussed earlier. (see PHOTOPERIODISM). The e.p. appears to be
the same one that entrains the daily rhythms of the adrenal corticoids and of locomotor activity (Meier, 1973) and is more sensitive to light in the house sparrow than the i.p. (Menaker & Eskin,
1967). Most of the evidence indicates that the eye is a part of
the e.p. in some mammals (Halberg, 1954; see DAILY RHYTHMS OF ADRE-
NAL CORTICOIDS) but not in many of the other vertebrates, including
fish (Erikson, 1972), amphibians (Adler, 1969), reptiles (Underwood et al., 1970), and birds (Menaker, 1968) in which enucleation
does not eliminate entrainment. Although removal of the frontal
organ (homologue of repilian parietal eye) of blinded green frogs
has been reported to cause them to free-run in the presence of an
L:D regimen (Adler, 1969), the question regarding the location of
the e.p. receptors must be considered open for investigation. Removal of the parietal eye of a lizard does not impair entrainment
(Underwood et al., 1970). As illustrated graphically by Menaker
(1972), light can penetrate deeply into tissue so that there is no
particular requirement for an external sense organ in most animals.
It may even be possible for the receptors to be located in other
areas of the body besides the head region. Blinded and hooded hens
can still be entrained by an L:D regimen (Harrison & Becker, 1969).

Pigeon hatchlings are also sensitive to light directed only to the body skin (Harth & Heaton, 1973).

Although numerous experiments have demonstrated that the pineal gland is not necessary for photoperiodic entrainment in the endothermic vertebrates (see Underwood et al., 1970), Wakahava (1972) has shown that pinealectomy obliterates the daily rhythm of mitotic rate in the epidermis of an amphibian larva subjected to a light-dark schedule. This effect appears to depend on the photoreceptors of the pineal and to be transmitted by way of the tractus pinealis, to the subcommissural organ (Dodt & Heerd, 1962; Oksche, 1962). However, further experiments are necessary to determine whether the effect is one involving entrainment or permission of a rhythm.

The inducing pathway (i.p.) has been studied most extensively in birds especially by Benoit and his coworkers (1961) who initiated their studies in ducks 40 years ago. Benoit concluded that photostimulation of the testes was possible in blinded ducks and that the pituitary, hypothalamus, and portions of the rhinencephalon may be involved in the photoperiodic response. The presence of the eyes is also not required for photostimulation of the reproductive system in house sparrows (Menaker & Keatts, 1968; Underwood & Menaker, 1970), Japanese quail (Sayler & Wolfson, 1968) or 2 species of Crowned sparrows (Gwinner et al., 1971). Using probes tipped with luminescent paint, Homma (1970) found photostimulatory areas for gonadal growth in the hypothalamus and on the olfactory and optic lobes of Japanese quail. The pineal does not appear to be part of the i.p. although some authors have reported that localized light in the pineal area can maintain the testes of Japanese quail transferred to short-day photoperiods (Kato et al., 1967; Oishi & Kato, 1968).

The pineal pathway (p.p.) (or more properly, pathway to the pineal) involves the eyes, inferior accessory optic tracts, and cervical sympathetic ganglia in mammals (Wurtman et al., 1968). The p.p. has also been investigated in birds (Axelrod et al., 1964; Quay, 1966; Sayler & Wolfson, 1969; Hedlund et al., 1971) but the data is difficult to interpret in view of the finding that pineal HIOMT activity (the enzyme supposedly responsible for melatonin synthesis and used extensively in the above experiments) bears no relation to pineal melatonin levels in quail and chickens (Lynch & Ralph, 1970).

ANNUAL CYCLES

Annual cycles are common among vertebrates. They include cylces of reproduction, migration, and hibernation. Annual cycles often have obvious ecological benefit enabling the animal to ex-

ploit times of abundance or avoid times of scarcity. The annual
cycle must involve the coordination of many physiological and behavioral mechanisms because the entire animal must be prepared for
reproduction, migration, or hibernation and the entire animal must
be integrated with its environment.

Annual cycles may be divided into 2 groups based on the amount
of control exercised by environmental cues, such as photoperiod and
temperature: 1) Exogenous control. This group of animals is almost totally dependent on its environment for the regulation of
the annual cycle. For example, reproduction may occur at all times
of the year when the photoperiod is sufficiently long. 2) Exogenous
and endogenous control. This group is responsive to environmental
cues in different ways during the year. That is, long photoperiods
may have stimulatory effects on the reproductive system at some
times of year but not at others.

Exogenous Control

Many vertebrates undergo annual changes that are directly related to day length or temperature. For example, some birds breed
whenever the day length is sufficient (Kirkpatric, 1959). See
PHOTOPERIODISM for a discussion of the photoperiodic mechanisms.
Temperature is more important in ectothermic than in endothermic
animals. In some animals, a combination of warm temperature and
long day length is necessary for reproductive stimulation. Although
temperature is generally believed to have only a permissive role,
the mechanism may be more complex. Licht (1966) demonstrated in a
lizard, Anolis carolinensis that the relation of warm temperature
in a daily thermoperiod (14 Warm: 10 Cold) with respect to a photoperiod may have important consequences. Warm temperatures (32°C)
resulted in a gonadal growth when it accompanied the photophase
(14L:10D) but not when it accompanied the dark phase. The alternate cold temperature was 20°C.

Exogenous and Endogenous Control

Another group of animals have annual or seasonal cycles, but
they do not appear to rely on either changes in day length or in
temperature. Many species of the tropical zone fall into this category. Often, reproduction is correlated with wet periods. For example, a sparrow endemic to Colombia (Zonotrichia capensis) has 2
annual breeding periods that are timed with the late parts of 2
rainy seasons (Miller, 1959). It appears that these animals are in
suspended state following a reproductive cycle and require an enviro-
mental cue to inititate a new cycle. There are some tropical fish
which can be induced to spawn by a substance that is leached out of

the soil during flooding (Lake, 1967). Thus the principal mechanism
is endogenous and is triggered by proximate environmental factors.

No studies are available concerning hormone rhythms in the
environmental triggering of reproduction or in the suspended state
of readiness. There are 2 hormones, though, that seem to warrant
further investigation in that regard, thyroxin and prolactin. Thyroidectomy prevents the normal seasonal regression of the reproductive system in some tropical birds (Thaplijal & Pandha, 1965). Prolactin has strong antigonadal effects in vertebrates (Meier & Dusseau
1968; Joseph & Meier, 1974), and is responsive to blood osmolarity
in fish (Ball, 1969) and mammals (Tyson et al., 1972).

Some of the hibernating animals also have seasonal cycles that
appear to be largely independent of the photoperiod. The control
mechanisms may be related to those discussed in the following
section.

Riley (1936) found that the reproductive system of the house
sparrow, Passer domesticus, though responsive to long day lengths
for most of the year, became refractory to stimulation by long day
lengths late in the summer. Similar findings for fish were reported
by Harrington (1959). A yearly cycle of photosensitivity and photorefractoriness has now been reported in species of all the major
vertebrate classes. The principal advantage of refractory periods,
apparently, is to prevent reproduction at a time when the care of
the young may conflict either with fall migration or with unfavorable
winter conditions.

In migratory birds, migration and reproduction are closely co-
ordinated events during the annual cycle suggesting that the control
mechanisms are also closely integrated. Premigratory fattening and
migratory restlessness, as well as gonadal recrudescence, are stimulated in the spring by the increasing day length. After the young
are raised, the birds become refractory to long days and the reproductive system regresses. Fall migratory events occur at a time of
decreasing day lengths but apparently are not dependent on them. An
intervening period of short days is necessary in some species for the
reestablishment of photosensitivity (reviews: Farner, 1964; Wolfson,
1964). Thus, photoperiodic cues are interpreted by the bird in
various ways during the year. Although annual changes in day length
set the times of migration and reproduction, an important timing
mechanism appears to be within the bird itself.

The timing mechanism for the annual cycle must include circadian
elements because both photostimulation (see PHOTOPERIODISM) as well
as the maintenance of photorefractoriness (Hamner et al., 1968;
Murton et al., 1970) involve circadian systems. It must also include neural and hormonal elements in order to be responsive to pho-

toperiodic cues and to influence reproductive, metabolic, and behavioral conditions. The mechanism for timing the annual cycle
must also be able to organize all of the events of the annual
cycle such as those associated with migration and reproduction.
All of these requirements appear to have been satisfied in a paradigm that assigns prominent roles to the daily rhythms of prolactin and adrenal corticoids (Meier et al., 1971; Meier & Mac-
Gregor, 1972).

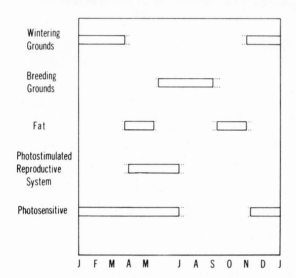

Fig. 19. Major events
and conditions of the
annual cycle of the
white-throated sparrow,
Zonotrichia albicollis.

The rationale for the circannual mechanism was developed as
a result of a series of experiments performed with the migratory
white-throated sparrow, Zonotrichia albicollis (Fig. 19). In an
initial experiment, daily injections of prolactin administered
during the afternoons of 16-hour photoperiods caused rapid increases in fat stores that were as high after one week of injections as those found in feral birds during the spring and fall
migrations (Meier & Davis, 1967). In addition to a stimulation
of fat storage, prolactin injections during the afternoon also
induced nocturnal restlessness in the nocturnal migrant (Meier,
1969b). However, injections of prolactin given early during the
photoperiod caused losses in fat stores and failed to induce
nocturnal activity. The injections of prolactin also had variable effects on the reproductive system augmenting or strongly
inhibiting gonadotropic activities depending on the time of injection (Meier, 1969a; Meier & MacGregor, 1972).

The existence of daily variations in reproductive, metabolic
and behavioral responses to prolactin suggested that another system
was influenced by photoperiodic cues and entrained the rhythms of
responses. The adrenal corticoids appear to be an extension of
this system in the white-throated sparrow. In both photosensitive
and photorefractory birds that were maintained in continuous
light in order to remove photoperiodic cues, prolactin injections
were administered daily at 0, 4, 8, 12, 16, or 20 hours after
injections of corticosterone. Various responses occurred depending on the temporal relations of the hormones. The most noteworthy
ones involved the injections of prolactin at 0, 4, or 12 hours after
injections of corticosterone. The 12-hour relation promoted growth
of the reproductive system, heavy fat stores, and nocturnal restlessness oriented to the north under the open sky; the 8-hour pattern
inhibited the reproductive system, decreased fat stores, and did not
induce nocturnal restlessness; and the 4-hour pattern of corticosterone and prolactin stimulated increases in fat stores and induced
noctrunal restlessness that was oriented to the south under the open
night sky (Neier & Martin, 1971; Meier et al., 1973; Meier, 1972,
1973a, 1973b; Meier & MacGregor, 1972; Martin & Meier, 1973). The

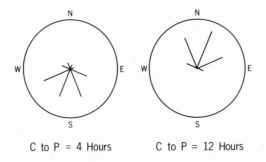

C to P = 4 Hours   C to P = 12 Hours

Fig. 20. The temporal relation of daily injections of corticosterone and prolactin control orientation in the migratory white-throated sparrow, Zonotrichia albicollis tested in orientation cages. The
intensity and compass orientation of the nocturnal activity of the
2 groups of birds receiving corticosterone (C) and prolactin (P)
are directly proportional to the lengths and directions of the
vectors, respectively. Derived from Martin & Meier (1973).

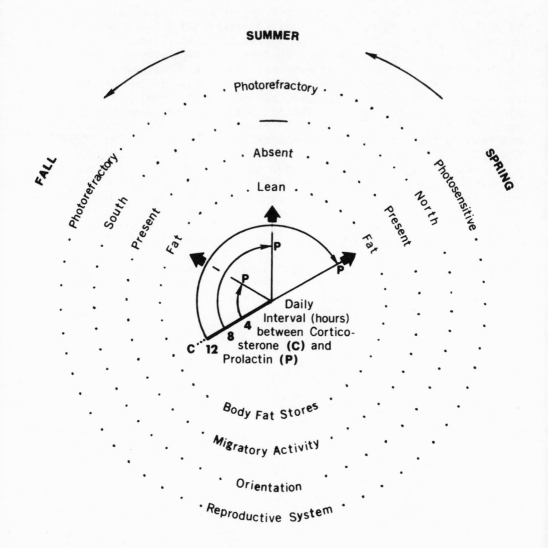

Fig. 21. Responses to exogenous corticosterone (C) and prolactin (P) vary depending on the temporal relation of the injections. Daily injection of prolactin administered 12 hours after corticosterone stimulate spring conditions of migration and reproduction. Similarly, an 8-hour pattern of hormone injections induces summer photorefractory conditions, and a 4-hour pattern of injections induces fall conditions. From Meier, American Scientist, 61:184-187 (1973).

conditions induced by the 12-, 8-, and 4-hour relations of hormone injections are similar to those found during the vernal migratory period, the summer photorefractory period, and the fall
migratory period, respectively (Figs. 20 & 21). The results produced by exogenous hormones may be correlated with studies of the
daily rhythms of endogenous corticosterone (Dusseau & Meier, 1971)
and prolactin (Meier et al., 1969) in the white-throated sparrow.
There is a 12-hour interval between the daily rise of plasma corticosterone and the release of pituitary prolactin during May when
the birds are in the vernal migratory condition and the gonads are
recrudescing, and an 8-hour interval between the hormones in August
when the birds are lean and reproductively photorefractory (Fig. 22).

The phases of the rhythms of corticosterone and prolactin
change from one season to another in the white-throated sparrow,
both with respect to each other and with respect to the daily photoperiod (Meier et al., 1969; Dusseau & Meier, 1971). The daily
rise of plasma corticosterone concentrations occurred near dawn in
May and early in the dark in August although the day-length was
approximately the same in the 2 months. The daily rise in pituitary prolactin content occurred at midday in both months but the decrease, or apparent release, of prolactin occurred during the afternoon in May and near dawn in August (Fig. 22). These findings suggest that the seasonal changes in the phases of the hormone rhythms
are parts of an endogenous mechanism that may be influenced by
changes in day length but might continue to produce seasonal variations in reproduction, metabolism, and behavior under conditions
of constant day lengths. The existence of a circannual rhythm of
metabolic and reproductive changes has been demonstrated in a number of animals maintained on constant photoperiods and temperatures
for more than a year. King (1970) reported that the expected
seasonal changes in fat stores persisted in a sparrow related to
the white-throated sparrow maintained for over a year in either
long or short daily photoperiods although the cycles varied by
several months from a year.

Thus, the control of the annual cycle in the white-throated
sparrow involves endogenous and exogenous components. The principal apparatus is endogenous and may be considered circannual. But
it can be influenced by day length which probably acts as a fine
adjustor in setting times for the seasonal events. The feedback
of other hormones may also be expected to influence this mechanism.
As discussed earlier, the thyroid hormones influence the rhythms
of adrenal corticoids (see DAILY RHYTHMS OF THYROID HORMONES) and
also influence avian reproduction (Thaplijal & Pandha, 1965). In
addition, the gonad must be present during the winter in the
white-throated sparrow for the photoperiodic induction of vernal
fattening (Weise, 1967). This finding may be analogous to the
role of estrogen in the estrous cycle in which estrogen is neces-

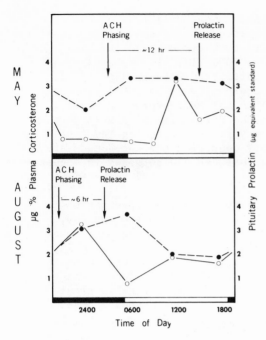

Fig. 22. Daily rhythms of plasma corticosterone and pituitary prolactin in photo-sensitive (May) and photo-refractory (August) <u>Zono-trichia albicollis</u> maintained on natural photoperiods. The closed circles represent the plasma concentrations of cor-ticosterone (ACH), and the open circles represent the amounts of pituitary pro-lactin. From Meier & Mac-Gregor, Am. Zoologist 12: 257-271 (1972).

sary for the continuation of the cycle and for the surge of pro-lactin on the evening of proestrus (see ESTRUS CYCLE).

SUMMARY AND CONCLUDING REMARKS

The neuroendocrine system provides the foundation and frame-work for the temporal organization of the vertebrate system. It regulates the cellular rhythms and integrates them so that behavior and metabolism support each other and the organism can function efficiently as an individual. The basic temporal unit of the neuroendocrine system is the circadian rhythm which exists with-out obvious external input. However, the neuroendocrine mechanism is responsive to environmental stimuli, especially the daily cycle of illumination, so that phases of the rhythms are set by the daily photoperiod. In turn the rhythms of the neuroendocrine system organize the entire animal so that it behaves in different ways during the course of a day. In addition the changing relations between hormone rhythms account for infradian cycles such as es-trous, lunar, and annual cycles.

The role of hormones in rhythms may be divided into 3 princi-pal categories: entrainers, modifiers, and inducers. The entrain-ers set the phases of the daily rhythms. The catecholamines and the adrenal corticoids acting separately and synergistically appear to be the principal hormonal agents of entrainment. The modifiers influence the amplitude of the rhythms, the relations of individual rhythms to each other, and the sensitivity of the entraining system to the environment. The hormones of the thyroid and the pineal are included in this category. The inducers act synergistically with the entraining hormones, stimulating those processes that are inducible at the time of day when the inducers are present. That is, the entrainers set rhythms of metabolic and behavioral responses to the inducers. The temporal relation of the daily rhythms of entrainers and inducers may change from day to day and produce the infradian cycles. Prolactin, growth hormone, insulin, and the hormones of the reproductive system often appear to act in the capacity of inducers.

Although many behaviors are clearly controlled directly and indirectly by the neuroendocrine system, there is also considerable evidence that specific behaviors may influence the rhythms of the neuroendocrine system and consequently many metabolic and reproductive conditions. It may well be possible to treat many physiological problems, such as obesity and infertility, by simple adjustments in our environment and in our daily schedule of activities. There is enormous potential in utilizing knowledge of circadian rhythms for improving the human condition.

REFERENCES

ADER, R., 1969, Early experiences accelerate maturation of the 24 hour adrenocortical rhythm, Science 163:1225.

ADER, R., FRIEDMAN, B., & GROTA, L. J., 1967, "Emotionality" and adrenal cortical function: Effects of strain and 24-hour corticosterone rhythm, Anim. Behav. 15:37.

ADLER, K., 1969, Extraoptic phase shifting of circadian locomotor rhythm in salamanders, Science 164:1290.

ALLEN, C., & KENDALL, J. W., 1967, Maturation of the circadian rhythm of plasma corticosterone in the rat, Endocrinology 80:926.

ALLEN, C., & KENDALL, J. W., & MONTE, A. G., 1972, The effect of surgical isolation of the basal hypothalamus on the nycthemeral rhythm of plasma corticosterone concentration in rats with hetero- topic pituitaries, Endocrinology 91:873.

ALLEVA, J. J., WALESKI, M. V., & ALLEVA, F. R., 1971a, A biological clock controlling the estrous cycle of the hamster, Endocrinology 88:1368.

ALLEVA, J. J., WALESKI, M. V., ALLEVA, F. R., & UMBERGER, C. J., 1968, Synchronizing effect of photoperiodicity on ovulation in hamsters, Endocrinology 82:1227.

ALVISI, C., & FERRARA, M., 1969, Contributo allo studio del ruolo delle strutture "limbiche" del lobo temporale nella regolazione del ritmo circadiano del cortisolo, G. Psichiat. Neuropat. 97:281.

ANDREWS, R. V., & FOLK, G. E., 1964, Circadian metabolic patterns in cultured hamster adrenal glands, Comp. Biochem. Physiol. 11: 393.

ARCANGELI, P., DIGIESI, V., MADEDDU, G., & TOCCAFONDI, R., 1973, Temporary displacement of plasma corticoid circadian peak in- duced by ablation of olfactory bulbs in dog, Experientia 29: 358.

ARIMURA, A., & SCHALLY, A. V., 1971, Augmentation of pituitary re- sponsiveness to LH-releasing hormone (LH-RH) by estrogen, Proc. Soc. Exp. Biol. Med. 136:290.

ARIMURA, A., DEBELJUK, L., & SCHALLY, A. V., 1972, LH release by
    LH-releasing hormone in golden hamsters at various stages of
    estrous cycle, Proc. Soc. Exp. Biol. Med. 140:609.

ARRINGTON, L. D., ABPLANALP, H., & WILSON, W. O., 1962, Experimental
    modification of the laying pattern in Japanese quail, Brit.
    Poultry Sci. 3:105.

ASCHOFF, J., 1955, Jahresperiodik der Fortpflanzung bei Warmblutern,
    Stud. Gena. 8:742.

AUERBACH, N., 1963, Diurnal variation in the level of serum protein-
    bound iodine in humans, Hartford Hosp. Bull. 18:168.

AXELROD, J., WURTMANN, R. J., & WINGET, C. M., 1964, Melatonin syn-
    thesis in the hen pineal gland and its control by light, Nature
    201:1134.

BACON, W., CHERMS, F. L., MACDONALD, G. J., & MCSHAN, H., 1969,
    Gonadotropin potency variation in anterior pituitaries from
    sexually mature male quail, Poul. Sci. 48:718.

BAGGERMAN, B., 1973, Report at symposium of Comp. Endocrinol., 1971.
    Gen. Comp. Endocrinol. Suppl. 3.

BAKKE, J. L., & LAWRENCE, N., 1965, Circadian periodicity in thyroid
    stimulating hormone titer in rat hypophysis and serum, Metabolism
    14:841.

BALL, J. N., 1969, Prolactin and growth hormone, in "Fish Physiology,"
    (W. S. Hoar & D. J. Randall, eds.), pp. 207-240, Academic Press,
    New York.

BARTTER, F. C., DELEA, C. S., & HALBERG, F., 1962, A map of blood
    and urinary changes related to circadian variations in adrenal
    cortical function in normal subjects, Ann. N. Y. Acad. Sci.
    98:969

BASTIAN, J. W., & ZARROW, M. X., 1955, A new hypothesis for the
    asynchronous ovulatory cycle of the domestic hen (Gallus domes-
    ticus), Poul. Sci. 34:776.

BENOIT, J., 1961, Opto-sexual reflex in the duck: physiological
    and histological aspects, Yale J. Biol. Med. 34:97.

BERSON, A., & YALOW, R. S., 1968, Radioimmunoassay of ACTH in plasma,
    J. Clin. Invest. 47:2725.

BINDON, B. M., & LAMOND, D. R., 1966, Diurnal component in response by the mouse to gonadotrophin, F. Reprod. Fert. 12:249.

BLUM, A. A., GREENSPAN, F. S., & MAGNUNS, J., 1968, Circadian rhythm of serum T.S.H. in normal human subjects, Proc. Intern. Congr. Endocrinol. 3rd, Mexico City 157:14.

BODENHEIMER, S., WINTER, J. S. D., & FAIMAN, C., 1973, Diurnal rhythms of serum gonadotrophin testosterone, estradiol and cortisol in blind men, J. Clin. Endocrinol. Metab. 37:472.

BOEHLKE, K. W., CHURCH, R. L., TIEMEIER, D. W., & ELEFTHERIOU, B. E., 1966, Diurnal rhythm in plasma glucocorticoid levels in channel catfish (lctalurus punctatus), Gen. Comp. Endocrinol. 7:18.

BOISSIN, J., BAYLE, J. D., & ASSENMACHER, I., 1971, Effets de la deconnexion hypothalamo-hypophysaire sur les rythmes circadiens de l'activite generale et de la corticosteronemie chez la Caille, C. R. Soc. Biol. 165:1382.

BOWERS, C. Y., FRIESEN, H. G., HWANG, P., GUYDA, H. J., & FOLKERS, K., 1971, Prolactin and thyrotropin release in man by sythetic pyroglutanyl-histidyl-prolinamide, Biochem. Biophys. Res. Commun. 45:1033.

BOYAR, R., PERLOW, M., HELLMAN, L., KAPEN, S., & WAITZMAN, E., 1972, Twenty-four hour pattern of luteinizing hormone secretion in normal men with sleep stage recording, J. Clin. Endocrinol. Metabl. 35:73.

BOYD, T. A. S., & MCLEOD, L. E., 1964, Circadian rhythms of plasma corticoid levels, intraocular pressure, and aqueous outflow facility in normal and glaucomatous eyes, Ann. N. Y. Acad. Sci. 117:597.

BUCKMAN, M. T., & PEAKE, G. T., 1973, Osmolar control of prolactin secretion in man, Science 181:755.

BULLOUGH, W. S., & LAWRENCE, E. B., 1964, Mitotic control by internal secretion. The role of the chalon-adrenalin complex, Exp. Cell Res. 33:176.

BUNNING, E., 1936, Die endogene Tagesrhythmik als Grundlage der photoperiodischen Reacktion. Ber. Deut. Botan. Ges. 54:590.

BUNNING, E., 1967, "The Physiological Clock," Springer-Verlag, New York.

BURNS, J. T., & MEIER, A. H., 1971, Daily variations in the pigeon crop sac response to prolactin, Experientia 27:572.

BUTCHER, R. L., FUGO, N. W., COLLINS, W. E., 1971, Semicircadian rhythm in plasma levels of prolactin during early gestation in the rat, Endocrinology 90:1125.

CHEIFETZ, P. N., GAFFUD, N., & DINGMAN, F., 1968, Effects of bilateral adrenalectomy and continuous light on the circadian rhythm of corticotrophin in female rats, Endocrinology 82:1117.

CHEIFETZ, P. N., GAFFUD, N. T., & DINGMAN, J. F., 1969, The effect of lysine vasopressin and hypothalamic extracts on the rate of corticosterone secretion in rats treated with dexamethasone and pentobarbitone, J. Endocrin. 43:521.

CLARK, R. H., & BAKER, B. L., 1964, Circadian periodicity in the concentration of prolactin in the rat hypophysis, Science 143:375.

COOVER, G. D., GOLDMAN, L., & LEVINE, S., 1971, Plasma corticosterone levels during performance and extinction of a lever-press response in hippocampectomized rats, Physiol. Behav. 7:727.

CRITCHLOW, V., LIEBELT, R. A., BAR-SELA, M., MOUNTCASTLE, W., & LIPCOMB, H. S., 1963, Sex difference in resting pituitary adrenal function in the rat, Amer. J. Physiol. 205:807.

DAVID-NELSON, M. A., & BRODISH, A., 1969, Evidence for diurnal rhythm of corticotropin-releasing factor (CRF) in the hypothalamus. Endocrinology 76:895.

DELACERDA, F. G., & STEBEN, R. E., 1974, The effect of an endurance type exercise program on the circadian rhythm of urine 17-ketosteroids, Med. Sci. in Sports (in press).

DENYES, A., & BAUMBER, J., 1964, Lipogenesis of cold-exposed and hibernating golden hamsters, Ann. Acad. Sci. Fenn. Ser. A, IV. 71:129.

DEVLAMING, V. L., & SAGE, M., 1972, Diurnal variation in fattening response to prolactin treatment in two cyprinodontid fishes, Cyprinodon variegatus and Fundulus similis, Marine Sci. 16:59.

DEWAN, E. M., 1967, On the possibility of a perfect rhythm method of birth control by periodic light stimulation, Am. J. Obstretr. Gynecol. 99:1016.

DODT, E., & HEERD, E., 1962, Mode of action of pineal nerve fibers in frogs, J. Neurophysiol. 25:405.

DONALDSON, E. M., & MCBRIDE, J. R., 1967, The effects of hypophysectomy in the rainbow trout Salmo gairdneiri (Rich.) with
special reference to the pituitary interrenal axis. Gen. Comp.
Endocrinol. 9:93.

DRAY, F., REINBERG, A., SEBOUN, J., 1965, Rhtyhme biologique de la
testosterone libre du plasma chez l'Homme adults sain: existence d'une variation circadienne, C. R. Acad. Sci. (D) (Paris).

D'TORIO, A., & LEDUC, J., 1960. The influence of thyroxine on the
omethylation of catecholamines, Dach. Biochem. 87:224.

DUNN, J. D., ARIMURA, A., & SCHEVING, L. E., 1972, Effect of stress
on circadian periodicity in serum L. H. and prolactin concentration, Endocrinology 90:29.

DUNN, J., BENNETT, M., & PEPPLER, R., 1972, Pituitary-adrenal function in photic and olfactory deprived rats, Proc. Soc. Biol.
Med. 140:755.

DUSSEAU, J., & MEIER, A. H., 1971, Diurnal and seasonal variations
of plasma adrenal steroid hormone in the white-throated sparrow
Zonotrichia albicollis, Gen. Comp. Endocrinol. 16:399.

EGAMI, N., 1954, Effect of artificial photoperiodicity on time of
oviposition in the fish, Oryzias latipes, Annot. Zool. Japan
27:57.

ELLIOTT, J. A., STETSON, M. H., & MENAKER, M., 1972, Regulation of
testis function in golden hamsters: A circadian clock measures
photoperiodic time, Science 178:771.

ERIKSSON, L. O., 1972, Die Jahresperiodik augen-und pineal-organloser
bachsaibling salvelinus fontinalis mitchell, Aquilo Ser. Zool.
13:8.

EVERETT, J. W., 1964, Central neural control of reproductive functions of the adenohypophysis, Physiol. Rev. 44:373.

EVERETT, J. W., & SAWYER, C. H., 1950, A 24-hour periodicity in the
"LH release apparatus" of female rats, disclosed by barbiturate
sedation. Endocrinology 47:198.

FAIMAN, C., & RYAN, R. J., 1967, Diurnal cycle in serum concentrations
of follicle-stimulating hormone in men, Nature 215:857.

FAIMAN, C., & WINTER, J. S. D., 1971, Diurnal cycles in plasma FSH,
testosterone and cortisol in men, J. Clin. Endocrinol. Metab.

33:186.

FARNER, D. S., 1964, The photoperiodic control of reproductive
cycles in birds, Amer. Scient. 52:137.

FARNER, D. S., 1965, Circadian systems in the photoperiodic responses of vertebrates, in "Circadian Clocks," (J. Aschoff,
ed.), pp. 357-369. North Holland Publ. Co., Amsterdam.

FENWICK, J. E., 1970, The pineal organ; photoperiod and reproductive cycles in the goldfish, J. Endocrinol. 46:101.

FERIN, M., RICHART, R. M., VANDEWIELE, R. L., 1974, "Biorhythms
and Human Reproduction," Wiley and Sons, Inc., New York.

FOLLETT, B. K., & SHARP. P. J., 1969, Circadian rhythmicity in
photoperiodically induced gonadotropin release and growth
in the quail, Nature 223:968.

FORSGREN, E., 1928, On the relationship between the formation of
bile and glycogen in the liver of rabbit, Skand. Arch. Physiol.
53:137.

FRANK, G., HALBERG, F., HARNER, R., 1966, Circadian periodicity,
adrenal corticosteroids, and the EEG of normal man, J. Psychiatric Res. 4:73.

FRANK, G., HARNER, R., MATTHEWS, J., JOHNSON, E., & HALBERG, F.,
1961, Circadian periodicity and the human electroencephalogram,
Proc. Ann. Meeting Am. Electroencephalog. Soc., 15th p. 24.

FRANKS, R. C., 1967, Diurnal variation of plasma 17-hydroxycortico-
steroids in children, J. Clin. Endocrinol. Metab. 27:75.

FRAPS, R. M., 1954, Neural basis of diurnal periodicity in release
of ovulation-inducing hormone in fowl, Proc. Natur. Acad. Sci.
U.S.A. 40:348.

FRAPS, R. M., 1955, Egg production and fertility in poultry, in
"Progress in the Physiology of Farm Animals," (J. Hammond,
ed.), vol. 2, pp. 661-740, Butterworths, London.

FRAPS, R. M., 1961, Ovulation in the domestic fowl, in "Control of
Ovulation," (C. A. Villee, ed.), pp. 135-167. Pergamon, London.

FRAPS, R. M., Fevold, H. L., & Neher, B. H., 1947, Ovulatory response
of the hen to presumptive luteinizing and other fractions from
fowl anterior pituitary tissue, Anat. Rec. 99:571.

FREEMAN, M. E., REICHERT, L. E., JR., & NEILL, J. D., 1972, Regulation of the proestrus surge of prolactin secretion by gonadotropin and estrogens in the rat, Endocrinology 90:232.

FULLERTON, D. T., 1968, Circadian rhythms of adrenal cortical activity in depression, Arch. Gen. Psychiatry 19:674.

FURR, B. J. A., BONNEY, R. C., ENGLAND, R. M., & CUNNINGHAM, F. J., 1973, Luetinizing hormone and progesterone in peripheral blood during the ovulatory cycle of the hen Gallus domesticus, J. Endocrinol. 57:159.

GAGLIARDINO, J. J., & HERNANDEZ, R. E., 1972, Circadian variation of the serum glucose and immunoreactive insulin levels, Endocrinology 88:1529.

GAMULIN, T., & HURE, J., 1956, Spawning of the sardine at a definite time of day, Nature 177:193.

GARCIA, L. E., & MEIER, A. H., 1973, Daily rhythms in concentration of plasma cortisol in male and female Gulf killifish, Fundulus grandis, Biol. Bull. 144:471.

GARNER, W. W., & ALLARD, H. A., 1920, Effect of relative length of day and night and other factors of the environment on growth and reproduction in plants, J. Agr. Res. 18:553.

GUILLEMAN, R., DEAR, W. E., & LIEBELT, R. A., 1959, Nycthemeral variations in plasma free corticosteroid levels of the rat, Proc. Soc. Exp. Biol. Med. 101:394.

GANONG, W. F., 1969, "Reveiw of Medical Physiology," Large Medical Publications, Los Altos, Calif.

GIRARD-GLOBA, A., & BOURDEL, G., 1973, Physiological regulation of the circadian rhythm in hepatic tyrosine tranaminase: Schedule of protein ingestion as a determinant factor, J. Nutrition. 103:251.

GLENISTER, D. W., & YATES, F. E., 1961, Sex difference in the rate of disappearance of corticosterone-4-C^{14} from plasma of intact rats: Further evidence for the influence of hepatic 4-steroid hydrogenase activity on adrenal cortical function, Endocrinology 68:747.

GREIG, F., & WEISZ, J., 1972, Preovulatory levels of luteinizing hormone, the critical period and ovulation in rats, J. Endocrinol. 57:235.

GWINNER, E. G., TUREK, F. W., & SMITH, S. D., 1971, Extraoccular light perception in photoperiodic responses of the white-crowned sparrow (Zonotrichia leucophrys) and of the golden-crowned sparrow (Zonotrichia atricapilla), Z. vergl. Physiol. 323-331.

HALASZ, B., 1969, In "Frontiers in Neuroendocrinology," (Ganong & Martini, eds.), pp. 307-342. Oxford University Press, New York.

HALASZ, B., SLUSHER, M. A., & GORSKI, R. A., 1967, Adrenocortico-trophic hormone secretion in rats after partial or total deafferentation of the medial basal hypothalamus, Neuroendocrinology 2:43.

HALBERG, F., 1953, Some physiological and clinical aspects of 24-hour periodicity, Lancet 73:20.

HALBERG, F., 1962, Discussion of glycogen metabolism, in "Mechanism of Regulation of Growth," pp. 31-32, Ross Conference on Pediatric Research, Ross Laboratories.

HALBERG, F., 1969, Chronobiology, Ann. Rev. Physiol. 31:675.

HALBERG, F., & VISSCHER, M. B., 1954, Temperature rhythms in blind mice, Fed. Proc. 13:65.

HALBERG, F., ALBRECHT, P. G., & BITTNER, J. J., 1959, Corticosterone rhythm of mouse adrenal in relation to serum corticosterone and sampling, Amer. J. Physiol. 197:1083.

HALBERG, F., & HOWARD, R. B., 1958, 24-hour periodicity and experimental medicine, Examples and interpretations, Postgraduate Med. 24:349.

HALBERG, F., ADKINS, G., & MARTE, E., 1962, Reserpine effect upon the variance spectrum of human rectal temperature, Fed. Proc. 21:347.

HALBERG, F., BARNUM, C. P., & VERMUND, H., 1953, Hepatic phospholipid metabolism and the adrenal, J. Clin. Endocrinol. Metab. 13:871.

HALBERG, F., PETERSON, R. E., & SILBER, R. H., 1959, Phase relations of 24-hour periodicities in blood corticosterone. Mitoses in cortical adrenal parenchyma, and total body activity, Endocrinology 64:222.

HALBERG, F., VISSCHER, M. B., & BITTNER, J. J., 1953, Eosinophil rhythm in mice, range of occurrence; effects of illumination feeding and adrenalectomy, Amer. J. Physiol. 174:109.

HALBERG, F., ZANDER, H. R., HOUGLUM, M. W., & MUHLEMANN, H. R., 1954,
Daily variations in tissue mitoses, blood eosinophils and rectal
temperature of rats, Amer. J. Physiol. 177:361.

HALBERG, F., FRANK, G., HARNER, R., MATHEYS, J., AAKER, H., GRAVEM,
H., & MELBY, J., 1961, The adrenal cycle in men on different
schedules of motor and mental activity, Experientia 17:1.

HAMNER, K. C., & TAKIMOTO, A., 1964, Circadian rhythms and plant
photoperiodism, Amer. Nat. 98:295.

HAMNER, W. M., 1963, Diurnal rhythm and photoperiodism in testicular
recrudescense of the house finch, Science 142:1294.

HAMNER, W. H., 1964, Circadian control of photoperiodism in the house
finch demonstrated by interrupted night experiments, Nature
203:1400.

HAMNER, W. M., 1965, Avian photoperiodic response-rhythms: Evidence
and inference, in "Circadian Clocks," (J. Aschoff, ed.), pp.
379-384, North-Holland, Amsterdam.

HAMNER, W. H., 1968, The photorefractory period of the house finch,
Ecology 49:211.

HARRINGTON, R. W., 1959, Effects of four combinations of temperature
and daylength on the ovogenetic cycle of a low latitude fish,
Fundulus confluentes, Zoologica 44:149.

HARRISON, T. S., 1964, Adrenal medullary and thyroid relationships,
Physiol. Rev. 44:161.

HARTH, M. S., & HEATON, M. B., 1973, Nonvisual photic responsiveness
in newly hatched pigeons (Columba livia), Science 180:753.

HAUS, E., 1964, Periodicity in response and susceptibility to environmental stimuli, Ann. N. Y. Acad. Sci. 117:292.

HAUS, E., LAKATUA, D., & HALBERG, F., 1967, The internal timing of
several circadian rhythms in the blinded mouse, Exper. Med.
Surgery 25:7.

HEDLUND, L., RALPH, C. L., CHEPKO, J., & LYNCH, H. J., 1971, Diurnal
serotonin cycle in the pineal body of Japanese quail: Photoperiod phasing and the effect of superior cervical ganglionectomy, Gen. Comp. Endocrinol. 16:52.

HELLMAN, L., FUJINORI, N., CURTI, J., WEITZMAN, E. D., KREAM, J.,
ROFFWARG, H., ELLMAN, S., FUKUSHIMA, D. K., GALLAGHER, T. F.,
Cortisol is secreted episodically by normal man, J. Clin.

Endocrinol. Metab. 30:411.

HICKMAN, P. E., HORTON, B. J., & SABINE, J. R., 1972, Effect of adrenalectomy on the diurnal variation of hepatic cholesterogenesis in the rat, J. Lipid Res. 12:17.

HIROSHIGE, T., & SAKAKURA, M., 1971, Circadian rhythm of corticotropin-releasing activity in the hypothalamus of normal and adrenolectomized rats, Neuroendocrinology 7:25.

HIROSHIGE, T., & SATO, T., 1970, Postnatal development of circadian rhythm of corticotropin-releasing activity in the rat hypothalamus, Endocrinol. Japan 17:1.

HIROSHIGE, T., KAZURO, A., WADA, S., & KANSKO, M., 1973, Sex difference in the rat hypothalamus, Neuroendocrinology 11:306.

HOFFMAN, R. A., 1964, Speculations on the regulation of hibernation, Ann. Acad. Sci. Fenn., Ser, A, IV. 71:199.

HOFFMAN, R. A., & REITER, R. J., 1966, Responses of some endocrine organs of female hamsters to pinealectomy and light, Life Sci. 5:1147.

HOKFELT, B., & LUFT, R., 1959, The effect of suprasellar tumours on the regulation of adrenocortical function, Acta endocr. 32:177.

HOLLWICH, F. VON, 1969, The influence of light via the eye on the endocrine system, Anales del Instituto Barraquer 9:133.

HOMMA, K., & SAKAKIBARA, Y., 1971, Encephalic photoreceptors and their significance in photoperiodic control of sexual activity in Japanese quail, in "Biochronometry," (M. Menaker, ed), pp. 333-341, Natl. Acad. Sci. Washington, D. C.

HONDA, Y., TAKAHASHI, K., TAKAHASHI, S., 1969, Growth hormone secretion during nocturnal sleep in normal subjects, J. Clin. Endocrinol. Metab. 29:20.

HUNTER, W. M., & RIGAL, W. M., 1966, The diurnal pattern of plasma growth hormone concentration in children and adolescents, J. Endocrinol. 34:147.

JACOBSSON, T., BLUMENTHAL, M., HAGNMAN, H., & HEILIKINEN, E., 1969, The diurnal variation of urinary excretion of 17-ketogenic steroids in the elderly (age group: 66-94 years), Acta. endocr. 66:25.

JENNER, C. E., & ENGLES, W. L., 1952, The significance of the dark period in the photoperiodic response of male juncos and white-throated sparrows, Biol. Bull. 103:345.

JOLIN, T., & MONTES, A., 1973, Daily rhythm of plasma glucose and insulin levels in rats, Hormone Res. 4:153.

JOHN, T. M., MEIER, A. H., & BRYANT, E. E., 1972, Thyroid hormones and the circadian rhythms of fat and crop sac reponses to prolactin in the pigeon, Physiol. Zool. 45:34.

JOHNSON, J. T., & LEVINE, S., 1973, Influence of water deprivation on adrenocortical rhythms, Neuroendocrinology 11:268.

JOHNSON, J. H., & SAWYER, C. H., 1971, Adrenal steroids and the maintenance of a circadian distribution of paradoxical sleep in rats, Endocrinology 89:507.

JORI, A., DISALLE E., & SANTIRI, V., 1971, Daily rhythmic variation and liver drug metaboliens in rats, Biochem. Pharmacol. 20:2965.

JORI, A., CACCIA, S., & DISALLE, E., 1973, Tissue catecholamines and daily rhythm of liver microsomal enxyme activity, European J. Pharmacology 21:37.

JOSEPH, M. M., & MEIER, A. H., 1971, Daily variations in the fattening response to prolactin in Fundulus grandis held on different photoperiods, J. Exp. Zool. 178:59.

JOSEPH, M. M., & MEIER, A. H., 1973, Daily rhythms in concentrations of plasma corticosterone in the common pigeon, Columba livia, Gen. Comp. Endocrinol. 20:326.

JOSEPH, M. M., & MEIER, A. H., 1974, Circadian component in the fattening and reproductive responses to prolactin in the hamster, Proc. Soc. Exp. Biol. Med. (in press)

JOUVET, M., 1969, Biogenic amines and the states of sleep, Science 163:32.

KACHI, T., MATSVOHIMA, S., & ITO, T., 1973, Diurnal variations in pineal glycogen content during the estrous cycle in female mice, Archivum histolgicum japonecum 35:153.

KALMUS, H., 1940, Diurnal rhythms in the axolotl larva and in drosophila, Nature 145:72.

KALRA, S. P., AJIKA, K., KRULICH, L., FAWCETT, C. P., QUIJADA, M., & MCCANN, S. M., 1971, Effects of hypothalamic and pre-optic electrochemical stimulation on gonadotropin and prolactin release in proestrous rats, Endocrinology 88:1150.

KAMBERI, I. A., MICAL, R. S., & PORTER, J. C., 1970, Effect of anterior pituitary perfusion and intraventricular injection of catecholamines and indolamines on LH release, Endocrinology 87:1.

KAMBERI, I. A., MICAL, R. S., & PORTER, J. C., 1971, Effects of melatonin and serotonin on the release of FSH and prolactin, Endocrinology 88:1288.

KAMIGOSHI, M., & TANAKA, K., 1969, Changes in pituitary FSH concentrations during ovulatory cycle of the hen, Poultry Sci. 48:2026.

KATO, M., KATO, Y., & OISHI, T., 1967, Radioluminous paints as activators of photoreceptor systems studies with swallowtail butterfly and quail, Proc. Jap. Acad. 43:220.

KAYSER, C., 1957, Le sommeil hivernal, probleme de thermoregulation, Rev. Can. Biol., 16:303.

KAYSER, C., 1961, "The Physiology of Natural Hibernation," Pergamon Press, New York.

KENT, G. C., JR., TURNBULL, J. G., & KIRBY, A. C., 1964, A daily rhythm in prolactin secretion on release in hamsters, Assoc. Southeastern Bio. Bull. 11:48 (Abstract)

KENT, G. C., 1967, Physiology of reproduction, in "The Golden Hamster: Its Biology and Use in Medical Research," Hoffman, Robinson & Magalhaus, p. 119, University Press, Ames, Iowa.

KIELY, M. J., & DOMM, L. V., 1973, Circadian uptake of H-thymidine in the rat incisor under the influence of cortisone, Proc. Soc. Exp. Biol. Med. 143:844.

KING, J. R., 1970, Photoregulation of food intake and fat metabolism in relation to avian sexual cycles, in "Coll. Intern. CN.R.S. No. 172," (P. Benoit & Assenmacher, eds.), pp. 365-385.

KIRKPATRICK, C. M., 1959, Interrupted dark period: tests for refractoriness in bobwhite quail hens, in "Photoperiodism and Related Phenomena in Plants and Animals," (R. B. Withrow, ed.), pp. 751-758, Amer. Ass. Advan. Sci. Washington.

KITAY, J. I., & ALSCHULE, M. D., 1954, "The Pineal Gland," Harvard Univ. Press, Cambridge, Massachusetts.

KOLODNY, R. C., JACOBS, L. S., & DAUGHADAY, W. H., 1972, Mammary stimulation causes prolactin secretion in non-lactating women. Nature 238:284.

KOPROWSKI, J. A., TUCKER, H. A., & CONVEY, E. M., 1972, Prolactin and growth hormone circadian periodicity in lactating cows, Proc. Soc. Exp. Biol. Med. 140:1012.

KRIEGER, D. T., & KRIEGER, H. P., 1967, The effect of short-term administration of CNS acting drugs on the circadian variation of the plasma 17-OHCS in normal subjects, Neuroendocrinology 2:232.

KRIEGER, D. T., ALLEN, W., PIZZO, F., & KRIEGER, H. P., 1961, Characterization of the normal temporal pattern of plasma corticosteroid levels, J. Clin. Endocr. 32:266.

KRIEGER, D. T., & KRIEGER, H. P., 1966, The circadian variation of the plasma 17-OHCS in central nervous system disease, J. Clin. Endocrinol. Metab. 26:939.

KRIEGER, D. T., KRIEGER, H. B., 1967, Circadian pattern of plasma 17-hydroxy corticosteroid alteration by anticholinergic agents, Science 155:1421.

KRIEGER, D. T., & KRIEGER, H. P., 1966, Adrenal function in central nervous system disease, Endocrines and the Central Nervous System 43:400.

KRIEGER, D. T., & KRIEGER, H. P., 1967, Circadian pattern of plasma 17-hydroxy-corticosteroid: alteration by anticholinergic agents, Science 155:1421.

KRIEGER, D. T., OSSOWSKI, R., FOGEL, M., & ALLEN, W., 1972, Lack of circadian periodicity of human serum FSH and LH levels, J. Clin. Endocrinol. Metab. 35:619.

KRIEGER, D. T., & PIZZO, D. P., 1971, Circadian periodicity of plasma 11-hydrosycorticosteroid levels in subjects with partial and absent light perception, Neuroendocrinology 8:165.

LAIRD, C. W., & FOX, R. R., 1970, Diurnal variations in rabbits: biochemical indicators of thyroid function, Life Sci. 9:191.

LAKE, J. S., 1967, Rearing experiments with five species of Australial freshwater fishes. I. Inducement to spawning, Australian J. Marine Freshwater Res. 18:137.

LEATHERLAND, J. F., & MCKEOWN, B. A., 1973, Circadian rhythm in the plasma levels of prolactin in goldfinch, Carassius auratus L., J. Interdiscipl. Cycle Res. 4:137.

LEE, R. W., & MEIER, A. H., 1967, Diurnal variations of the fattening response to prolactin in the golden topminnow, Fundulus chrysotus, J. Exptl. Zool. 166:307.

LEVINE, R. J., OATES, J. A., VENDSALU, A., & SJOERDSAM, A., 1962, Studies on the metabolism of aromatic amines in relation to altered thyroid function in man, J. Clin. Endocrin. 22:1242.

LICHT, P., 1966, Reproduction in lizards: Influence of temperature on photoperiodism in testicular recrudescence, Science 154:1668.

LISK, R. D., 1969, Cyclic fluctuations in sexual responsiveness in the male rat, J. Exp. Zool. 171:313.

LITTMANN, K. P., & GERDES, H., 1972, Testosterontagesrhythmic and HCG-Stimulation bei akuten und chronischen leberkronkungen, Klin. Wechr. 50:1123.

LOFTS, B., & MURTON, R. K., 1968, Photoperiodic and physiological adaptations regulating avian breeding cycles and their ecological significance, J. Zool. (London) 155:327.

LYNCH, H. J., & RALPH, C. L., 1970, Diurnal variation in pineal melatonin and its non-relationship to H1OMT activity, Amer. Zool. 10:300.

MACGREGOR, R., III, 1972, Avian reproduction systems: daily variations in responses to hormones, Proc. Int. Symp. Biological Rhythms, Little Rock, Ark. (in press).

MANN, D. R., & BARRACLOUGH, C. A., 1973, Changes in peripheral plasma progesterone during the rat 4-day estrous cycle: an adrenal diurnal rhythm, Proc. Soc. Exp. Biol. Med. 135:934.

MACROVITCH, S., 1924, The migration of the aphidas and the appearance of the sexual forms as affected by the relative length of daily light exposure, J. Agr. Res. 27:513.

MARSHALL, J. A., 1967, Effect of artificial photoperiodicity on the time of spawning in Trichoposis vittatus and T. pumilis (Pisces, Belontiidae) Anim. Behav. 15:510.

MARTIN, D. D., & MEIER, A. H., 1973, Temporal synergism of corticosterone and prolactin in regulating orientation in the migratory white-throated sparrow (Zonotrichia albicollis), Condor 75:369.

MARTIN, M., & HELLMAN, D. E., 1963, Temporal variation in Su-4885 responsiveness in man: Evidence in support of circadian variation in ACTH secretion, J. Clin. Endocrinol. Metab. 24:243.

MARTIN, M. M., MINTZ, D. H., & TAMAGAKI, H., 1963, Effect of altered thyroid function upon steroid circadian rhythms in man, Clin. Res. 10:35.

MASON, J. W., 1968, A review of psychoendocrine research on the pituitary-adrenal cortical system, Psychosom. Med. 30:576-6

MAYHEW, W. W., 1964, Photoperiodic responses in three species of the lizard genus Uma, Herpetologica 20:95.

MCCARTHY, J. ., CORLEY, R. C., & ZARROW, M. X., 1960, Diurnal rhythms in plasma corticosterone and lack of diurnal rhythm in plasma compound F-like material in the rat, Proc. Soc. Exp. Biol. 104:786.

MCCORMACK, C. E., & MEYER, R. K., 1962, Ovulation induced by progesterone in immature rats pretreated with pregnant mare serum gonadotropin, Gen. and Comp. Endocrinol. 3:300.

MCDONALD, R. K., EVANS, F. T., WEISE, V. K., & PATRICK, R. W., 1959, Effects of morphine on ACTH production, J. Pharmacol. 125:241.

MEHRLE, P. M., & FLEMING, W. R., 1970, The effect of early and mid-day prolactin injection on the lipid content of Fundulus kansae held on a constant photoperiod, Comp. Biochem. Physiol. 36:597.

MEIER, A. H., 1969a, Diurnal variations of metabolic responses to prolactin in lower vertebrates, Gen. Comp. Endocrinol. Suppl. 2:55.

MEIER, A. H., 1969b, Antigonadal effects of prolactin in the white-throated sparrow, Zonotrichia albicollis, Gen. Comp. Endocrinol. Suppl. 13:222.

MEIER, A. H., 1970, Thyroxin phases the circadian fattening response to prolactin, Proc. Soc. Exp. Biol. Med. 133:1113.

MEIER, A. H., 1972, Temporal synergism of prolactin and adrenal steroids, Gen. Comp. Endocrinol. Suppl. 3:499.

MEIER, A. H., 1973, Temporal synergism of corticosterone and prolactin controlling seasonal conditions in the white-throated sparrow, Zonotrichia albicollis, Int. Symp. Biological Rhythms, Little Rock, Ark. (in press).

MEIER, A. H., 1973, Daily hormone rhythms and seasonal conditions in a sparrow, Amer. Scientist 61:184.

MEIER, A. H., BURNS, J. T., & DUSSEAU, J. W., 1969, Seasonal variations in the diurnal rhythms of pituitary prolactin content in the white-throated sparrow, Zonotrichia albicollis, Gen. Comp. Endocrinol. 12:282.

MEIER, A. H., BURNS, J., T., DAVIS, K. B., & JOHN, T. M., 1971, Circadian variations in crop sac and fat responses to prolactin in the pigeon, J. Interdisciplinary Cycles Res. 2:161.

MEIER, A. H., & DAVIS, K. B., 1967, Diurnal variations of the fattening response to prolactin in the white-throated sparrow, Zonotrichia albicollis, Gen. Comp. Endocrinol. 8:110.

MEIER, A. H., & DUSSEAU, J. W., 1968, Prolactin and the photoperiodic gonadal response in several avian species, Physiol. Zool. 41:95.

MEIER, A. H., & DUSSEAU, J. W., 1973, Daily entrainment of the photoinducible phases for photostimulation of the reproductive system in the sparrows, Zonotrichia albicollis and Passer domesticus, Biol. Reproduction 8:400.

MEIER, A. H., GARCIA, L. E., & JOSEPH, M. M., 1971a, Corticosterone phases a circadian waterdrive response to prolactin in the spotted newt, Notophthalmus viridescens, Biol. Bull, 141:331.

MEIER, A. H., JOHN, T. M., JOSEPH, M. M., 1971d, Corticosterone and the circadian pigeon crop sac response to prolactin, Comp. Biochem. Physiol. 40:459.

MEIER, A. H., & MACGREGOR, R., III, 1972, Temporal synergism of corticosterone and prolactin controlling fat storage in the white-throated sparrow, Zonotrichia albicollis, Gen. Comp. Endocrinol. 17:311.

MEIER, A. H., & MARTIN, D. D., 1971, Temporal synergism of corticosterone and prolactin controlling fat storage in the white-throated sparrow, Zonotrichia albicollis, Gen. Comp. Endocrinol. 17:311.

MEIER, A. H., MARTIN, D. D., & MACGREGOR, R., III, 1971b, Temporal synergism of corticosterone and prolactin controlling gonadal growth in sparrows, Science 173:1240.

MEIER, A. H., TROBEC, T. N., JOSEPH, M. M., & JOHN, T. M., 1971c, Temporal synergism and adrenal steroids in the regulation of fat stores, Proc. Soc. Exp. Biol. Med. 137:408.

MEIER, A. H., TROBEC, T. N., HAYMAKER, H. G., MACGREGOR, R., III., & RUSSO, A. C., 1973, Daily variations in the effects of handling on fat storage and testicular weights in several vertebrates, J. Exp. Zool. 184:281.

MENAKER, M., 1965, Circadian rhythms and photoperiodism in Passer domesticus, in "Circadian Clocks," (J. Aschoff, ed.), pp. 385-395, North Holland Publ. Co., Amsterdam.

MENAKER, M., 1968, Extraretinal light perception in the sparrow, I. Entrainment of the biological clock, Proc. Nat. Acad. Sci. 59:414.

MENAKER, M., 1972, Nonvisual light reception, Sci. Amer. 226:22.

MENAKER, M., & ESKIN, A., 1967, Circadian clock in photoperiodic time measurement: A test of the Bünning Hypothesis, Science 157:1182.

MENAKER, M., & KEATTS, H., 1968, Extraretinal light perception in the sparrow, Proc. Nat. Acad. Sci. 60:146.

MIGEON, C. J., TYLER, J., MAHONEY, P., FLORENIN, A. A., CASTLE, H., BLISS, E. L., & SAMUELS, L. T., 1956. The diurnal variations of plasma levels and urinary excretion of 17-hyroxy-corticosteroids in normal subjects, night workers and blind subjects, J. Clin. Endocrinol. 16:622.

MILLER, A. H., 1959, Reproductive cycles in an equatorial sparrow, Proc. Nat. Acad. Sci. 45:1095.

MILLS, J. N., 1966, Human circadian rhythms, Physiol. Rev. 46:128.

MOLNAR, G. D., TAYLOR, W. F., LANGWORTHY, A., FATOURECHI, V., 1972, Diurnal growth hormone and glucose abnormalities in unstable diabetics: Studies of ambulatory-bed subjects during continuous blood glucose analysis, J. Clin. Endocronol. Metab. 34:837.

MORIN, L. P., 1973, Ovulatory and body weight response of the hamster to constant light or pinealectomy, Neuroendocrinology 12:192.

MULLER, E. E., GUISTINA, F., MIEDICO, P., PACILE, A., COCCHI, D., & KING, F. W., 1970, Circadian pattern of bioassayable and radioimmunoassayable growth hormone in the pituitary of female rats, Proc. Soc. Exp. Biol. Med. 135:934.

MURTON, R. K., BAGSHAWE, K. D., & LOFTS, B., 1969, The circadian basis of specific gonadotrophin release in relation to avian spermatogenesis, J. Endocrinol. 45:311.

MURTON, R. K., LOFTS, B., ORR, A. A., 1970, The significance of circadian based photosensitivity in the house sparrow, Passer domesticus, ibis. 112:448.

MURTON, R. K., LOFTS, B., & WESTWOOD, N. J., 1970b, Manipulation of photorefractoriness in the house sparrow (Passer domesticus) by circadian light regimes, Gen. Comp. Endocrinol. 14:107.

NAKAGAWA, K., 1971, Probable sleep dependency of diurnal rhythm of plasma growth hormone response to hypoglycemia, J. Clin. Endocrinol. Metab. 33:854.

NALBANDOV, A. V., 1961, Neuroendocrine reflex mechanisms: bird ovulation, in "Comparative Endocrinology," (A. Gerbman, ed.) pp. 161-173, Wiley, New York.

NANKIN, H. R., & TROEN, P., 1972, Repetitive luteinizing hormone elevations in serum of normal men, J. Clin. Endocrinol. Metab. 33:558.

NATHANIELSZ, P. W., 1969, A circadian rhythm in the disappearance of thyroxine from the blood in the calf and the thyroidectomized rat, J. Physiol. (Lond.) 204:79.

NEILL, J. D., & REICHERT, L. E., JR., 1971, Development of a radioimmunoassay for rat prolactin and evaluation of the NIAMD rat prolactin radioimmunoassay, Endocrinology 88:548.

NOKIN, J., VEKEMANS, M., L'HERMITE, M., & ROBYN, C., 1972, Circadian periodicity of serum prolactin concentration in man, Brit. Med. Jour. 3:561.

ODELL, W. D., & MOXER, D. L., 1971, "Physiology of Reproduction," Mosby, St. Louis.

OGURI, M., OMURA, Y., HIBIYA, T., 1968. Uptake of ^{14}C-labelled 5-hydroxy tryptamine into the pineal organ of rainbow trout, Bull. Japan Soc. Sci. Fisheries 34:687.

OISHI, T., & KATO, M., 1968, Pineal organ as a possible photoreceptor in photoperiodic testicular response in Japanese quail, Mem. Fac. Sci. Kyoto Univ., Ser. Biol. 2:12.

OKSCHE, A., 1962, Histologische, histochemische und experimentelle studien am subcommissura lorgon von Anuren (mit Hinweisen auf den Epiphysenkomplex), Z. Zellforsch. 57:240.

OKSCHE, A., & KIRCHSTEIN, H., 1967, Die ultrastruktur der sinneszellen in pineal-organ von Phoxinus laevis, Z. Zellforsch. Mikroshop Anat. 78:151.

OKSCHE, A., KIRCHSTEIN, H., KOBAYASHI, H., & FARNER, D. S., 1972,
Electron microscopic and experimental studies of the pineal
organ in the white-crowned sparrow, Zonotrichia leucophgys
gambeli, Z. Zellforsch. 124:247.

OPEL, H., 1966, The timing of oviposition and ovulation in the
quail (Coturnix coturnix japonica), Br. Poultry Sci. 7:29.

OPPENHEIMER, J. H., FISHER, L. V., & JAILER, J. W., 1961, Disturbance
of the pituitary-adrenal interrelationship in diseases of the
central nervous system, J. Clin. Endocrinol. Metab. 21:1023

ORTAVANT, R., MAULEON, P., & THIBAULT, C., 1964, Photoperiodic
control of gonadal and hypophyseal activity in domestic mammals, Ann. N. Y. Acad. Sci. 117:157.

ORTH, D. M., & ISLAND, D. P., 1969, Light synchonization of the
circadian rhythms in plasma cortisol (17-OHCS) concentration
in man, J. Clin. Endocrinol. 29:479.

ORTH, D. N., ISLAND, D. P., & LIDDLE, G. W., 1967, Experimental
alternation of the circadian rhythm in plasma cortisol (17-OHCS)
concentration in man, J. Clin. Endocrinol. Metab. 27:549.

OSTERMAN, P. O., LUNDBERG, P. O., & WIDE, L., 1973, The level and
circadian rhythm of plasma free 11-hydroxycorticoids in patients
with localized intracranial processes, especially of the sellar
region, Acta Neural Scandinav. 49:115.

PALKA, Y., COYER, D., & CRITCHLOW, V., 1969, Effects of isolation
of medial basal hypothalamus on pituitary-adrenal and pituitary-
ovarian functions, Neuroendocrinology 5:333.

PARKER, D. C., ROSSMAN, L. G., & VANDERLAAN, E. F., 1973, Sleep-re-
lated, nyctohemeral and briefly episodic variation in human
plasma prolactin concentrations, J. Clin. Endocrinol. Metab.
36:1119.

PERKOFF, G. T., EIK-NEA, K., 1959, Studies of the diurnal variation
of plasma 17-hydroxycorticosteroids in man, J. Clin. Endocrinol.
Metab. 19:432.

PINCUS, G., 1943, A diurnal rhythm in the excretion of urinary ketosteroids by young men, J. Clin. Endocrinol. 3:195.

PITTENDRIGH, C. S., 1966, The circadian oscillation in Drosophila
pseudoobscura pupae: A model for the photoperiodic scale,
Z. Plorzerphysiol. 54:275.

POPOVIC, P., 1956, Thyroidectomy and rhythms of oxygen consumption and temperature in rats, Compte. Rend. Soc. Biol. Paris 150:1249.

POPOVIC, V. P., 1960, Endocrines in hibernation, Bull. Mus. Comp. Zool. Haw., 124:105.

QUABBLE, H. J., SCHILLING, E., & HELGE, H., 1966, Pattern of growth hormone secretion during a 24-hour fast in normal adults, J. Clin. Endocrinol. Metab. 26:1173.

QUAY, W. B., 1963, Circadian rhythm in rat pineal serotonin and its modifications by estrous cycle and photoperiod, Gen. Comp. Endocrinol. 3:473.

QUAY, W. B., 1965, Regional and circadian differences in cerebral cortical serotonin concentration. Life Sciences 4:379.

QUAY, W. B., 1966, Rhythmic and light-induced changes in levels of pineal S-hydroxyindoles in the pigeon (Columba livia), Gen. Comp. Endocrinol. 6:371.

RADZIALOWSKI, F. M., & BOUSQUET, W. F., 1967, Circadian rhythm in hepatic drug mobilizing activity in the rat, Life Sci. 6:2545.

RADZIALOWSKI, F. M., & BOUSQUET, W. F., 1968, Daily rhythmic variation in hepatic drug metabolism in the rat and mouse. J. Pharmacol. Exptl. Ther. 163:229.

RALPH, C. L., & FRAPS, R. M., 1959, Effect of hypothalamic lesions on progesterone-induced ovulation in the hen, Endocrinology 65:819.

RAMALEY, J. A., 1973, The development of daily changes in serum corticosterone in pre-weanling rats, Steroids 21:433.

RAPOPORT, M., FEIGIN, R. D., BRUTON, J., & BEISEL, W. R., 1966, Circadian rhythm for tryptophan pyrrolase activity and its circulating substrate, Science 153:1642.

RAPS, D., BARTHE, P. L., & DESSAULES, P. A., 1971, Plasma and adrenal corticosterone levels during the different phases of the sexaul cycle in normal female rats. Experientia 27:399.

REINBERG, A., 1969, Rhythmes circadiens du metabolisme du potassium chez l'homme, in "Le Potassium et La Vie," pp. 103-104, Presses Universitaries de France, Paris.

REINBERG, A., 1969, Biorhythmes et chronolobiologie, Presse Medicale 77:877.

REINBERG, A., 1965, "Biological Rhythms," Walker & Son, New York.

REINBERG, A., & SIDI, E., 1966, Circadian changes in the inhibitory
    effects of an antihistaminic drug in man, J. Invest. Dermatol.
    46:415.

REINBERG, A., HALBERG, F., GHATA, J., 1969, Rhythm circadien de
    diverses fonctions physiologiques de l'Homme adulte sain, actif
    et au repos (pouls, pression arterielle excretions urinaires
    des 17OHCS des catecholamines et du potassium), J. Physiol.,
    Paris 61:383.

REINBERG, A., SIDI, E., & GHATA, J., 1965, Circadian reactivity
    rhythms of human skin to histamine or allergen and the adrenal
    cycle, J. Allergy 36:273.

REINGERG, A., HALBERG, F., GHATA, J., & SIFFRE, M., 1966, Spectre
    thermique (rhythmes de la temperature rectale) d'une femme
    adulte saine avant, pendant, apres on isolement souterraine de
    trois mois, Compt. Rend. Acad. Sci., 262:782.

REINBERG, A., GHATA, J., & HALBERG, F., 1970. Rhythmes circadiens
    du pouls, de la pression arterielle, des excretions urinaires
    en 17-hydroxycorticosteroides catecholamines et potassium chez
    l'homme adulte sain, actif et au repos, Ann. Endocrinol. (Paris)
    31:277.

REIS, D. J., & WURTMANN, R. J., 1968, Diurnal changes in brain nor-
    adrenalin, Life Sciences 7:91.

REIS, D. J., WEINBREN, M., & CORVELLI, A., 1968, A circadian rhythm
    of norepinephrine regionally in cat brain: its relationship
    to environmental lighting and to regional diurnal variations
    in brain serotonin, J. Pharmacol. Exper. Therap. 164:135.

REITER, R. J., & HESTER, R. J., 1966, Interrelationships of the
    pineal gland, the superior cervical ganglic and the photoperiod
    in the regulation of the endocrine systems of hamsters, Endo-
    crinology. 79:1168.

RESKO, J. A., & EIK-NES, K. B., 1966, Diurnal testosterone levels
    in peripheral plasma of human male subjects, J. Clin. Endocrinol.
    Metab. 26:573.

RETIENNE, K., ZIMMERMANN, W. J., SCHINDLER, C. J., & LIPSCOMB, H. S.,
    1968, A correlative study of resting endocrine rhythms in rats,
    Acta Endocrinol. 57:615.

RIDDLE, O., 1963, Prolactin in vertebrate function and organization, J. Natl. Cancer Inst. 31:1039.

RIDDLE, O., BATES, R. W., & DYKSHORN, S. W., 1932, A new hormone of the anterior pituitary, Proc. Soc. Exp. Biol. Med. 29:1211.

RILEY, G. M., 1936, Light regulation of sexual activity in the male sparrow (Passer domesticus), Proc. Soc. Exptl. Biol. Med. 34:331.

RILEY, G. M., 1937, Experimental studies on spermatogenesis in the house sparrow, Passer domesticus (L.), Anat. Rec. 67:327.

ROBINSON, E. J., & RUGH, R., 1943, The reproductive processes of the fish, Oryzias latipes, Biol. Bull. 84:115.

ROTH, J., GLICK, S. M., YALOW, R. S., & BERSON, S. A., 1963, Hypoglycemia: A potent stimulus to secretion of growth hormone, Science 140:987.

ROTHCHILD, I., & FRAPS, R. M., 1949, The interval between normal release of ovulating hormone and ovulation in the domestic hen, Endocrinology 44:134.

ROWAN, W., 1926, On photoperiodism, reproductive periodicity, and the annual migrations of birds and certain fishes, Proc. Boston Soc. Natl. Hist. 38:147.

RUBIN, R. T., GOVIN, P. R., ARENANDER, A. T., & POLAND, R. E., 1973, Human growth hormone release during sleep following prolonged flurazepam administration, Res. Comm. Chem. Path. Pharm. 6:331.

RUBIN, R. T., KALES, A., ADLER, R., FEGAN, T., & ODELL, W., 1972, Gonadotropin secretion during sleep in normal adult men, Science 175:196.

SABA, G. C., CARNICELLI, A., SABA, P., & MARESCOTTI, V., 1963, Diurnal rhythm in the adrenal cortical secretion and in the rate of metabolism of corticosterone in the rat, Acta Endocr. 44:413.

SABA, G. C., SABA, P., CARNICELLI, A., & MARESCOTTI, V., 1963, Diurnal rhythm in the adrenal cortical secretion and in the rate of metabolism of corticosterone in the rat, Acta Endocr. 44:409.

SASSIN, J. F., FRANTY, A. G., WEITZMAN, E. D., & KAPEN, S., 1972, Human prolactin: 24-hour pattern with increased release during sleep, Science 177:1205.

SATO, T., & GEORGE, J. C., 1973, Diurnal rhythm of corticotropin-releasing factor activity in the pigeon hypothalamus, Can. J. Physiol. Pharmacol. 51:743.

SEXENA, B. B., DEMURA, H., GAUDY, H. M., & PETERSON, R. E., 1968, Radio-immunoassay of human follicle stimulating and luteining hormones in plasma, J. Clin. Endocr. 28:519.

SAYLER, A., & WOLFSON, A., 1968, Influence of the pineal gland on gonadal maturation in the Japanese quail, Endocrinology 83:1237.

SAYLER, A., & WOLFSON, A., 1969, Hydroxyindole-O-methyl transferase (HLOMT) activity in the Japanese quail in relation to sexual maturation and light, Neuroendocrinology 5:322.

SCAPAGNINI, U., VAN LOON, G. R., MOBERG, G. P., & GANONG, W. F., 1970, Effect of α-methyl-p-tyrosine on the circadian variation of plasma corticosterone in rats, Eur. J. Pharmacol. 11:266.

SCHOOLEY, J. P., & RIDDLE, O., 1938, The morphological basis of pituitary function in pigeons, Amer. J. Anat. 62:313.

SEABLOOM, R. W., 1965, Daily motor activity and corticosterone secretion in the meadow vole, J. Mammal. 46:286.

SEIDEN, G., & BRODISH, A., 1972, Persistence of a diurnal rhythm in hypothalamus corticotrophin-releasing factor (CRF) in the absence of hormone feedback, Endocrinology 90:1401.

SINGH, D. V., PANDA, J. N., ANDERSON, R. R., & TURNER, C. W., 1967, Diurnal variation of plasma and pituitary thyrotropin (TSH) of rats, Proc. Soc. Exp. Biol. Med. 126:553.

SRIVASTAVA, A. K., & MEIER, A. H., 1972, Daily variation in concentration of cortisol in plasma in intact and hypophysectomized Gulf killifish, Science 177:185.

STOKES, J. A., CHERNIK, D. A., & PANDY, G., 1972, Effects of diazepam on growth hormone release during sleep, Sleep Res. 1:190.

STROEBEL, C. F., 1967, A biologic rhythm approach to psychiatric treatment, in "Proceedings of the Seventh Medical Symposium," pp. 215-241, IBM Press,

STROEBEL, C. F., 1967, Biochemical, behavioral, and clinical models of drug interactions, in "Proceedings of the Fifth International Colloquium of Neuropsychopharmalogicum," "Excerpta Medica," Washington, D. C.

SWANSON, L. V., & HAFS, H. D., 1971, LH and prolactin in blood serum
    from estrous to ovulation in holstein heifers, J. Anim. Sci.
    33:1038.

TAKEBE, K., SAKAKURA, M., HORIUCHI, Y., & MASHIMO, K., 1971, Per-
    sistence of diurnal periodicity of CRF activity in adrenalectom-
    ized and hypophysectomized rats, Endocrinol. Jap. 18:451.

TANAKA, K., WILSON, W. O., MATHER, F. B., & MCFARLAND, L. Z., 1966,
    Diurnal variation in gonadotropic potency of the adenohypophysis
    of Japanese quail (Coturnix coturnix japonica), Gen. Comp.
    Endocrinol. 9:374.

TAYA, K., & IGARASHI, M., 1973, Changes in F.S.H., LH and prolactin
    secretion during estrous cycle in rats, Endocrinologia Japonica
    20:205.

THAPLIYAL, J. P., & PANDHA, S. K., 1965, Thyroidgonal relationship
    in spotted munia, Uroloncha punctulata, J. Exp. Zool. 158:253.

THOMPSON, W. F., 1919, The spawning of the grunion (Leuresthes tenuis),
    Calif. Fish Game Comm., Fish. Bull. 3:1.

TOPEL, D. G., WEISS, G. M., SIERS, D. G., & MAGILTON, J. H., 1973,
    Comparison of blood source and diurnal variation on blood hy-
    drocortisone growth hormone, lactate, glucose and electrolytes
    in swine, J. Anim. Sci. 36:531.

TROBEC, T. N., 1974, Daily rhythms in the hormonal control of fat
    storage in lizards, Proc. Int. Soc. Study Biol. Rhythms (in
    press).

TYSON, J. E., FRIESON, H. G., & ANDERSON, M. S., 1972, Human lacta-
    tional and ovarian response to endogenous prolactin release,
    Science 177:897.

ULRICH, R. S., & YUWILER, A., 1973, Adrenocortical influences on the
    development of the diurnal rhythm in hepatic tyrosine transamin-
    ase, Endocrinology 89:936.

ULRICH, R. S., & YUWILER, A., 1973, Failure of 6-hyroxydopamine to
    abolish the circadian rhythm of serum corticosterone, Endocrin-
    ology 92:611.

UNDERWOOD, H., & MENAKER, M., 1970, Photoperiodically significant
    photoreception in sparrows: is the retina involved? Science
    167:298.

UNGAR, F., 1964, In vitro studies of adrenal-pituitary circadian rhythm in the mouse, Ann. N. Y. Acad. Sci. 117:374.

VANHAELST, L., VAN COUTER, E., DE GOUTE, J. P., & GOLSTEIN, J.,
    1972, Circadian variations of serum thyrotropin levels in man,
    J. Clin. Endocrinol. Metab. 35:479.

VAN LOON, G., SCAPAGNINI, R., COHEN, R., & GANONG, W. F., 1971,
    Effects of intraventricular administration of adrenergic
    drugs on the adrenal venous 17-hydroxycorticosteroid response
    to surgical stress in the dog, Neuroendocrinology 8:257.

VAN TIENHOVEN, A., 1961, Endocrinology of reproduction in birds,
    in "Sex and Internal Secretions," (W. C. Young, ed.), Vol. 2,
    pp. 1088-1169, Williams & Wilkins, Co., Baltimore.

VAN TIENHOVEN, A., NALBANDOV, A. V., & NORTON, H. W., 1954, Effect
    of dibenamine or progesterone-induced and 'spontaneous' ovula-
    tion in the hen, Endocrinology 54:605.

VERNIKOS-DANIELLIS, J., LEACH, C. S., WINGET, C. M., Rambaut, P. C.
    & MACK, P.B., 1972, Thyroid and adrenal cortical rhythmicity
    during bed rest, J. Applied Physiology 33.

WAHLSTROM, G., 1965, The circadian rhythm of self-selected rest
    and activity in the canary and the effects of barbiturates,
    reserpine, monoamine oxidase inhibitors and enforced, dark
    periods, Acta Physiologica Scand. 65 (Supplementum 250):1-67.

WAKAHURA, M., 1972, Daily variation in mitotic rate in tail-fin epi-
    dermis of larval Xenopus laevis and its modification by pineal
    organ-subcommissural organ system and photoperiods, Neuroendo-
    crinology 9:267.

WALDSTEIN, S., 1966, Thyroid-catecholamine interrelations, A. Rev.
    Med. 17:123.

WALFISH, P. G., BRITTON, A., & MELVILLE, P. H., 1961, A diurnal
    pattern in the rate of disappearance of 1^{131}-labeled 1-thyroxin
    from the serum, J. Clin. Endocrinol. Metab. 21:582.

WALKER, B. W., 1952, A guide to the grunion, Calif. Fish Game 38:
    409.

WEISE, C. M., 1967, Castration and spring migration in the white-
    throated sparrow, Condor 69:49.

WEITZMANN, E. D., SCHAUMBURG, H., & FISHBEIN, W., 1966, Plasma
    17-hydroxycorticosteroid levels during sleep in man, J. Endo-
    crinol. Metab. 26:121.

WEITZMANN, E. D., GOLDMACHER, D., KRIPKE, D., MACGREGOR, P., KREAM, J., & HELLMAN, L., 1968, Reversal of sleep-waking cycle - effect on sleep pattern and certain neuroendocrine rhythms, Trans. American Neurological Association 93:153.

WILSON, W. O., & HUANG, R. H., 1962, A comparison of the time of oviposition for Coturnix and chicken, Poult. Sci. 41:1843.

WOLFSON, A., 1964, Role of day length and the hypothalmo-hypophysial system in the regulation of annual reproductive cycles, Excepta Medica Intern. Congr. Series, Amsterdam 83:183.

WOLFSON, A., 1965, Circadian rhythm and the photoperiodic regulation of the annual reproductive cycle in birds, in "Circadian Clocks," pp. 370-378, North Holland Publ. Co., Amsterdam.

WOODBURY, D. M., TIMARAS, P. S., & VERNADAKIS, A., 1957, "Hormones, Brain Function, and Behavior," (H. Hoagland, ed.), pp. 27-50, (Conference on Neuroendocrinology, Harrison, New York, 1956), Influence of adrenocortical steroids on brain function and metabolism, Academic Press, Inc., N. Y.

WEBSTER, B. R., GUANSING, A. R., & PIERCE, J. C., 1972, Absence of diurnal variation of serum TSH, J. Clin. Endocrinol. Metab. 34:899.

WURTMAN, R. J., & AXELROD, J., 1967, Daily rhythmic changes in tryosine transaminase activity in the rat liver, Proc. Nat. Acad. Sci. 57:1594.

WURTMAN, R. J., AXELROD, J., & KELLY, D. E., 1968, "The Pineal," Academic Press, N. Y.

WURTMAN, R. J., AXELROD, J., SNYDER, S. H., & CHU, E. W., 1965, Changes in the enzymatic synthesis of melatonin in the pineal during the estrous cycle, Endocrinology 76:798.

CHAPTER 14

HORMONES, PHEROMONES AND BEHAVIOR

John G. Vandenbergh, Ph.D.
Division of Research
North Carolina Department of Mental Health
Raleigh, North Carolina   27602

CONTENTS

INTRODUCTION

The relationship between hormones and behavior is never direct
in the sense that a hormone causes a behavior as the weight of an
apple causes a limb to bend. Rather, the hormone acts upon a number
of structures and functions which, in turn, result in the expression
of a behavior. The actions of hormones are limited to target organs
within the body but, through influencing the expression of specific
behaviors and external secondary sexual characteristics, the effects
of hormones can be communicated to other individuals. The release
of substances from the body which are produced as a result of hormonal metabolism or hormonal effects on target tissue can also result in the communication of information. Such substances and
their relationship to endocrine function and behavioral expression
are the subject of this discussion.

Based on extensive study of chemical communication in insects,
Karlson & Butenandt (1959) coined the word "pheromone" to describe
"...substances that are secreted by an animal to the outside and
cause a specific reaction in a receiving individual of the same
species, e.g., a release of a certain behavior or a determination
of a physiologic development," (p. 39). Expanding on Karlson &
Butenandt's thoughts, Wilson & Bossert (1963) suggested that pheromones be classified into two types: "releaser" and "primer." The
releaser type of pheromone induces immediate behavioral responses
mediated by the central nervous system and the primer type induces
longer-term endocrine or other physiological responses mediated
either through the CNS or by direct effects on the organs involved.
In extending the pheromone concept from insects to mammals, Bronson
(1968) has suggested that the term "releaser pheromone" is inap-
propriate because it denotes a rigidity of response which is probably not applicable to mammals. He suggests the term "signalling
pheromone" be used in this context for the excellent reason that
it implies only that information is being transferred and does
not designate the nature of the response. In this review I will
examine both priming and signalling pheromones of mammals, focusing
on those related to endocrine function.

PHEROMONES AND MARKING BEHAVIOR

Only specific aspects of scent marking in mammals will be examined because the literature on this subject is far too extensive
to be covered within the confines of this chapter and because a
number of excellent reviews of this topic have appeared recently
to which the reader can refer. For example, Wilson & Bossert (1963)
and Wilson (1970) describe the physical characteristics of chemical
transmission through the environment, with emphasis on invertebrate
pheromones. The occurrence and distribution of skin glands involved

in scent marking are described by Mykytowycz (1970), with particular reference to his own extensive work on rabbits. The reviews of Ralls (1971), Eisenberg & Kleiman (1972), and Johnson (1973) provide thoughtful analyses of the social functions of scent marking in mammals.

In this discussion, I will focus on those few species in which the interrelationships between hormones, pheromones and marking behavior have been demonstrated or in which progress has been made in chemically identifying the pheromone involved in scent marking.

The most intense investigations of the endocrine variables associated with scent marking behavior have been directed toward the Mongolian gerbil (<u>Meriones unguiculatus</u>). The gerbil possesses a mid-ventral sebaceous gland which, in the adult male, is a large, actively secreting pad of tissue on the mid-ventral line but, in the female, is somewhat smaller and more variable in size (Mitchell, 1965; Glenn & Grey, 1965). Castration causes the gland to involute and the effect of castration can be reversed by testosterone administration (Mitchell, 1965; Thiessen <u>et al</u>., 1968). The effect of castration is also partly reversible by either estradiol or progesterone (Glenn & Grey, 1965), indicating that the gland is responsive to a number of steroids.

Mongolian gerbils utilize this gland to mark low-lying objects in their environment with an odiferous, oily secretion (Thiessen <u>et al</u>., 1969). Male gerbils mark about twice as frequently as females and the marking behavior appears to be androgen dependent because castration of a male results both in atrophy of the gland and a decline in marking behavior (Blum & Thiessen, 1971; Thiessen <u>et al</u>., 1971). The marking behavior can be restored with testosterone propionate injections in proportion to the dose of hormone administered (Blum & Thiessen, 1971) as well as by hypothalamic implants of testosterone (Thiessen & Yahr, 1970). Androgen control over marking behavior in the male is thus quite clear but, in the female, the relationship to endocrines is less certain. In one study ovariectomy failed to eliminate the onset of marking behavior in developing females nor did ovariectomy of adults reduce marking behavior (Whitsett & Thiessen, 1972). Yet, in a subsequent study ovariectomy did reduce marking behavior when only females showing high frequencies of marking behavior preoperatively were selected (Wallace <u>et al</u>., 1973). Additional evidence that ovarian secretions are probably not involved in the control of female marking behavior was presented by Owen & Thiessen (1973) when they showed that ovariectomized females marked only slightly less than intact, non-selected, controls. It thus seems likely that the ovaries are not involved in the marking behavior of gerbils except under unusual conditions. Estradiol benzoate and progesterone alone or in combination do not modify female marking behavior but testosterone

proprionate does result in above normal levels of marking behavior
(Thiessen & Lindzey, 1970; Thiessen et al., 1971; Owen & Thiessen,
1973). Androgens of adrenal origin are apparently uninvolved since
adrenalectomy in addition to ovariectomy has no effect on marking.

The social function of marking behavior is as yet unclear. It
may, as Thiessen et al. (1969) state, "...be used to aggregate con-
specifics, to disperse members of a population, to attract members
of the opposite sex, and to afford cues for individual recognition,
as well as to mark the home territory of a gerbil or group of gerbils." Some evidence suggests that the marking may be related to
territoriality (Thiessen, 1968) but, in the absence of observational
data on gerbils in the wild, conclusions as to its social significance will remain speculative. The recent finding that phenylacetic
acid is the active ingredient in the sebum of the ventral gland
which elicits a behavioral response in a conditioned task and in a
stimulus preference stituation may permit experimentation to un-
cover the pheromone's social significance (Thiessen et al., 1974).

Progress has also been made in understanding the social functions of scent marking in ungulates. Müller-Schwarze and his associates, focusing on the black-tailed deer and pronghorn antelope,
have revealed not only the important role olfactory communication
plays in these species but have been able to identify at least one
of the pheromones used by these ungulates. In the black-tailed
deer, scent from the tarsal gland is important for short-range
sex, age, and individual recognition (Müller-Schwarze, 1971). Sex,
age, and individual differences in the composition of tarsal gland
secretion were confirmed by gas chromatography. Other scents produced by the black-tailed deer include a metatarsal scent which is
discharged in fear-inducing situations and a component of female
urine which attracts males.

Olfactory signals also serve important social functions in the
pronghorn antelope, and recently one of the scents has been chemically identified (Müller-Schwarze et al., 1974). Vegetation marked
with the secretion of the subauricular glands by one pronghorn is
sniffed, licked, and thrashed by other males. By testing a number
of fractions of the subauricular gland secretion, the active ingredient was found to be isovaleric acid. Isovaleric acid is also one
of the components of the pheromone which apparently induces mounting behavior in male rhesus monkeys (Curtis et al., 1971), and it
is possible that short-chain fatty acids may act as signalling pheromones in a number of species.

PHEROMONES AND AGGRESSIVE BEHAVIOR

A role for olfaction in communicating a number of social mes-

sages has been strongly suggested in many studies of mammals in natural or semi-natural environments. Experimental evidence identifying olfaction as the dominant sense in such communication or reveal-
ing the physiological basis for production or reception of the scent
is often lacking. In mice, however, the role of olfaction in aggressive behavior has been extensively investigated in the laboratory,
and the results of these studies are relevent to this review of hor-
mone-pheromone-behavior interactions. Although it is apparent from
a number of studies that odors play a role in eliciting or suppressing aggressive interactions in mice, an understanding of the relationship between a specific odor and a specific aggressive response
has not been achieved.

In paired encounters male mice have been repeatedly observed
to sniff one another before and during bouts of fighting (Finsburg
& Allee, 1942; Banks, 1962; Clark & Schein, 1966), thus suggesting
that odors can provide information leading to attack or flight.
Mackintosh & Grant (1966) examined the effect of strange vs. familiar
male odors on aggression between males in established pairs. In
their study, replacing one of a pair of males with a strange male resulted in five times more aggression than when one of the paired
males was briefly removed and then returned. Introducing a stranger
scented with the original partner's odor or the original partner
scented with a stranger's odor increased fighting three-four fold
compared to the level of fighting resulting from introducing the
original partner rubbed with water. Moving a pair of mice from
their home cage to a cage previously inhabited by another pair of
mice also results in increased fighting between the pair (Archer,
1968). These results indicate that strange mice elicit attack and
that olfaction is important to the mouse in detecting strangness.

A relationship between olfaction and aggression was also suggested by the finding that fighting in previously aggressive mice
was abolished by olfactory bulbectomy (Ropartz, 1968a). The effect
bulbectomy had on aggression was not mediated by endocrine mechanisms because injecting bulbectomized mice with testosterone propionate failed to restore aggressive behavior (Rowe & Edward, 1971).
Although these results indicate a possible role for olfaction, other
information suggests that a relationship between odors and fighting
is certainly not direct. Male mice made peripherally anosmic with
a ZnSO4 flush of the nasal epithelium attacked castrates only
slightly less than normal males indicating that the "...sense of
smell is not a necessary condition for the display of aggressive
behavior in male mice" (Edwards et al., 1972). Zinc-sulfate-treat-
ed males took longer than normal males to initiate an attack, suggesting that the smell of an opponent may potentiate the arousal
necessary for aggression. Thus, fighting behavior may not be "released" by an odor but specific odors may act to bring opponents into close proximity, and tactile or other close-range interactions may
then escalate into an attack.

Another complexity added to the odor-aggression relationship is that aggression is not a unitary phenomenon. There are many kinds of aggression, as Moyer (1968) has described and, when aggressive behavior is absent in one context, it may be elicited in another. An excellent example of context specific aggression was provided by Rowe & Edwards (1971) when they found that bulbectomized males failed to attack castrates in a paired encounter, but, when the bulbectomized males were deprived of food for 48 hours and paired in the presence of a pellet of food, 70% of the bulbectomized males fought for control of the food pellet. Thus, aggression is abolished in certain contexts by olfactory bulbectomy but not in others.

By examining aggression in one context in a series of experiments, Mugford and associates have been able to show that castrates scented with male urine elicit more aggression from intact male mice than do castrates daubed with water (see Table 1 for references). Urine from females, on the other hand, tends to reduce aggression toward a castrate male. In a study examining whether scents may effect aggressive behavior indirectly by eliciting competing responses rather than by directly stimulating or inhibiting aggressive responses, Connor (1972) found that male mice displayed increased sexual behavior and decreased aggression toward male intruders scented with female urine. Conversely, females scented with male urine received more aggressive attention and less sexual attention from the resident. Finding that the resident's behavior can be diverted from aggression to sex or from sex to aggression depending upon the nature of the scent may help to explain the increases and decreased in aggression noted by Mugford and his associates (Table I).

The presence of odors in the urine of male mice having a potentiating influence on aggressive behavior are dependent upon androgen levels. Urine from castrate males fails to elicit aggression (Mugford & Nowell, 1970) while urine from spayed females treated with testosterone produces an increase in aggression toward castrated males scented with such urine (Mugford & Nowell, 1971a; 1971b). The presence of odors in the urine of female mice which reduce aggressive behavior, on the other hand, seems to be independent of ovarian hormones. In one experiment, urine from spayed females was found to have no effect, but in a second experiment urine apparently collected from the same females resulted in decreased aggression (Mugford & Nowell, 1971b). Such conflicts, especially within the same set of experiments, indicate that the relationships between hormones, pheromones and aggressive behavior are extremely complex and require a good deal of additional experimentation before definitive conclusions can be drawn.

The complex manner in which pheromones may mediate the relationship between hormones and aggressive behavior may indicate that an array of odors are involved and that the odors may be derived

Table I. A summary of the effects of scents from different donor
mice on the aggressive response of an intact male to a castrate male
scented with the odor of a donor compared to the response toward a
castrate male daubed with water.

Scent Donor	Status	Effect on Aggression	Reference
Male	Socially dominant	Increase	Mugford & Nowell, 1970
Male	Socially subordinate	Increase	
Male	Castrate	No change	
Female	Adult, normal	Decrease	
Female	Spayed, TP injected	Increase	Mugford & Nowell, 1971a
Female	Spayed, TP injected plus preputialectomy	Increase	
Female	Estrous	Decrease	Mugford & Nowell, 1971b
Female	Dietrous	Decrease	
Female	Spayed	No change	
Female	Intact + TP	No change	
Female	Adult, normal	Decrease	
Female	Spayed	Decrease	
Female	Spayed + TP	Increase	
Female	Spayed + estrogen	No change	
Male	Intact	Increase	Jones & Nowell, 1973b
Male	Intact + preputial secretion	Increase	
Male	Intact + coagulating gland secretion	No change	
Male	Water + preputial secretion	Increase	
Male	Water + coagulating gland secretion	No change	

from more than one source. No attempts have yet been reported to
identify the source of the pheromone produced by female mice which
results in reduced aggression, but in males the possibility that an
androgen-dependent organ may be the source of the pheromone enhancing aggression has been examined in a number of studies.

The preputial gland is one such androgen-dependent organ that
has been considered as a possible source of odors involved in aggression. The preputial of the male mouse had already been shown
to secrete material attractive to female mice (Bronson & Caroom,
1971) making the gland a reasonable candidate as the source of such
an aggression-related pheromone. McKinney & Christian (1970) examined this possibility by pairing previously isolated male mice
after one member of the pair was preputialectomized. They found a
decrease in latency of attack and an increase in both total fights
and accumulated attacking time among such pairs of males compared
to pairs of sham operated males or pairs of preputialectomized
males. Although these measures indicated a relationship between
the preputial and aggression, the social rank between members of a
pair was independent of the presence or absence of the preputial
gland.

In a replicate of the McKinney & Christian (1970) study
Mugford (1973) claims to have found just the reverse effect of
preputialectomy. The same measures of aggression taken on similarly constituted pairs revealed a decrease rather than an increase in
the level of aggression. Close inspection of the results indicates
that the decrease was evident only when the males were placed in a
clean cage. When placed in a cage previously occupied by fighting
males no differences in levels of aggression are apparent. Another
inconsistency in findings concerning the preputial gland is that
Jones & Nowell (1973a) report that no differences in aggression
toward castrates are apparent when castrates are scented with male
urine collected from males with the preputial intact or removed.
Yet in another study (Jones & Nowell, 1973b) secretions of the
preputial added to bladder urine from intact males enhanced aggression. In view of such complex and conflicting findings a role
for the preputial in mediating aggressive responses can not be
assigned at this time.

Other glands which may be involved in the production of a pheromone inhibiting aggression are the seminal vesicles and coagulating
glands. Haug (1971) found that males in which these glands had been
removed elicited more attacks from other males than sham controls.
Jones & Nowell (1973a) examined the role of these glands by testing
urine collected from testosterone treated males following removal of
the coagulating glands and following removal of both the coagulating
glands and the seminal vesicles. Castrate males scented with urine
from both groups of glandectomized males elicited more aggression

from intacts than did the urine from non-glandectomized males. Since removal of the coagulating glands alone resulted in the absence of the aggression-inhibiting pheromine, Jones & Nowell (1973b) conclude that these glands are the source of this pheromone. To term the pheromone an aggression-inhibitor may be somewhat misleading because when coagulating gland secretions are tested against water, no dimunition of aggression occurs (Jones & Nowell, 1973b, see Table I) but when tested against bladder urine a dimunition does occur. Thus the effect of the coagulating gland secretion may be to mask or to counteract the urinary substance which induces aggression rather than to actively inhibit aggressive responses.

In addition to the pheromones described above which have a signalling function, a priming pheromone related to aggression may also exist in the mouse. This priming function was discovered by Ropartz (1968b; 1968c) in a series of experiments designed to examine the causal basis for the adrenal enlargement noted when male mice are grouped under dense conditions (Christian & Davis, 1964). He first noted that exposing a group of male mice to air scented with the odors from another cage containing a group of males or with just the urine of such males resulted in an increase in locomotor activity within the group (Ropartz, 1968b). Additional work (Ropartz, 1968c, 1968d; Archer, 1969) has shown that urinary odors from grouped male mice induces adrenal hypertrophy and ascorbic acid depletion in males receiving the odors and that the effect can be blocked by olfactory bulbectomy. Furthermore, the urine from a group of castrated male mice fails to induce adrenal hypertrophy, but the urine from intact males does induce the effect on isolated castrates. These results indicate that production but not reception of this priming pheromone is androgen dependent.

The effect of group odor on isolate castrate mice is particularly significant because it suggests that the pheromone has a true priming effect. That is, the odor is not having its effect on the adrenal through a signalling function by increasing the level of aggression within a group but rather, is directly affecting the male mouse in the absence of opponents. It is possible that the signalling pheromone which induces aggression and the priming pheromone inducing adrenal hypertrophy may be the same substance, but if it is, it is having a dual effect.

SEX RECOGNITION AND ATTRACTION

The term "pheromone" was first coined to describe chemical messengers involved in sex attraction among insects (Karlson & Butenant, 1959). A number of insect sex attractants have been identified and some are being prepared synthetically and used to lure males of pest species to traps or disrupt normal mating behavior

(Bierl et al., 1970; Law & Regnier, 1971; Cameron et al., 1974). Mammals must also find and recognize a sexually active member of the opposite sex to breed and, like insects, a number of species have evolved a system of chemical signals to aid in sex attraction and sex recognition.

Observation of domestic animals indicates that olfaction plays at least a contributory role in recognition of estrus females by males. In cattle, Hart et al. (1946) concluded that the smell of the estrous cow was of prime importance in arousing the bull. Hale (1966) failed to confirm this finding when visual and other stimuli were held constant. In reviewing a number of studies, Hafez et al. (1969) concluded that smell is probably secondarily associated with sexual arousal in the bull. A similar situation may hold for horses because olfactory stimuli from the mare are capable of inducing mounting behavior in young stallions, but adult stallions mount even though anosmic (Wierzbowski, 1959). In sheep, olfactory cues do seem critical for rams to identify an estrus ewe because anosomic rams fail to distinguish estrous from anoestrous ewes in a flock. They approach all ewes and mount only those which fail to move away whereas normal males only approach the estrous ewes in a block (Lindsay, 1965). A considerable amount of work has been done on the role of olfaction in the mating behavior of pigs. In association with other stimuli the odor of the boar elicits the immobilization reflex in sows so that they stand rigidly for the mount (Signoret & du Mesnil du Buisson, 1961).

As any owner of a bitch can attest, an estrus bitch can attract male dogs from considerable distances. The attractiveness of the female is probably due to a substance in her urine because male are highly attracted to urine from an estrous female compared to urine from anoestrous females (Beach & Gilmore, 1949). More recently evidence has been presented to suggest that the sex attractant substance of the dog is contained in the anal sac (Donovan, 1969).

Naturalistic observations of wild mammals often suggest that pheromones are involved in attracting males to receptive female (see reviews by Johnson, 1973 and Eisenberg & Kleiman, 1972), but in only a few cases have experiments been conducted to verify that olfaction is the dominant modality involved in sexual recognition or attraction and fewer yet to identify the source of the pheromone or its chemical identity. A number of experimental studies on rodents, however, have investigated whether olfactory cues are sufficient for sex recognition and whether the ability to detect the odors is hormone dependent.

Using a test in which only odor could provide the sensory cue, Bowers & Alexander (1967) demonstrated that the male house mouse could discriminate between the odors of males and females.

Gerbils and rats demonstrate the same ability (Dagg & Windsor,
1971; Le Magnen, 1952; Carr _et al._, 1965). In addition to dis-
criminating between the sexes, rats have also been shown to discriminate estrous from anestrous females. Water-deprived male
rats, either gonadally intact or prepuberally castrated, could
be trained to discriminate between estrous and anestrous females
when water was used as a reward (Carr & Caul, 1962). The rate
at which the olfactory discrimination was established as well as
the accuracy of responses were similar whether the rats were
trained to respond to odors from either estrous or anestrous females. Using a different learning paradigm, Carr _et al._ (1962)
confirmed that the ability to discriminate the sexual state of the
female is independent of the male's gonadal state, and further,
that both intact and castrate males have similar thresholds for
responding to female odors. In a more recent study Stern (1970)
found that castration did reduce the amount of time male rats
investigated odors from estrous females but attributed this difference to the reduction in overall activity shown by castrate
males. In a study conducted on two related species of _Peromyscus_,
Doty (1972) showed that endocrine factors can influence a female's
ability to respond to male odors. He tested the preferences of
estrous and anestrous _P. maniculatus bairdi_ females for the odors
from males of the same species versus odors from males of a closely related species, _P. leucopus noveboracensis_. Only when in
estrus did _P. m. bairdi_ show a distinct preference for odors from
males of their own species. These results strongly suggest that
olfaction could play an important role in sexual isolation between
two species which often come into contact at the periphery of their
ranges. Additional evidence that olfactory communication can play
a role in species identification was presented by Bowers & Alexander (1967) and Mainardi (1963) for the house mouse, _Mus musculus_.
A species' preference for its own odor appears to be the result of
olfactory experiences encountered early in development (Mainardi,
1963; Quadagno & Banks, 1970).

The source of the odor which permits sex identification has
not been identified in rodents, but secretions from the preputial
gland are likely candidates. Bronson & Caroom (1971) found that female mice are attracted to secretions of the preputial. Additional
evidence suggesting the preputial gland is the source of sex-
identity pheromones was recently provided by Orsulak & Gawienowski
(1972). Odors from saline homogenates of adult male preputial
glands were highly preferred by female rats to odors from homogenates
of muscle and liver. The reverse also proved to be true when adult
males showed a distinct preference for female preputial odors. Homogenates of other glandular tissue such as salivary glands and foot
pads from the opposite sex were not preferred by either sex. Although these studies strongly indicate that, in rodents, the preputial is the source of a pheromone which permits each sex to iden-

tify the other, a more convincing demonstration would be to find
that sex could not be identified if the stimulus animal was preputialectomized. Should the preputial gland prove to be the source
of sex specific odors in mice, another connection could be made
between hormones and pheromones because the preputial is an androgen
dependent organ in rodents. In the guinea pig sex identification
may depend upon complex differences in the components of urine.
Male guinea pigs can distinguish between male and female urine and
are highly attracted to female urine. Testing fractions of urine
using a number of chemical procedures revealed that the preference
is based on a pattern of components having widely different chemical characteristics (Beruter et al., 1973).

Attempts to relate electrophysiological changes in the brain
to specific sex odors known to be identificable in behavior tests
have not yielded conclusive results. In a series of experiments,
Pfaff & Pfaffman (1969) found that sexually experienced male rats
could discriminate the odor of estrous female urine from the odor
of urine from ovariectomized females. After castration the males
failed to show the discrimination. When unit recordings were made
from the preoptic area and the olfactory bulb of males during exposure to these odors, both odors induced over 80% of the units
to respond and no differences could be attributed to the odor. A
similar experiment was conducted on mice (Scott & Pfaff, 1970) but
this time units in a number of areas of the female brain were sur-
veyed for a differential response to the urinary odors from gonadally intact and castrate males and two control substances. No neurons were observed to respond exclusively to urine odors, and only
a few neurons showed consistently different responses to the odors
from normal and castrated males.

Once proximity between opposite sexed animals has been achieved,
a number of interactions between the male and female are necessary
to effect successful mating. Olfactory signals may play an important role in such interactions in a number of species.

A common experimental procedure used to investigate the role
of odors in mating behavior is to induce anosmia by surgical removal of the olfactory bulbs and to observe the anosmic animal in
mating tests. In male hamsters and mice, such a procedure results
in the abolition of mating behavior (Murphy & Schneider, 1970; Rowe
& Edwards, 1972). In male rats olfactory bulbectomy has less severe
effects on mating behavior. Some investigators report essentially
no decrement in male sexual behavior (Stone, 1923; Beach, 1942),
whereas others have reported at least partial deficits following
olfactory bulb destruction (Bermant & Taylor, 1969; Heimer & Larsson, 1967). An interaction between early social experience and the
effects of olfactory bulbectomy has been described by Wilhelmsson
& Larsson (1973). Male rats made anosmic at 30 days of age and
reared in groups showed deficits in sexual behavior when compared

with intact, group-reared males. However, when reared in isolation, anosmic males failed to display any sex behavior. Unfortunately, no measures of endocrine status were made of the males so that the effects could have been mediated by a physiological effect of either the isolation or the surgical treatment. Further studies are necessary to clarify this point.

In addition to rendering the animal anosmic, removal of the olfactory bulbs may also disrupt CNS connections essential for the expression of normal mating behavior and thus anosmia may not be the cause of the decrement in sexual behavior. In an attempt to separate the effects of anosmia from the CNS insult caused by olfactory bulbectomy, two studies comparing the effects of peripherally induced anosmia with olfactory bulbectomy have been conducted with hamsters. Powers & Winans (1973), using an intranasal flush of $ZnSO_4$ to temporarily destroy the olfactory epithelium (Alberts & Galef, 1971), found no deficit in mating behavior of male hamsters. Doty & Anisko (1973), utilizing intranasal procaine hydrochloride to block olfactory sensitivity, found just the opposite; mating behavior was abolished in treated hamsters. In both studies olfactory bulbectomy abolished male mating behavior confirming the earlier finding of Murphy & Schneider (1970). Furthermore, the peripherally anosmic hamsters in both experiments failed olfactory discrimination tests. In view of such conflicting data it is impossible at present to separate central from peripheral olfactory mechanisms in the mediation of mating behavior in this rodent. The recent findings by Margolis (personal communication) that intranasal treatment with $ZnSO_4$ causes a decrement in olfactory bulb weight and destruction of olfactory glomeruli of mice may indicate that a technique thought only to produce peripheral anosmia may in fact induce CNS damage thus further complicating this very interesting issue.

The effects of anosmia on the expression of female sexual behavior have also been examined and, in general, the effects are considerably less severe than in the male (Bermant & Taylor, 1969; Donovan & Kopriva, 1965; Moss, 1971; Thompson & Edwards, 1972). In female hamsters, olfactory bulbectomy or anosmia induced by an intra-nasal flush with $ZnSO_4$ fails to reduce normal levels of lordosis behavior in pairing with a male (Carter, 1973). In females treated with testosterone immediately after birth, however, sexual behavior is suppressed by olfactory bulbectomy later in life indicating that the involvement of an intact olfactory system is dependent upon early masculinization (Doty et al., 1971).

In addition to the studies using anosmia as a variable, a number of investigators have tested the male's sexual responses to specific odors or secretions from the female. Murphy (1973), for example, has shown that male hamsters actively sniff and lick the vaginal discharge from estrous female hamsters during mating episodes

and will mount other males scented with the female vaginal discharge. Unscented males are also mounted but less frequently
than scented males indicating that female odors have an additive
effect on other stimuli which induce mounting behavior.

Studies by Michael and co-workers have shown that a primate,
the rhesus monkey, may also utilize the olfactory sense in coordin-
ating mating behavior. The suggestion that olfaction played a role
in mating behavior of rhesus monkeys stems from an experiment by
Michael & Keverne (1968). In the experiment male monkeys were
found to bar press for access to a female rhesus monkey held in an
adjacent, but visually isolated cage. Ovariectomized, and therefore unreceptive, females failed to induce consistent bar pressing
by the male but, when the female was treated with estrogen, the
male responded with high rates of bar pressing. The males were
then made anosmic by the insertion of plugs into the nasal olfactory area. When such an anosmic male was tested with an estrogen
treated female, he failed to work consistently for access to the
female. Following removal of the block the male again responded
to the female. These results suggested that olfaction played a
role in the male's attraction to the female but were not conclusive because the male capable of smelling could have been responding to the female's vocal signals or, alternatively, the loss of
the anosmic male's responsivity could be explained by the male's
discomfort due to the insertion of plugs. However, further studies
testing the male's response to vaginal secretions from the estrogen
treated female confirm the involvement of pheromones.

Males were shown to bar press repeatedly for access to an
ovariectomized female scented with vaginal secretions collected
from estrogen treated females (Michael & Keverne, 1970). The active ingredient in the vaginal secretions of receptive females
was found to be extractable with ether (Keverne & Michael, 1971)
and has been chemically identified as a complex of the five short-
chain fatty acids: acetic, propionic, isobutyric, n-butyric and
isovaleric (Curtis et al., 1971). A synthetic mixture of these
acids matching the concentration found in vaginal washings of receptive females induced high rates of mounting attempts by male
monkeys when paired with females scented with the mixture. This
pheromone has been named "Copulin" by Michael & Keverne (1970).
Evidence has recently appeared that the short-chain fatty acids
comprising Copulin result from bacterial action upon vaginal secretions rather than the secretions themselves (Michael et al.,
1972). The amount of fatty acids found in vaginal washings was
reduced in the presence of penicillin and was eliminated if the
washings were autoclaved. Behavioral tests of vaginal washings
from females treated systemically or intravaginally with an anti-
microbial agent have not yet been reported.

The vaginal washings of a number of other primates including the human contain the same fatty acids as the rhesus monkey although the concentrations of the five acids differ among species (Michael et al., 1972). Baboon vaginal washings taken during the receptive period of the female's cycle were effective in inducing male rhesus monkeys to mount ovariectomized female rhesus scented with the baboon washings. This finding suggests that the pheromone is of a rather non-specific nature, certainly in comparison to the high degree of species specificity seen in insect pheromones.

Among macaques, olfactory examination by males of females' genitalia has been commonly noted (Jay, 1965; Rahaman & Parthasarathy, 1971), and it is quite possible that a signalling pheromone may be involved in the mating activities of a number of macaque species. However, given the remarkable adaptability of macaques and in view of the fact that they possess keen auditory, visual and tactile senses, it would seem likely that olfaction plays a contributory rather than obligatory role in their mating activities. The identification of the pheromone, Copulin, in laboratory experiments should facilitate studies of olfactory communication of rhesus monkeys under naturalistic conditions so that the relative role of olfaction can be studied in a more complex social environment.

PHEROMONAL INFLUENCES ON OVARIAN FUNCTION

In addition to contributing to the identification of sex and the expression of sexual behavior in mammals, pheromones have a strong, though indirect, effect on sexual behavior by modifying ovarian function. The effect is indirect in the sense that the pheromone acts upon the endocrine mechanism controlling ovarian function and the ovarian hormones, in turn, influence the expression of sex behavior. Pheromonal control over reproductive events in the female house mouse has received the greatest attention and pheromones have been demonstrated to influence both the development and adult functioning of the ovary in this species.

Although I violate the sequence in which such priming pheromones have been discovered, it seems more logical to present them in the order in which they play their role in the reproductive development of the female. Thus, pheromonal control over puberty will be described first, followed by pheromonal control over adult estrous cyclicity, and lastly pheromonal influences on pregnancy in the mouse.

Pheromones and Puberty

The control exerted by a priming pheromone over the rate of

sexual maturation in female mice has been extensively investigated in recent years and the findings demonstrate quite clearly the interrelatedness of pheromones, hormones and sexual behavior. Vandenbergh (1967) noted that female mice attained puberty twenty days earlier if reared with an adult male than if reared in all female groups from weaning. Simultaneously, Castro (1967) noted that vaginal opening occurred earlier in mixed sexed groups than in all female groups. The stimulus provided by the male was shown to be chemical in nature and probably airborne since bedding material soiled by a male and transferred to a cage containing females induced early onset of first estrus and since a wire mesh barrier separating the sexes failed to interfere with the male's effect on the young females (Vandenbergh, 1969). More recently, male urine has been shown to be the source of the puberty-accelerating pheromone (Cowley & Wise, 1972; Colby & Vandenbergh, 1974).

The presence of a male has been shown to hasten the onset of puberty by two weeks in another rodent, the collared lemming (Dicrostonyx Groenlandicus) (Hasler & Banks, ms. in prep.), and in the pig by about one month (Brooks & Cole, 1970). Additional experimentation may reveal that a male pheromone is responsible for the accelerated sexual maturation noted in these studies.

The proper hormonal condition in the male mouse is necessary for production of the pheromone because castrates are without effect when physically present with females (Vandenbergh, 1969) and because urine from castrates also fails to hasten puberty (Colby & Vandenbergh, 1974). Prior sexual experience of the male, however, seems to be unimportant for production of the pheromone because Eisen (1973) has shown that female mice matured equally rapidly when paired with a virgin or an experienced adult male.

The effects of the presence of a male on endocrine changes leading to puberty in the female have been examined recently. The pairing of an adult male with a 24 to 25-day old female resulted in detectable uterine growth within 24 hours after exposure to the male (Bronson & Stetson, 1973). In the same study, LH concentrations in the female remained constant while FSH levels appeared to be depressed for the first 48 hours after exposure. By 60 hours, however, LH surged to a level commonly seen in adult females at proestrus. In a follow-up study in which all subject females were rigorously selected to be within a 1 g weight range and 15% of the subjects were discarded as non-responders, ovarian steroids in addition to gonadotropin levels were assayed (Bronson & Desjardens, 1974). The first event observed following exposure to an adult male was a four-five fold rise in circulating levels of LH within 1-3 hours followed three hours later by a 15-20 fold increase in estradiol. Estradiol peaked again on the second day but not until the third day did adult-like periovular changes in LH, FSH and pro-

gesterone concentrations occur. The rapidity and magnitude of the
endocrine response reveals the remarkable effect the male, or a
factor produced by the male, has on initiating ovarian function in
the mouse.

Among priming pheromones, the substance causing accelerated
female development displays the longest interval between presentation of the stimulus and production of its effect. Exposing female mice to the presence of an adult male from two days after birth
to 21 days of age resulted in first estrus occurring 11.3 days earlier than among females not exposed to a male (Vandenbergh, 1967).
The onset of puberty among such male-exposed females occurred at
43.6 days, 12.6 days after separation from the male. Fullerton
& Cowley (1971) reported similar findings following preweaning exposure to the presence of a male. The physical presence of the
male during the preweaning period is not necessary for inducing the
effect; Kennedy & Brown (1970) report acceleration of sexual maturation of female mice caged immediately adjacent to an adult male
for four hours per day between the ages of four and 18 days. Male
urine applied directly to the nares of females prior to weaning
also induced accelerated sexual development (Cowley & Wise, 1972),
indicating that the stimulus was probably the same as in the previous experiments utilizing post-weaning exposure to a male.

In addition to being subject to acceleratory substances from
the male, the sexual maturation of female mice is also subject to
inhibitory substances from the female. This effect was noted by
Vandenbergh et al. (1972) when isolated female mice were found to
attain puberty earlier than grouped females. Drickamer (1974) has
recently confirmed the effect of grouping on female sexual maturation and further shown that the effect is pheromone mediated since
bedding material soiled by a group fo females and transferred to
a cage containing an isolated female induced delayed sexual maturation. Furthermore, Drickamer's work indicated that the inhibitory
substance is only produced when females are in a group. This finding by Drickamer adds another level of complexity to the pheromone-
behavior system because it suggests that a behavioral interaction
is necessary to promote the production of a pheromone which, in turn,
affects the endocrine underpinnings of another individual's sexual
behavior.

Yet another interesting interaction between pheromones and
hormones has been revealed by a series of studies conducted by
Zarrow and his coworkers. In this case a pheromone from a male
mouse was shown to facilitiate gonadotropin induced ovulation in
juvenile female mice (Zarrow et al., 1970). Males from two of
five strains of mice have failed to show the ability to facilitate
hormone induced ovulation (Zarrow et al., 1972). By testing hybrids between strains of mice with and without the ability to
produce the pheromone, it appears that only one gene may control

the male's ability to produce the pheromone (Eleftheriou et al.,
1972). Among the strains tested no strain-related differences
in the female's responsivity to the pheromone were noted.

Pheromones and Adult Ovarian Cyclicity

Not only are pheromones important in the development of the
ovary of the mouse and perhaps other species, but they are also a
potent influence on adult ovarian cyclicity as well. (See reviews
by Whitten, 1966 and Whitten & Bronson, 1970). The discovery
that the ovarian cycle of the adult mouse was subject to pheromonal
influences originated in the observation that estrous cycles ceased
among female mice housed in dense, all-female groups (Whitten, 1957;
Lamond, 1959). Two earlier reports (Merton, 1938; Andervont, 1944)
suggested that grouping of female mice may prolong the estrous cycle
but neither stimulated an inquiry into the mechanisms involved.
Whitten (1959), however, followed up his work by demonstrating
that females in a dense group remain in diestrus for as long as
40 days and that this suppression continues when the females are
blinded or when they are held within the group cage but separated
from each other by partitions to eliminate tactile stimulation.
Deafened mice also show suppression of estrous when grouped (Whitten, 1966). Thus, by default, olfaction seems to be the sense necessary for responding to grouping. A direct test of the importance
of olfaction is not possible because olfactory bulbectomy or destruction of the olfactory mucosa suppress normal ovarian functioning in the mouse (Whitten, 1956; Lamond, 1958; Vandenbergh, 1973).
Evidence is quite strong that chemical communication is involved
because Champlin (1971) showed that estrus could be suppressed in
isolated females by exposure to soiled bedding material from a group
of females.

The suppression of adult female ovarian cyclicity in the
presence of grouped females may be the same phenomenon as the inhibition of sexual maturation in grouped female mice (Vandenbergh
et al., 1972; Drickamer, 1974). A specific factor produced by
grouped females has not yet been isolated, and a definitive test
of whether both phenomena are due to the same substance awaits its
isolation.

Estrus suppression among grouped female mice is half of what
has become known as the "Whitten effect." The remaining portion
of the Whitten effect is that once female suppression of estrus
cyclicity is produced, estrus cycles can resume following isolation
from grouping and, in the presence of an adult male mouse, will
resume in a synchronous fashion (Whitten, 1958; 1959; Lamond, 1958).
A disproportionate number of females ovulate on the night of the
third day following removal from a group and exposure to a mature

male.   The substance causing this effect is present in the urine
of the male because when male urine is applied to the nares of females two days prior to removal from a group, a high proportion of
the females ovulate on the first or second night after being placed
with the male (Marsden & Bronson, 1964).   Subsequent work has shown
that the estrus-accelerating pheromone is present in bladder urine
and that its presence is dependent upon androgen (Bronson & Whitten,
1968).   The substance can be carried in a stream of air for at
least 3 m as shown by Whitten et al. (1968) and thus seems to be
an olfactorally perceived pheromone.   It is possible, however, because of the wind-tunnel device used by Whitten et al. (1968),
that the pheromone may have been carried as an aerosol and perceived
by the female mice as a gustatory stimulus.   Tests of the pheromone's
volatility in relatively still air have not been made, therefore,
transmission through mechanisms other than olfaction can not be excluded at present.

The Whitten effect is found not only in the laboratory mouse
but in another small rodent and, in a modified form, in sheep and
goats as well.   The female deermouse (Peromyscus mainiculatus
bairdii) displays suppressed estrus cyclicity when grouped and
synchronous estrus when paired with a male or exposed to male deermouse urine (Bronson & Marsden, 1964).   The male urinary pheromone
seems to be species specific because male deermouse urine does not
synchronize estrus of female house mice (Marsden & Bronson, 1965)
nor does urine of male house mice synchronize estrus of female deermice (Bronson & Dezell, 1968).   Estrus synchrony is not found in all
rodents, however, because attempts to induce synchronous estrus in
laboratory rats and guinea pigs have failed (Whitten & Bronson, 1970;
Harned & Casida, 1972).

Synchronization of estrus due to the presence of a male had
been demonstrated in sheep more than a decade before the phenomenon
was described in mice (Underwood et al., 1944 quoted in Hulet,
1966).   Sheep breed with a seasonal rhythm, with ewes coming into
estrus at intervals during the autumn mating period.   Schinckel
(1954) found that the presence of a vasectomized ram in a flock of
ewes for 14 days just prior to the breeding season leads to the ewes
in the flock coming into estrus synchronously during the first seven
days after a fertile ram is introduced.   Similar results have been
obtained in goats (Sheldon, 1960).   The synchronization of estrus in
sheep and goats is similar to that found in mice; in both, suppression of ovarian function prior to induction of estrus is necessary.
In the mouse the suppression results from stimuli from a dense group
of females and in sheep and goats from seasonal factors which cause
ovarian quiescence.

Pheromonal Influences on Pregnancy

In addition to influencing the development and adult functioning of the house mouse ovary, pheromones also are involved in gestational processes in this species. Bruce (1959) observed that pregnancy was blocked in about 80% of newly inseminated female mice
when they were exposed to an adult male from a different genetic
strain. Estrus promptly resumed among females exposed to the alien
male and, if fertile matings occurred with the second male, all offspring were the result of the second male's sperm. Males from the
same strain as the original stud male block only about 30% of the
pregnancies (Parkes & Bruce, 1961). The alien male is only effective
in blocking pregnancy if exposed to the female during the first four
days following the initial insemination (Bruce, 1961). A maximum
number of pregnancies were blocked following 48 hours of exposure
to the alien male but a 12 hour exposure induces a measurable effect.
Repeated short exposures to the male of 15 min per day for four days
are also capable of blocking pregnancy (Chipman et al., 1966). The
fact that pregnancy can be blocked only during the four day period
following insemination suggests that the corpora lutea fail to develop normally and, consequently, an insufficient amount of progesterone is available for normal implantation to occur (Parkes &
Bruce, 1961). Injection of prolactin to maintain corpora lutea
function over the three day period in which the females are exposed
to an alien male prevents the block to pregnancy, thus indicating
that the male's blocking effect operates via inhibition of prolactin
release in the female (Bruce & Parkes, 1960; Parkes & Bruce, 1961;
Dominic, 1966). More recently, Chapman et al. (1970) suggested
that an LH release triggered by the alien male may be the primary
factor in pregnancy blockage. An LH surge may be the more satis-
factory description of the mechanism because it can result in the
reappearance of estrus noted as a part of the pregnancy block phenomenon. In fact, pregnancy blockage may be simply a side effect of
the induction of estrus by the alien male.

Dominic has shown that the substance inducing pregnancy block
is contained in male urine and that spayed, androgen treated female mice equal intact males in their ability to block pregnancy
(Dominic, 1964; 1965; 1966). The male's ability to block pregnancy
develops at puberty, is abolished by castration either before or
after puberty, and can be restored by testosterone injections (Bruce,
1965; Dominic, 1965). That the pregnancy block effect, or "Bruce
effect," is due to a male pheromone was demonstrated when the pregnancies of newly mated females were blocked by exposure to cloth
or bedding material soiled by strange males (Bruce, 1960; Parkes &
Bruce, 1962). The mode of communication of the pheromone is apparently olfactory since the pregnancies of anosmic females are
not blocked by stimuli from strange males (Bruce & Parrot, 1960).

The pregnancy-block effect appears to be limited to wild-type or non-inbred laboratory mice because studies using inbred strains or hybrid crosses between inbred strains failed to demonstrate the effect (Marsden & Bronson, 1965; Chipman & Bronson, 1968). Among other species, the pregnancy-block effect has been demonstrated only in the deermouse, P. m. bairdii (Bronson & Eleftheriou, 1963).

Summary of Priming Pheromones

As has become obvious to the reader, a number of "effects" relating to reproductive functions can be produced by priming pheromones in the house mouse and a few other species such as deermice, pigs, sheep and goats. In diagrammatic form (Fig. 1) I have summarized these effects as they relate to the house mouse. Both male and female mice produce one or more pheromones, found in urine or in soiled bedding material, which produce an array of stimulatory and inhibitory effects on female reproductive functions. As yet a specific pheromone which induces a specific effect has not been purified or identified. It is unlikely that the same pheromone is produced by both males and females because of basic differences in their reproductive physiology and because the male-induced effects are stimulatory whereas the female-induced effects are inhibitory. It is possible, as Bronson (1971) suggests, that the male produces one pheromone which induces all three male effects, but evidence to support this suggestion is not yet available. Work is in progress in a number of laboratories to isolate active components of male urine and success in these investigations will greatly facilitate answering this question as well as the many others that remain in this field.

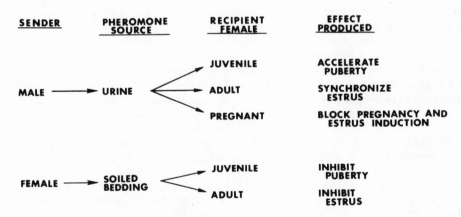

Fig. 1. A diagram of primer pheromone effects influencing reproductive functions of female house mice.

The primer effects are of particular interest in the context of this volume because they most clearly reveal the close inter-relationship between hormones, pheromones, and behavior. In the acceleration of puberty effect, for example, appropriate levels of androgen are necessary for the male mouse to produce a substance in his urine which, when perceived by the female, induces a prompt release of LH and consequent elevation of estradiol levels. Such endocrine changes, in turn, are essential for ovulation and the expression of behavioral receptivity which signal the onset of puberty in the female.

OVERVIEW AND FUTURE DIRECTIONS

Turner, in the third edition of his textbook: General Endocrinology (1960, p. 8), notes three points in the development of endocrinology. An examination of these points is particularly relevant because there is already some analogy between the early history of endocrinology and the current field of pheromonology. Since endocrinology has a considerably longer history, researchers studying pheromones may profit by the experiences of endocrinologists.

The first point of Turner's is that endocrinology advanced as a medical specialty before the basic aspects had received adequate attention. In a sense, a similar statement applies to the study of pheromones because much of the impetus in the field derived from the work of economic entomologists. The remarkable success in identifying insect pheromones and their utility to solve practical problems gave hope to those interested in mammalian chemical communication that meaningful progress could be made.

In his second point, Turner states that: "In all instances a substantial amount of physiological experimentation preceded the chemical identification of a hormone." We need only add "behavioral" to "physiologic experimentation" to see the relevance of this point to mammalian pheromone research. Many observations have been made both in laboratories and under naturalistic conditions of behavioral and physiological processes thought to be influenced by pheromones but as yet few actual substances have been isolated.

The third relevant point made by Turner needs no modification: "The announcement of new hormones has usually been followed by exaggerations and oversimplifications of their roles in the organism." Researchers investigating pheromones have as yet had little time to fall into this trap and it may be possible to avoid repeating some of the history of endocrinology. As pheromones are announced it is essential that results be replicated in other laboratories and that the pheromone be tested under a variety of conditions to determine the limits of its action. Proof of a pheromone's activity in a highly controlled environment only reveals that the pheromone may be having a communicatory effect under more natural conditions. As yet we know little about the relative contribution of pheromones as signals between individuals in which other communicatory signals are also present.

Confirmation of the pheromonal action of a compound or a specific mixture of compounds is a difficult step but is only the beginning of research to examine the complexities of pheromone production and reception. If the study of pheromones parallels that of the development of endocrinology, we can expect that future research on pheromones will not only reveal the complexities of their production and reception but how they fit into the overall scheme of intra-specific communication as well.

ACKNOWLEDGEMENTS

Work from the author's laboratory is supported in part by grant MH 16870 from the U.S.P.H.S.

REFERENCES

ALBERTS, J. R., & GALEF, B. G., JR., 1971, Acute anosomia in the rat: A behavioral test of a peripherally-induced olfactory deficit, Physiol. Behav. 6:619.

ANDERVONT, H. B., 1944, The influence of environment on mammary cancer in mice, J. Nat. Cancer Inst. 4:579.

ARCHER, J., 1968, The effect of strange male odor on aggressive behavior in male mice, J. Mammal. 49:572.

ARCHER, J. E., 1969, Adrenocortical responses to olfactory social stimuli in male mice, J. Mammal. 50:839.

BANKS, E. M., 1962, A time and motion study of prefighting behavior of mice, J. Gent. Psychol. 101:165.

BEACH, F. A., 1942, Analysis of the stimuli adequate to elicit mating behavior in the sexually inexperienced male rate, J. Comp. Psychol. 33:163.

BEACH, F. A., & GILMORE J., 1949, Response of male dogs to urine from females in heat, J. Mammal. 30:391.

BERMANT, G., & TAYLOR, ., 1969, Interactive effects of experience and olfactory bulb lesions in male rat copulation, Physiol. Behav. 4:13.

BERUTER, J., BEAUCHAMP, G. K., & MUETTERTIES, E. L., 1973, Complexity of chemical communication in mammals: Urinary components mediating sex discrimination by male guinea pigs, Biochem. Biophys. Res. Comm. 53:264.

BIERL, B. A., BEROZA, M., & COLLIER, C. W., 1970, Potent sex attractant of the gypsy moth: its isolation, identification, and synthesis, Science 170:87.

BLUM, L., & THIESSEN, D. D., 1971, The effect of different amounts of androgen on scent marking in the male mongolian gerbil, Horm. Behav. 2:93.

BOWERS, J. M., & ALEXANDER, B. K., 1967, Mice: Individual recognition by olfactory cues, Science 158:1208.

BRONSON, F. H., 1968, Pheromonal influence on mammalian reproduction. in "Reproduction and Sexual Behavior," (M. Diamond, ed,), pp 341-361, Indiana University Press, Bloomington.

BRONSON, F. H., 1971, Rodent pheromones, Biol. Reprod. 4:344.

BRONSON, F. H., & CAROOM, D., 1971, Preputial gland of the male mouse: Attractant function, J. Reprod. Fertil. 25:279.

BRONSON, F. H., & DESJARDINS, C., 1974, Circulating concentrations of FSH, LH, estradiol, and progesterone associated with the acute, pheromonal induction of puberty in female mice, Endocrinol. (in press).

BRONSON, F. H., & DEZELL, H. E., 1968, Studies on the estrus-inducing (pheromonal) action of male deermouse urine, Gen. Comp. Endocrinol. 10:339.

BRONSON, F. H., & ELEFTHERIOU, B. E., 1963, Influence of strange males on implantation in the deermouse, Gen. Comp. Endocrinol. 3:515.

BRONSON, F. H., & MARSDEN, H. M., 1964, Male-induced synchrony of estrus in deermice, Gen. Comp. Endocrinol. 4:634.

BRONSON, F. H., & STETSON, M. H., 1973, Gonadotropin release in prepubertal female mice following male exposure: A comparison with the adult cycle. Biol. Reprod. 9:449.

BRONSON, F. H., & WHITTEN, W. K., 1968, Oestrus-accelerating pheromone of mice: Assay, androgen-dependency and presence in bladder urine, J. Reprod. Fertil. 15:131.

BROOKS, P. H., & COLE, D. J. A., 1970, The effect of the presence of a boar on the attainment of puberty in gilts, J. Reprod. Fertil. 23:435.

BRUCE, H. M., 1959, An exteroceptive block to pregnancy in the mouse, Nature 184:105.

BRUCE, H. M., 1960, A block to pregnancy in the mouse caused by the proximity of strange males, J. Reprod. Fertil. 1:96.

BRUCE, H. M., 1961, Time relations in the pregnancy block induced in mice by strange males, J. Reprod. Fertil. 2:138.

BRUCE, H. M., 1965, Effect of castration on the reproductive phero- mones of male mice. J. Reprod. Fertil. 10:141.

BRUCE, H. M., & PARKES, A. S., 1960, Hormonal factors in exterocep- tive block to pregnancy in mice, J. Endocrinol. 20:24.

BRUCE, H. M., & PARROTT, D. M. V., 1960, Role of olfactory sense in pregnancy block by strange males, Science 131:1126.

CAMERON, E. A., SCHWALBE, C. P., BEROZA, M., & KNIPLING, E. F., 1974, Disruption of gypsy moth mating with microencapsulated disparlure, Science 183:972.

CARR, W. J., & CAUL, W. F., 1962, The effect of castration in the rat upon the discrimination of sex odours, Anim. Behav. 10:20.

CARR, W. J., SOLBERG, B., & PFAFFMANN, C., 1962, The olfactory threshold for estrous female urine in normal and castrated male rats, J. Comp. Physiol. Psychol. 55:415.

CARR, W. J., LOEB, L. S., & DISSINGER, M. L., 1965, Responses of rats to sex odors, J. Comp. Physiol. Psychol. 59:370.

CARTER, C. S., 1973, Olfaction and sexual receptivity in the fe- male golden hamster, Physiol. Behav. 10:47.

CASTRO, B. M., 1967, Age of puberty in female mice: Relationship to population density and the presence of adult males, An. Acad. Brasil. C. 39:289.

CHAMPLIN, A. K., 1971, Suppression of oestrus in grouped mice: The effects of various densities and the possible nature of the stimulus, J. Reprod. Fertil. 27:233.

CHAPMAN, V. M., DESJARDINS, C., & WHITTEN, W. K., 1970, Pregnancy block in mice: Changes in pituitary LH and LtH and plasma progestin levels, J. Reprod. Fertil. 21:333.

CHIPMAN, R. K., & BRONSON, F. H., 1968, Pregnancy blocking capacity and inbreeding in laboratory mice, Experientia 24:199.

CHIPMAN, R. K., HOLT, J. A., & FOX, K. A., 1966, Pregnancy failure
    in laboratory mice after multiple short-term exposure to
    strange males, Nature 210:653.

CHRISTIAN, J. J., & DAVIS, D. E., 1964, Endocrines, behavior, and
    population, Science 146:1550.

CLARK, L. H., & SCHEIN, M. W., 1966, Activities associated with
    conflict behavior in mice, Anim. Behav. 14:44.

COLBY, D. R., & VANDENBERGH, J. G., 1974, Regulatory effects of
    urinary pheromones on puberty in the mouse, Biol. Reprod.
    (in press).

CONNOR, J., 1972, Olfactory control of aggressive and sexual behavior
    in the mouse (Mus musculus L.), Psychonom. Sci. 27:1.

COWLEY, J. J., & WISE, D. R., 1972, Some effects of mouse urine on
    neontal growth and reproduction, Anim. Behav. 20:499.

CURTIS, R. F., BALLANTINE, J. A., KEVERNE, E. B., BONSALL, R. W.,
    & MICHAEL, R. P., 1971, Identification of primate sexual phero-
    mones and the properties of synthetic attractants, Nature 232:396.

DAGG, A. I., & WINDSOR, D. E., 1971, Olfactory discrimination limits
    in gerbils, Canad. J. Zool. 59:283.

DOMINIC, C. J., 1964, Source of the male odour causing pregnancy-
    block in mice, J. Reprod. Fertil. 8:266.

DOMINIC, C. J., 1965, The origin of the pheromones causing pregnancy
    block in mice, J. Reprod. Fertil. 10:469.

DOMINIC, C. J., 1966, Block to pseudopregnancy in mice caused by
    exposure to male urine, Experientia 22:534.

DONOVAN, B. T., & KOPRIVA, P. C., 1965, Effect of removal or stimu-
    lation of the olfactory bulbs on the estrous cycle of the guinea
    pig, Endocrinol. 77:213.

DONOVAN, C. A., 1969, Canine anal glands and chemical signals (Phero-
    mones), J. Amer. Vet. Med. Assoc. 155:1995.

DOTY, R. L., 1972, Odor preferences of female Peromyscus maniculatus
    bairdii for male mouse odors of P. m. bairdii and P. leucopus
    noveboracensis as a function of estrous state, J. Comp. Physiol.
    Psychol. 81:191.

DOTY, R. L., & ANISKO, J. J., 1973, Procaine hydrochloride olfactory
    block eliminates mounting in the male golden hamster, Physiol.
    Behav. 10:395.

DOTY, R. L., CARTER, C. S., & CLEMENS, L. G., 1971, Olfactory control
    of sexual behavior in the male and early-androgenized female
    hamster, Horm. Behav. 2:325.

DRICKAMER, L. C., 1974, Social inhibition of sexual maturation,
    Develop. Psychobiol. (in press).

EDWARDS, D. A., THOMPSON, M. L., & BURGE, K. G., 1972, Olfactory
    bulb removal vs. peripherally induced anosmia: Differential
    effects on the aggressive behavior of male mice, Behav. Biol.
    7:823.

EISEN, E. J., 1973, Genetic and phenotypic factors influencing
    sexual maturation of female mice, J. Anim. Sci. 37:1104.

EISENBERG, J. F., & KLEIMAN, D. G., 1972, Olfactory communication
    in mammals, in "Annual Review of Ecology and Systematics,"
    (R. F. Johnson, ed.), vol. 3, pp. 1-32, Annual Reviews Inc.,
    Palo Alto, California.

ELEFTHERIOU, B. E., BAILEY, D. W., & ZARROW, M. X., 1972, A gene
    controlling male pheromonal facilitation of PMSG-induced ovula-
    tion in mice, J. Reprod. Fertil. 31:155.

FULLERTON, C., & COWLEY, J. J., 1971, The differential effect of
    the presence of adult male and female mice on the growth and
    development of the young, J. Genet. Psychol. 119:89.

GINSBURG, B., & ALLEE, W. C., 1942, Some effects of conditioning on
    social dominance and subordination in inbred strains of mice,
    J. Physiol. Zool. 15:485.

GLENN, E. M., & GRAY, J., 1965, Effect of various hormones on the
    growth and histology of the gerbil (Meriones unguiculatus)
    abdominal sebaceous gland, Endocrinol. 76:1115.

HAFEZ, E. S. E., SCHEIN, M. W., & EWBANK, R., 1969, The behavior of
    cattle, in "The Behaviour of Domestic Animals," (E. S. E.
    Hafez, ed.), pp. 235-295, Williams & Wilkins Co., Baltimore.

HALE, E. B., 1966, Visual stimuli and reproductive behavior in
    bulls. J. Anim. Sci. 25:36.

HARNED, M. A., & CASIDA, L. E., 1972, Failure to obtain group syn-
    chrony of estrus in the guinea pig, J. Mammal. 53:223.

HART, G. H., MEAD, S. W., & REGAN, W. M., 1946, Stimulating the sex drive of bovine males in artificial insemination, Endocrinol. 39:221.

HAUG, M., 1971, Comportement agressif des souris males anosmiques traitées avec un androgene de synthese, C. R. Acad. Sci. (Paris) 272:3188.

HEIMER, L., & LARSSON, K., 1967, Mating behavior of male rats after olfactory bulb lesions, Physiol. Behav. 2:207.

HULET, C. V., 1966, Behavioral, social and psychological factors affecting mating time and breeding efficiency in sheep, J. Anim. Sci. 25:5.

JAY, P., 1965, The common langur of North India, in "Primate Behavior," (I. DeVore, ed.) pp. 197-249, Holt, Rinehart and Winston, New York.

JOHNSON, R. P., 1973, Scent marking in mammals. Anim. Behav. 21:521.

JONES, R. B., & NOWELL, N. W., 1973a, The coagulating glands as a source of aversive and aggression-inhibiting pheromone(s) in the male albino mouse, Physiol. Behav. 11:455.

JONES, R. B., & NOWELL, N. W., 1973b, Effects of preputial and coagulating gland secretions upon aggressive behaviour in male mice: A confirmation, J. Endocrinol. 59:203.

KARLSON, P., & BUTENANDT, A., 1959, Pheromones (ectohormones) in insects, Ann. Rev. Entomol. 4:39.

KENNEDY, J. M., & BROWN, K., 1970, Effects of male odor during infancy on the maturation, behavior, and reproduction of female mice, Develop. Psychobiol. 3:179.

KEVERNE, E. B., & MICHAEL, R. P., 1971, Sex-attractant properties of ether extracts of vaginal secretions from rhesus monkeys, J. Endocrinol. 51:313.

LAMOND, D. R., 1958, Infertility associated with extirpation of the olfactory bulbs in female albino mice, Aust. J. Expt'l. Biol. Med. Sci. 36:103.

LAMOND, D. R., 1959, Effect of stimulation derived from other animals of the same species on oestrous cycles in mice, J. Endocrinol. 18:343.

LAW, J. H., & REGNIER, F. E., 1971, Pheromones, Ann. Rev. Biochem.

40:533.

LEMAGNEN, J., 1952, Les phénomenes olfactosexuels chez l'homme, Arch. des Sci. Physiol. 6:125.

LINDSAY, D. R., 1965, The importance of olfactory stimuli in the mating behavior of the ram, Anim. Behav. 13:75.

MACKINTOSH, J. H., & GRANT, E. C., 1966, The effect of olfactory stimuli on the agonistic behaviour of laboratory mice, Z. Tierpsychol. 23:584.

MAINARDI, D., 1963, Eliminazione della barriera etologica all' isolamento riproduttive tra Mus musculus domesticus e M. m bactricimus mediante azione sull'apprendimento infantile, Instituto Lombardo-Accademia di Scienze e Lettere 97:291.

MARSDEN, H. M., & BRONSON, F. H., 1964, Estrous synchrony in mice: Alteration by exposure to male urine, Science 144:3625.

MARSDEN, H. M., & BRONSON, F. H., 1965, Strange male block to pregnancy: Its absence in inbred mouse strains, Nature 207:878.

MCKINNEY, T. D., & CHRISTIAN, J. J., 1970, Effect of preputialectomy on fighting behavior in mice, Proc. Soc. Exp. Biol. Med. 134:291.

MERTON, H., 1938, Studies on reproduction in the albino mouse, Proc. R. Soc. Edinb. 58:80.

MICHAEL, R. P., & KEVERNE, E. B., 1968, Pheromones in the communication of sexual status in primates, Nature 218:746.

MICHAEL, R. P., & KEVERNE, E. B., 1970, Vaginal origin of primate sex pheromones, Nature 225:84.

MICHALE, R. P., ZUMPE, D., KEVERNE, E. B., & BONSALL, R. W., 1972, Neuroendocrine factors in the control of primate behavior, Rec. Prog. Horm. Res. 28:665.

MITCHELL, O. G., 1965, Effect of castration and transplantation on ventral gland of the gerbil, Proc. Soc. Expt'l. Biol. Med. 119:953.

MOSS, R. L., 1971, Modification of copulatory behavior in the female rat following olfactory bulb removal, J. Comp. Physiol. Psychol. 74:374.

MOYER, K. E., 1968, Kinds of aggression and their physiologic basis, Comm. Behav. Biol. 2:65.

MUGFORD, R. A., 1973, Intermale fighting affected by home-cage odors of male and female mice, J. Comp. Physiol. Psychol. 84:289.

MUGFORD, R. A., & NOWELL, N. W., 1970, Pheromones and their effect on aggression in mice, Nature 226:967.

MUGFORD, R. A., & NOWELL, N. W., 1971a, The preputial glands as a source of aggression-promoting odors in mice, Physiol. Behav. 6:247.

MUGFORD, R. A., & NOWELL, N. W., 1971b, Endocrine control over production and activity of the anti-aggression pheromone from female mice, J. Endocrinol. 49:225.

MÜLLER-SCHWARZE, D., 1971, Pheromone in black-tailed deer (Odocoileus hemionus columbianus), Anim. Behav. 19:141.

MÜLLER-SCHWARZE, D., MÜLLER-SCHWARZE, C., SINGER, A. G., & SILVERSTEIN, R. M., 1974, Mammalian pheromone: Identification of active component in the subauricular scent of the male pronghorn, Science 183:860.

MURPHY, M. R., 1973, Effects of female hamster vaginal discharge on the behavior of male hamsters, Behav. Biol. 9:367.

MURPHY, M. R., & SCHNEIDER, G. E., 1970, Olfactory bulb removal eliminates mating behavior in the male golden hamster, Science 167:302.

MYKYTOWYCZ, R., 1970, The role of skin glands in mammalian communication, in "Communication by Chemical Signals," (J. W. Johnston, Jr., D. G. Moulton, & A. Turk, eds.), vol. 1, pp. 327-360, Appleton-Century-Crofts, New York.

ORSULAK, P. J., & GAWIENOWSKI, A. M., 1972, Olfactory preferences for the rat preputial gland, Biol. Reprod. 6:219.

OWEN, K., & THIESSEN, D. D., 1973, Regulation of scent marking in the female mongolian gerbil Meriones unguiculatus, Physiol. Behav. 11:441.

PARKES, A. S., & BRUCE, H. M., 1961, Olfactory stimuli in mammalian reproduction, Science 134:1049.

PARKES, A. S., & BRUCE, H. M., 1962, Pregnancy-block in female mice place in boxes soiled by males, J. Reprod. Fertil. 4:303.

PFAFF, D., & PFAFFMANN, C., 1969, Behavioral and electrophysiological responses of male rats to female rat urine odors, in "Olfaction and Taste," (C. Pfaffmann, ed.), pp. 258-267, The Rockefeller University Press, New York.

POWERS, J. B., & WINANS, S. S., 1973, Sexual behavior in peripherally anosmic male hamsters, Physiol. Behav. 10:361.

QUADAGNO, D. M., & BANKS, E. M., 1970, The effect of reciprocal cross fostering on the behavior of two species of rodents, Mus musculus and Baiomys taylori ater, Anim. Behav. 18:379.

RAHAMAN, H., & PARTHASARATHY, M. D., 1971, The role of the olfactory signals in the mating behavior of bonnet monkeys, Comm. Behav. Biol. 6:97.

RALLS, K., 1971, Mammalian scent marking, Science 171:443.

ROPARTZ, P., 1968a, The relation between olfactory stimulation and aggressive behaviour in mice, Anim. Behav. 16:97.

ROPARTZ, P., 1968b, Demonstration of an increase of locomotor activity of groups of female mice in response to the odor of a group of strange males, C. R. Hebd, Seances Acad. Sci. Ser. D Sci. Natur. 267:2341.

ROPARTZ, P., 1968c. Olfaction and social behavior among the rodents, Mammalia 32:550.

ROPARTZ, P., 1968d, Étude du determinisme olfactif de l'effet de groupe chez la souris male, Rev. du Comportement Anim. 2:35.

ROWE, F. A., & EDWARDS, D. A., 1971, Olfactory bulb removal: Influences on the aggressive behaviors of male mice, Physiol. Behav. 7:889.

ROWE, F. A., & EDWARDS, D. A., 1972, Olfactory bulb removal: Influences on the mating behavior of male mice, Physiol. Behav. 8:37.

SCHINCKEL, P. G., 1954, The effect of the ram on the incidence and occurrence of oestrus in ewes, Austr. Vet. J. 30:189.

SCOTT, J. W., & PFAFF, D. W., 1970, Behavioral and electrophysiological responses of female mice to male urine odors, Physiol. Behav. 5:407.

SHELTON, M., 1960, Influence of the presence of a male goat on the initiation of oestrus, cycling and ovulation of the angora doe, J. Anim. Sci. 19:368.

SIGNORET, J. P., & DU MESNIL DU BUISSON, F., 1961, Étude du comporte-
    ment de la truie en oestrus, in "Proc. IV Int. Cong. Anim. Re-
    prod," vol. 2, pp. 171-175, The Hague.

STERN, J. J., 1970, Responses of male rats to sex odors, Physiol.
    Behav. 5:519.

STONE, C. P., 1923, Further study of sensory functions in the activ-
    ation of sexual behavior in the young male albino rat, J. Comp.
    Psychol. 3:469.

THIESSEN, D. D., 1968, The roots of territorial marking in the mongo-
    lian gerbil: A problem of species-common topography, Behav.
    Res. Meth. Instrum. 1:70.

THIESSEN, D. D., & LINDZEY, G., 1970, Territorial marking in the fe-
    male mongolian gerbil: Short-term reactions to hormones, Horm.
    Behav. 1:157.

THIESSEN, D. D., & YAHR, P., 1970, Central control of territorial
    marking in the mongolian gerbil, Physiol. Behav. 5:275.

THIESSEN, D. D., FRIEND, H., & LINDZEY, G., 1968, Androgen control of
    territorial marking in the mongolian gerbil (Meriones unguicula-
    tus), Science 160:432.

THIESSEN, D. D., BLUM, S. L., & LINDZEY, G., 1969, A scent marking
    response associated with the ventral sebaceous gland of the
    mongolian gerbil (Meriones unguiculatus), Anim. Behav. 18:26.

THIESSEN, D. D., OWEN, K., & LINDZEY, G., 1971, Mechanisms of ter-
    tritorial marking in the male and female mongolian gerbil
    (Meriones unguiculatus), J. Comp. Physiol. Psychol. 77:38.

THIESSEN, D. D., REGNIER, F. E., RICE, M., GOODWIN, M., ISAACKS, N.,
    & LAWSON, N., 1974, Identification of a ventral scent marking
    pheromone in the male mongolian gerbil (Meriones unguiculatus),
    Science 184:83.

THOMPSON, M. L., & EDWARDS, D. A., 1972, Olfactory bulb ablation and
    hormonally induced mating in spayed female mice, Physiol. Behav.
    8:1141.

TURNER, C. D., 1960, "General Endocrinology," W. B. Saunders Co.,
    Philadelphia.

VANDENBERGH, J. G., 1967, Effect of the presence of a male on the
    sexual maturation of female mice, Endocrinol. 81:345.

VANDENBERGH, J. G., 1969, Male odor accelerates female sexual maturation in mice, Endocrinol. 84:658.

VANDENBERGH, J. G., 1973, Acceleration and inhibition of puberty in female mice by pheromones, J. Reprod. Fertil. 19:409.

VANDENBERGH, J. G., DRICKAMER, L. C., & COLBY, D. R., 1972, Social and dietary factors in the sexual maturation of female mice, J. Reprod. Fertil. 28:397.

WALLACE, P., OWEN, K., & THIESSEN, D. D., 1973, The control and function of maternal scent marking in the mongolian gerbil, Physiol. Behav. 10:463.

WHITSETT, J. M., & THIESSEN, D. D., 1972, Sex difference in the control of scent-marking behavior in the mongolian gerbil (Meriones unguiculatus), J. Comp. Physiol. Psychol. 78, 381.

WHITTEN, W. K., 1956, The effect of removal of the olfactory bulbs on the gonads of mice, J. Endocrinol. 14:160.

WHITTEN, W. K., 1957, Effect of exteroceptive factors on the oestrous cycle of mice, Nature 180:1436.

WHITTEN, W. K., 1958, Modification of the oestrous cycle of the mouse by external stimuli associated with the male, J. Endocrinol. 13:399.

WHITTEN, W. K., 1959, Occurrence of anoestrus in mice caged in groups, J. Endocronol. 18:102.

WHITTEN, W. K., 1966, Pheromones and mammalian reproduction, in "Advances in Reproductive Physiology," (A. McLaren, ed.), vol. 1, pp. 155-177, Academic Press, London.

WHITTEN, W. K., & BRONSON, F. H., 1970, The role of pheromones in mammalian reproduction, in "Communication by Chemical Signals," (J. W. Johnston, Jr., D. G. Moulton, & A. Turk, eds.), vol. 1, pp. 309-325, Appleton-Century-Crofts, New York.

WHITTEN, W. K., BRONSON, F. H., & GREENSTEIN, J. A., 1968, Estrus-inducing pheromone of male mice: Transport by movement of air, Science 161:584.

WIERZBOWSKI, S., 1959, The sexual reflexes of stallions, Roczn. Nauk Roln. 73-B-4:753.

WILHELMSSON, M., & LARSSON, K., 1973, The development of sexual behavior in anosomic male rats reared under various social conditions, Physiol. Behav. 11:227.

WILSON, E. O., 1970, Chemical communication within animal species, in "Chemical Ecology," (E. Sondheimer & J. B. Simeone, eds.), pp. 133-155, Academic Press, New York.

WILSON, E. O., & BOSSERT, W. A., 1963, Chemical communication among animals, Rec. Prog. Horm. Res. 19:673.

ZARROW, M. X., ESTES, S. A., DENENBERG, V. H., & CLARK, J. H., 1970, Pheromonal facilitation of ovulation in the immature mouse, J. Reprod. Fertil. 23:357.

ZARROW, M. X., ELEFTHERIOU, B. E., & DENENBERG, V. H., 1972, Pheromonal facilitation of HCG-induced ovulation in different strains of immature mice, Biol. Reprod. 6:277.

CHAPTER 15

NEURAL AND HORMONAL BASIS OF MATERNAL BEHAVIOR IN THE RAT

Burton M. Slotnick, Ph.D.

The American University
College of Arts and Sciences
Department of Psychology
Washington, D. C. 20016

CONTENTS

INTRODUCTION

Maternal behavior encompasses activities concerned with the birth, maintenance, nutrition, and protection of the young. Although the form of these behaviors is closely related to physiological and ecological adaptations of the particular species, the variety and extent of maternal or parental care patterns in various orders of vertebrates is truly astonishing. For example, some viviparous and oviparous species of fish show no maternal interest in their young or eggs, whereas in others, such as the cichlids, the construction of a nest, care of eggs, and protection of young

rival in complexity many advanced forms of mammalian maternal care
(Noble & Curtis, 1939; Innes, 1966). Reptiles are not known to act
maternally toward their young, although oviparous species use protected natural sites or excavate nests for depositing eggs and some
show rudimentary incubation of their eggs (Noble & Mason, 1933). In
many species of birds both the male and female participate in nest
building, incubation of eggs, and rearing of the young. For pen-
guins, which reproduce under relatively adverse climatic conditions,
maternal care may be communal activity and a dozen or more adults
may take turns at incubation of eggs and feeding of the young. Some
species of birds such as the cowbird and cuckoo, are not maternal
but parasitic and simply deposit their eggs in the nest of other
birds.

Considerably less variability in maternal behavior exists in
mammals, and reproduction is characterized by a fertile mating,
pregnancy, and then birth (except for the egg laying monotremes),
nourishment, and protection of the young. The duration and extent
of postpartum maternal care in mammals is a function of the behavioral capacities of the young at birth and the rate at which they develop. The young of precocial species such as the guinea pig are
well developed at birth and may be nutritionally independent of the
mother in a few days. In altricial species such as rats, mice, and
hamsters, the young are physically immature when born and are totally dependent upon maternal care for the first three weeks of life.
For these species, a nest, lair, or burrow is essential and provides
a protected site for the expression of maternal behavior and serves
to confine and protect the otherwise defenseless litter.

Although there are excellent descriptive accounts of maternal
behavior for a number of mammalian species, the neural, endocrinological, and behavioral aspects have been studied intensively only
for the white laboratory rat. For this reason, the present review
is limited primarily to a consideration of studies on the rat. It
is hoped, of course, that the endocrinological and neural mechanisms elucidated through studies on the rat will provide a basis for
understanding the maternal behavior of other species. However,
the fact that most studies have concentrated on the rat has a number of disadvantages. The maternal behavior of the rat and other
rodents extends only to weaning, and its repertoire of maternal activities within this period is actually quite limited. Other laboratory species (such as the dog or rhesus monkey) show a far richer
pattern of maternal care that extends well beyond weaning and has
a strong modifying influence on the development of the infants' behavior.

Also, maternal behavior of the rat is difficult to observe under natural conditions because it generally takes place in a burrow
or other protected site. It is impractical to simulate these con-

ditions in the laboratory, and thus most investigators study rodents
in relatively small cages provided only with food, water, and materials for nesting. It is not known what limitations such restricted
test environments may impose on the expression of maternal care.

Lockard (1968) criticized the use of the laboratory rat for
psychological and endocrinological studies because of behavioral
and physiological changes that have occurred as a function of domestication. Although Boice (1973) has argued that changes produced
by domestication are not "degenerative" but adaptive to conditions
of captivity, some alterations in species-typical behavior and endocrine mechanisms have nevertheless occurred (Lockard, 1968).

The existence of species differences in maternal care patterns
and in hormonal mechanisms of pregnancy, parturition, and lactation
further limits the generalizability of studies on the rat. Indeed,
behavioral and endocrinological differences are demonstratable even
between phylogenetically closely related forms, and homologous behaviors (such as nest-building in rats, mice, and rabbits) may depend upon quite different patterns of hormonal stimulation (see reviews by Zarrow et al., 1972; Moltz, 1971). Species differences
may also extend to the neural control of maternal behavior (Slotnick & Nigrosh, 1974) and neural pathways mediating neuroendocrine
reflexes (Cowie & Tindal, 1971). Differences among species in neural
hormonal and behavioral factors underlying reproductive activities
are pervasive, and considerable caution must be exercised in general-
izing results obtained with the laboratory rat to other species.

In spite of these limitations, a large amount of new and exciting research on the hormonal and neural aspects of maternal behavior
in rodents has emerged in the last decade. Many formerly unresolved
problems have been answered; neural, endocrine, and behavioral mechanisms have been elucidated; and new techniques have been developed
to investigate maternal behavior. Like all productive research,
these studies have frequently raised new problems, some of which
would not have been contemplated only a few years ago.

MATERNAL BEHAVIOR IN THE RAT

Nesting

The intricacies of nest-building behavior are well illustrated
by Calhoun's study of wild Norwegian rats (1962). Rats were maintained in a semi-natural environment where they constructed complex
burrow systems consisting of tunnels, interconnecting passages, and
cavities. Preparturient females made nests in enlarged underground
cavities connected to the burrow system or in harborage boxes located
above ground. The nests had a distinctive structure. Vines, straw,

and grass were tightly interwoven to form a cup that rested on a
2-4 inch-high pad made of leaves and other flat material. Frequently, the inside of the nest was lined with finer textured grass or
paper and the entire nest was covered over and provided with a single narrow entrance. Simpler nests, consisting of only a flat pad
or cup were made by males and nonpregnant and non lactating females.

In most laboratory studies of maternal behavior, rats have been
given neither enough space nor appropriate materials to assess their
full capacity to build a nest. Generally, hay or strips of soft
paper toweling are provided for nesting. One portion of the cage
may be partitioned off or a small nest box provided. In unpartitioned
cages, rats generally construct a nest in the darkest corner or the
one furthest from the cage door. The quality of the nest is assessed
by the amount of available material used, the presence of a floor or
base, and the height of the walls. If an unlimited supply of nesting material is available (as in the studies of Richter, 1955), the
amount of material used provides a quantitative measure. When only
a fixed amount of material is given, rats may reinforce the nest
structure with food pellets and even feces. Several methods for
assessing "motivation" for gathering nesting material have been
described. In one study (Slotnick, 1963), rats were given 15-minute
tests with cotton string. When tested on days 14 and 20 of pregnancy, they pulled only a few feet of string into the cage and usually
did not retrieve it to the nest area. When tested after parturition,
the animals pulled in several hundred feet of string, brought it
directly to the nest area, and immediately began constructing a
nest. In another study (Oley & Slotnick, 1970), bar-pressing by
rats resulted in delivery of paper strips on a fixed-ratio schedule.
This operant procedure allowed nesting behavior to be monitored
continuously and demonstrated a sharp increase in responding prior
to parturition. Tests such as these might provide valuable ancillary measures of nesting behavior.

Behavior during parturition

Nagasawa & Yanai (1972) continuously observed 49 rats during
parturition. Their observations indicate that birth of the first
pup usually occurs on day 22 or 23 of pregnancy, and the entire litter is delivered within 2 hours. Definite evidence of labor is observed one to six hours before the birth of the first pup. During
parturition, periodic waves of contractions along the abdominal wall
occur, and the female stretches forward with her body pressed a-
gainst the floor. As the first fetus begins to emerge, the mother
assumes a "head between the heels" position, licks the fetus, and
pulls it forward. After the fetus emerges- she frees it of birth
membranes and eats the placenta and umbilical cord. Subsequent
fetuses are delivered with less effort, and birth may occur when

the female is stretching forward or licking a previously born pup.
During the period of parturition, and even directly after the birth
of the first pup, the female may engage in all components of maternal behavior including retrieving pups to the nest, arranging them
in a pile, licking them, assuming a nursing position over them, and
(more rarely) repair and improvement of the nest. Nagasawa & Yanai
(1972) report that some pups begin to suckle 15 to 20 minutes after
birth, although suckling is frequently interrupted by the birth of
the next fetus. A more detailed account of behavior during parturition in the rat is provided by Rosenblatt & Lehrman (1963).

Nursing and other pup care activities

In nursing, the dam adopts a distinct stance over the pups;
the back is arched and the outstretched fore and hind feet strad-
dle the litter. She may assume this position spontaneously or in
response to suckling initiated by pups while she is resting in the
nest. During the first one to two weeks of lactation, the dam generally initiates bouts of nursing soon after she enters the nest.
Nursing is frequently preceded by a complex of activities including
repairing the nest, arranging pups in a pile, licking them, and self-
grooming. The dam quickly returns stray pups to the pile; she may
also lick or otherwise care for some pups while others suckle.

The duration of individual nursing bouts has not been systematically studied, although unpublished observations in our laboratory
indicate that the dam may remain crouched quietly over the pups for
an hour or more at a time. Using a two-compartment cage that allowed automatic recording of the time spent in the nest compartment, Grota (1973) found that in the first postpartum week dams
spent 85 percent of their time or more in the nest area with their
litter. A definite rhythmicity in time spent with the litter was
also observed (Ader & Grota, 1970). Under a regimen of 12 hours
each of light and dark, dams spent the most time with the litter
during the middle of the light period and the least during the middle of the dark period. This cicardian rhythm probably reflects
the rat's normal activity cycle but may also be related to a diurnal
change in maternal responsiveness.

Retrieving and other tests of maternal behavior

Perhaps the most important measure of maternal behavior is the
survival and growth of the young. Most studies reviewed below, however, deal with the onset or short-term maintenance of maternal behavior rather than the adequacy of maternal care. Also, many of
these studies are concerned with the induction of maternal behavior
in pregnant, virgin female, or male rats rather than with the abil-

ity of the animal to adequately care for young. In these studies, the most commonly used measure of maternal behavior or maternal responsiveness is the retrieval of pups to the nest.

Generally, a "retrieving test" involves scattering the litter about the cage and recording the animal's behavior for 10 to 30 minutes. For dams in the first postpartum week, retrieving is generally initiated within 30 seconds and all the pups are brought back to the nest in one to two minutes. The disturbance provided by such a retrieving test appears to stimulate further maternal activity such as arranging pups within the nest, licking them, self-grooming, nest building, and, finally, adopting the nursing position. The amount of postretrieval maternal care may vary widely among individual animals and even in the same animal in repeated daily tests.

In a study of 32 primiparous rats tested 10 to 18 hours after parturition, Slotnick (1967a) found that different aspects of maternal care may vary independently. Measures of nesting, pup licking, and nursing were only weakly correlated with one another and not related to the time to retrieve pups. These data indicate that maternal behavior is not a unitary behavioral process and that the use of only one or two measures is insufficient to fully assess maternal care activities.

In spite of the low correlations between measures of maternal behavior, sequential analysis reveals sources of order in maternal responding. A sequential analysis of behavior during a typical retrieving test is shown in Fig. 1. The figure is based on data obtained from the first postpartum test of normal primiparous rats (Slotnick, 1969). At the beginning of the test, the dam sniffs one or two pups, then begins to retrieve pups but does not engage in other pup care activities. After the last pup has been retrieved there is a short bout of investigating and then the rat returns to the nest and remains with the litter. As discussed in the section on brain mechanisms and maternal behavior, this kind of analysis has proved useful in characterizing the types of deficits in maternal behavior resulting from brain lesions. Unfortunately, many studies simply characterize animals as "maternal" or "not maternal" and do not provide detailed analysis of behavior.

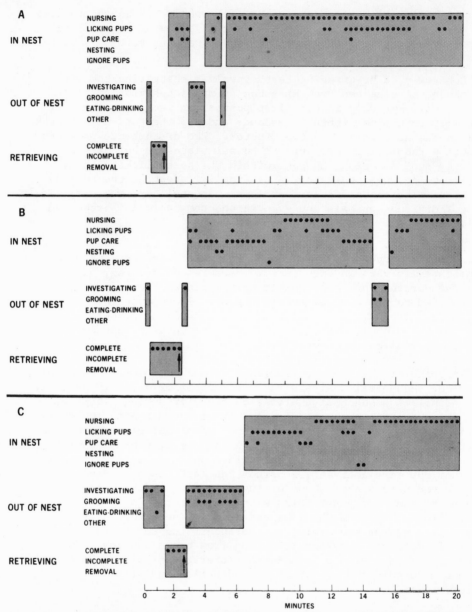

Fig. 1.   Sequential analysis of maternal behavior during a pup retrieving test on postpartum day 1 for each of 3 primiparous rats.
Maternal behavior was recorded by an observer using a panel of
switches connected to a multiple-pen event recorder.   For purposes
of illustration, the dominant activity for each 20 sec. period of
the test was determined and assigned to one of 3 mutually exclusive
categories (Retriving, Out of Nest, and In Nest).

HORMONAL FACTORS IN PREGANANCY, PARTURITION, AND LACTATION

Table 1 lists the primary hormones involved in pregnancy and lactation and briefly summarizes their actions. Because changes during pregnancy and lactation are complex and probably involve the entire endocrine system, the information in this table and in the following discussion is somewhat simplified. Additional details are provided by recent reviews of reproductive endocrinology (McCann et al., 1967; Catchpole, 1969; Nalbandov, 1973).

Pregnancy

Copulation in the rat generally precedes ovulation; pregnancy begins shortly after ovulation and terminates approximately 22 days later. Sperm motility and uterine contractions help to transport sperm to the oviduct where fertilization occurs. The ova begin cell division in the oviduct but enter the uterus at the 9 to 16 cell stage (3 to 4 days after ovulation), distribute themselves along the uterine wall, and become attached to the endometrial surface (implantation). By the fifth day of pregnancy placental formation has begun. By the time of birth, the conceptual mass may represent more than 30 percent of the total body weight of the pregnant animal.

The period of pregnancy can be divided into pregestational, gestational, and prepartum stages. These stages are based on major changes in endocrine control and merge into one another as pregnancy progresses. The pregestational (or preimplantation) stage lasts four to six days. During this time the corpus luteum of the ovary is formed and begins to secrete progesterone. Although estrogen production is largely suppressed, there is a brief estrogen surge on day four; the stimulus for this sudden increase is unknown, but it is necessary for ova implantation (Psychoyos, 1967).

During the gestational phase, the ovary secretes large amounts of progesterone which is vital to the maintenance and continuation of pregnancy. However, full expression of almost all of its many actions requires the presence of small quantities of estrogen. Estrogen appears to prepare tissue for the action of progesterone or increase the utilization or incorporation of progesterone into target organs. When the ratio of progesterone to estrogen is high, as it is in early and middle pregnancy, the two hormones act synergistically to stimulate growth of the uterus and the alveoli and ducts of the mammary gland to inhibit the contractile elements of the myometrium (muscular wall of the uterus). This latter action is especially important in producing a quiescent and relaxed uterus, thus allowing implantation of the ova and growth of the placenta and preventing expulsion of the embryos. Removal of progesterone by ovariectomy at any stage of pregnancy (except perhaps the last one to two days when progesterone levels are very low) results in absorption (early pregnancy) or abortion of the embryos. Maintenance of pregnancy to term after ovariectomy can be achieved by daily injections of two to four mg of progesterone and one ug of estrogen (Pepe & Rothchild, 1973).

The formation of a corpus luteum and secretion of progesterone depend upon stimulation of the ovary by pituitary gonadotropic hormones, particularly prolactin and lutenizing hormone (LH). A phasic release of these hormones follows mating (Linkie & Niswender, 1972; Morishige et al., 1973). An elevation of prolactin appears necessary for initiation of the luteal phase of ovarian function in the rat, and its relase from the pituitary is partly dependent upon vaginal stimuli during mating (Spies & Niswender, 1971). LH further stimulates the synthesis and secretion of progesterone, and low but tonic levels of LH during the first half of pregnancy are apparently necessary to maintain corpus luteum activity (Raj & Moudgal, 1970). Deprivation of LH, by administration of an LH antiserum for even a few hours interferes with corpora luteum activity and may result in death and resportion of the fetuses. This dependence upon LH apparently accounts for the fact that hypophysectomy before day 12 of gestation invariably results in termination of pregnancy. After days 11-12, hypophysectomy no longer terminates pregnancy because by this time the placentas produce sufficient luteotropic substances to maintain ovarian function.

Some of the recent data on serum levels of prolactin, LH, progesterone, follicle-stimulating hormone, (FSH), and estrogen during pregnancy are summarized in Fig. 2. The luteotropic surges responsible for initiating corpus luteum activity are reflected by the initial increase in LH and prolactin. The drop in LH on days 12 and 13 is correlated with an increase in gonadotropic stimulation by the placenta and may reflect a negative feedback by placental secretions on LH release. The precipitous decline in progesterone on days 16 to 18 signals the beginning of the preparturient phase of pregnancy. Removal of the progester-

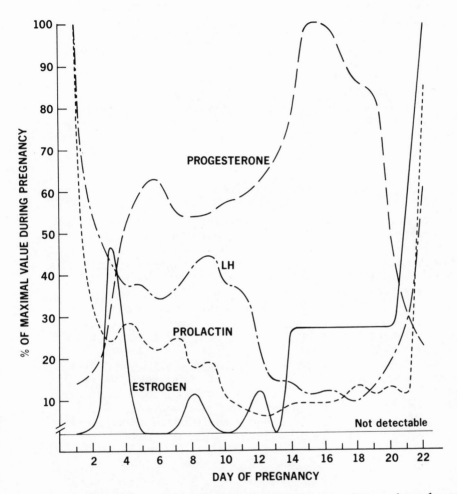

Fig. 2. Serum levels of progesterone, estrogen, LH, and prolactin during pregnancy. Serum levels are presented as a per cent of the highest level achieved during pregnancy. Calculations are based on data presented by Morishige et al. (1973) and Yoshinaga et al (1969).

one "block" to uterine myometrial activity is necessary for initiation of parturition. Exogenous progesterone given at this time will prolong pregnancy, and continued administration may produce fetal death. The factors that lead to the normal decrease in progesterone are not well understood. In some species, including the rat, the decrease in progesterone near term appears to be governed by the appearance of uterine enzymes with luteolytic properties (Flint & Armstrong, 1973). Other factors, including an increase in estrogen or chemical signals from the embryo and placenta, have also been implicated. However, the mechanisms that control the life-span of the corpus luteum -- and hence, the duration of pregnancy -- are still largely undetermined (Nalbandov, 1973).

Parturition

With the sudden decline in progesterone, spontaneous uterine activity increases and uterine tone and contractions are further stimulated by estrogen. This uterine activity coupled with increased intrauterine pressure (due primarily to rapid growth of the fetuses near term) decreases arterial blood pressure at placental sites. Uterine contractions at the beginning of labor further increase placental hypoxia and stimulate detachment of the placenta from the uterine wall. Strong, regular uterine contractions in the first stage of labor are probably stimulated by oxytrocin released from the neurohypophysis. Uterine musculature, relatively insensitive to oxytocin until shortly before term, becomes sensitive as progesterone is withdrawn and stimulation by estrogen increases. Fuchs & Saito (1971) found that uterine contractions and initiation of parturition could be induced by infusion of oxytocin into pregnant rats on day 21 or 22.

Lactation

Nourishment of young by milk secretion from mammary glands is a universal and distinguishing feature of the class Mammalia. In the rat there are six mammary glands on either side of the ventral thorax and abdomen. These are relatively flat sheets of tissues made up of parenchyma (glandular tissue) and stroma

or supportive tissue. Small sacs (alveoli) arranged in clusters
make up the secretory portion of the gland. Each alveolus consists of a single layer of milk-secreting epithelial cells
surrounded by a network of contractile myoepithelial (basket)
cells. The alveoli open into small ducts; these join a common
duct or glactophore that leads directly to the nipple (Fig. 3).
Milk secreted by the epithelial cells is stored in the lumen
of the alveolus. Contractions of the basket cells force milk
into the ducts and make it available to the suckling young.

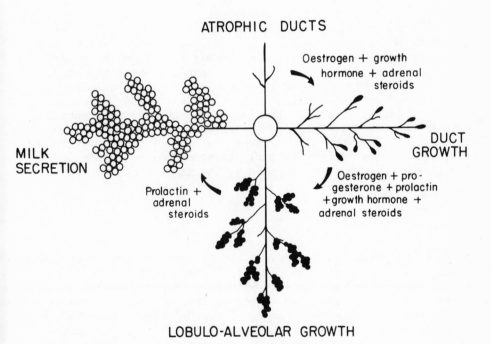

Fig. 3. Schema showing some of the hormones that influence
mammary growth and lactation. (From Cowie, 1972).

Hormonal requirements for growth and secretory function of the mammary gland have been studied extensively by determining the effects of various hormones in triply operated (hypophysectomized, ovariectomized, and adrenalectomized) rats and mice. A summary of these results is given in Fig. 3. Prelactational growth of the lobuloalveolar system requires a complex of hormones including ovarian estrogen and preogesterone, adrenal steroids, and pituitary prolactin and growth hormone (GH).

Lactation consists of two processes: (1) the formation and secretion of milk and (2) the release of milk into the glactophore and its removal by the young. Although prolactin is generally considered the primary lactogenic hormone, it exerts its full effect on milk secretion only in synergy with pituitary growth hormone and adrenal steroids (corticoids). The hormones comprise a "lactogenic complex" (Lyons, 1958). In the pregnant rat, lactogenic agents may also be produced by the placenta.

A complex relationship exists between the lactogens and estrogen and progesterone. By midpregnancy, stimulation by the ovarian hormones and the lactogenic complex results in growth of the mammary gland to a prelactational but not full secretory state. The high levels of progesterone during pregnancy inhibit milk secretion, partly by blocking alveolar synthesis of lactose, while the progesterone-estrogen combination partly suppresses lactogen release. At the end of pregnancy, when progesterone levels are low, estrogen stimulates prolactin release. The lactogenic complex then exerts its full influence on further proliferation of alveolar cells and stimulation of milk synthesis. Ovarian hormones inhibit mammary gland secretion; ovariectomy as early as midpregnancy results in a rapid increase in protein secreted by the mammary gland (Liu & Davis, 1967).

Neuroendocrine control of lactation

Before the relationship between the nervous and endocrine systems was understood, hormonal regulation was generally viewed in terms of a simple feedback between pituitary tropic hormones and their respective target organs. However, the discovery of neurosecretory cells in the hypothalamus, of the dependence of anterior pituitary function on hypothalamic secretions in the portal circulation, and the pervasive effects of environmental stimuli on reproductive endocrinology made it clear that hormonal regulation involved neurohumoral factors (see reviews by Everett, 1964; McCann & Dhariwal, 1966; Scharrer & Scharrer, 1963). Although all hormonal influences on behavior are mediated by the nervous system, the best understood neuroendocrine interactions in regard to mater-

nal behavior concern oxytocin and prolactin. These hormones
are necessary for lactation, and the control of their release involves interactions between the dam and her young.

The release of these hormones is controlled by neurons in the
hypothalamus, but the mechanisms are different in each case. Oxytocin is produced in cells of the paraventicular nucleus and stored
in secretory granules (Knaggs et al., 1971). The secretory material is transported down the axons of the paraventricular tract,
which courses through the median eminence and terminates as enlarged dilations on capillary perivascular spaces in the neurohypophysis (Fig. 4). The hormonal substances in the granules are
released from the terminal after axonal depolarization and diffuse
into the capillaries. These neurosecretory paraventricular cells
thus resemble other cells in the brain except that their axons terminate on perivascular spaces rather than on dendrites or soma of
other neurons and their secretory product is a hormone released into
the circulation rather than a neurotransmitter released at a synaptic junction.

Release of prolactin and other hormones produced in the anterior
lobe of the pituitary is controlled by another class of neurosecretory neurons in the tuberal region of the hypothalamus. Substances
released into the portal circulation in this part of the hypothalamus
act to regulate the release or production of anterior pituitary tropic hormones (McCann & Dhariwal, 1966). Fig. 4 illustrates the
anatomic relationships between the various hypothalamic neurosecretory neurons and the pituitary gland. The release of each of the
pituitary tropic hormones except prolactin, is stimulated by secretion of a specific hypothalamic releasing factor (Table 1). The
regulatory hormone for prolactin inhibits its release and has therefore been named prolactin inhibitory factor (PIF). Recent investigations of hypothalamic regulatory hormones have been reviewed by Schally et al., (1973).

The neuronal link in the regulation of pituitary hormone release provides the anatomical basis for the various effects external
stimuli have on the endocrine system and, consequently, on reproductive behavior. Fig. 5, adapted from the monograph of Scharrer &
Scharrer (1963), diagrams some of the potential feedback mechanisms
between the nervous and endocrine systems. Such interactions involve neuroendocrine reflexes in which neural stimuli causing the
release of a hormone are the afferent component and the hormone acting on its target tissue is the efferent component.

Several relatively simple neuroendocrine reflexes involving
oxytocin and prolactin occur as a function of the interaction between the lactating animal and her litter (also see section on
suckling and associated stimuli). In the case of milk release by

Table I.   MAJOR REPRODUCTIVE HORMONES IN PREGNANCY AND LACTATION

Hormone	Source	Principal Actions
Luteinizing Hormone (LH)	Basophylic cells of anterior pituitary	Stimulates ovulation of prepared ovarian follicles; stimulates synthesis of progesterone by corpus luteum and maintains secretion of progesterone for the first half of pregnancy. Postovulatory surge stimulated by mating. Steroidogenic effect requires prior priming by FSH and prolactin. Also implicated in luteolysis at end of pregnancy.
Follicle-Stimulating Hormone (FSH)	Basophylic cells of anterior pituitary	Stimulates growth of ovarian follicles and, with LH, stimulates estrogen secretion and ovulation.
Prolactin	Acidophylic cells of anterior pituitary	Stimulates movement of cholesterol into developing corpus luteum, making it available for steroidogenic effects of LH. Prolongs the life of the corpus luteum during pregnancy. With progesterone, stimulates lobulo-alveolar growth of the mammary gland. In synergy with adreno-corticosteroids, and growth hormone stimulates the synthesis and secretion of milk by the mammary gland alveolar epithelium just prior and after parturition. Post ovulatory surge stimulated by mating. Release of lactogenic hormones and continued production of milk postpartum is dependent upon suckling stimulation.
Follicle-Stimulating Hormone Releasing Factor (FSH-RF)	Tuberal region of hypothalamus	Stimulates the synthesis and release of FSH by the anterior pituitary.
Luteinizing Hormone Releasing Factor (LH-RF)	Tuberal region of hypothalamus	Stimulates the synthesis and release of LH by the anterior pituitary.
Prolactin Release Inhibiting Hormone (PRIH or PIF)	Tuberal region of hypothalamus	Inhibits the release of prolactin by the anterior pituitary.
Oxytocin	Paraventricular nucleus of hypothalamus; stored in the posterior pituitary	Acts on myometrium to stimulate uterine contractions during parturition. Stimulates contraction of mammary gland myoepithelial cells, forcing milk into the ducts (milk ejection).
Estrogen	Follicular cells in ovary	Stimulates ovarian and uterine blood flow, enhances incorporation of progesterone into uterine endometrium. Acts synergistically with progesterone to stimulate growth of the uterus in early pregnancy and growth of the mammary gland alveoli and ducts. Stimulates the release of luteotrophins from the anterior pituitary.
Progesterone	Corpus luteum in ovary	Acts synergistically with estrogen to stimulate growth of the uterine endometrium, and alveoli and ducts of the mammary glands. Prepares endometrium for implantation of blastocytes, inhibits uterine contractions, blocks the release of oxytocin and prolactin and inhibits milk metabolism in the mammary gland during early pregnancy.

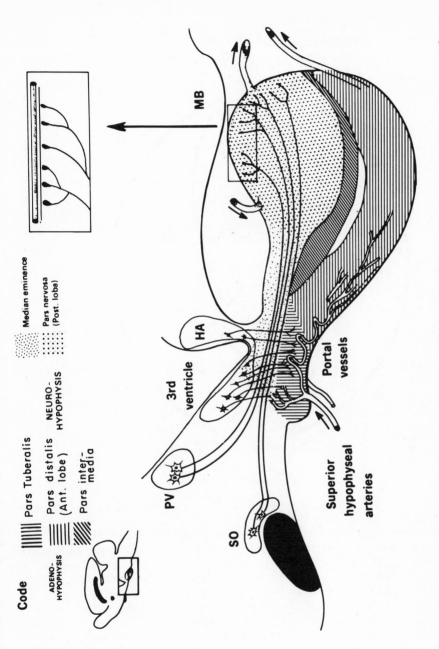

Fig. 4. Schematic representation of the hypothalamic-hypophyseal neurosecretory system of mammals. HA, hypophysiotropic area of hypothalamus, MB, mammillary body; OC, optic chiasm; PV, paraventricular nucleus; SO, supraoptic nucleus. (Modified after Flerko, 1966, and Reichlin, 1963).

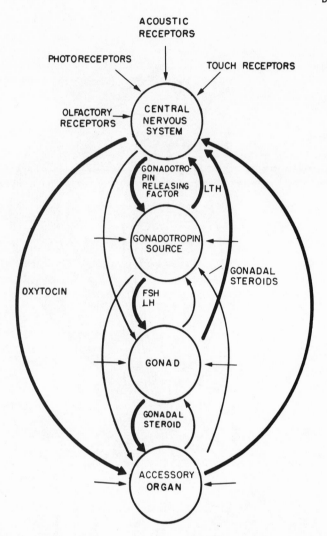

Fig. 5.   Illustration of the integration of neural and hormonal mechanisms in the control of reproductive processes.   A variety of afferent extrinsic stimuli (odor, light, sound, touch, etc.) directed towards the central nervous system may influence activity of neurosecretory neurons in the hypothalamus.   Hormones may reach their target organs directly (heavy arrows), as is the case in the effect of oxytocin on the uterus and mammary glands.   Other substances, also produced by nerve cells, reach the adenohypophysis which in turn acts through FSH, LH, and prolactin on the gonads.   The latter, by means of gonadal steroids, affect accessory sex organs.   Each of the organs constituting the chain may return nervous and hormonal stimuli, thus influencing central nervous system functions.   (After Scharrer & Scharrer, 1963).

oxytocin, the reflex is initiated by stimulation of sensory receptors in the teat by the suckling young. This afferent stimulus pro-
jects via a multisynaptic pathway to the paraventricular nuclei in
the hypothalamus. Oxytocin, released from the posterior pituitary,
forces milk in the mammary gland ducts by stimulating contraction
of the basket cells surrounding the mammary gland alveoli.

The brainstem and diencephalic pathways mediating the afferent
component of this reflex have been studied by electrical brain stimulation in lactating guinea pigs and rabbits (Tindal et al., 1967,
1969; Tindal & Knaggs, 1971; also see reviews by Beyer & Mena, 1966;
Cowie & Tindal, 1971). Increase in intramammary pressure served as
an assay for the release of oxytocin. The pathway ascends in the
caudal midbrain as a compact bundle in the lateral tegmentum; its
rostral extension is more diffuse but appears to project through
the medial and lateral hypothalamus to the paraventricular nuclei.

In addition to the afferent pathway described by Tindal and
co-workers, other, more rostral portions of the brain may be involved in oxytocin release. Stimulation of the limbic cortex, hippocampal rudiment, diagonal band of Broca and the septum results in
the release of oxytocin in the rabbit (Cross, 1961; Aulsbrook & Holland, 1969a), and Beyer et al., (1961) reported oxytocin release
from stimulation of the cingulate cortex in cats. Additional studies have shown that many of these limbic structures as well as effective stimulation points in the brain stem project directly to
the paraventricular nuclei (Woods et al., 1969).

Stimulation of certain brian areas, including the superior
colliculus, periaqueductal gray, tectoreticular tract, and portions
of the tegmental reticular formation, causes inhibition of oxytocin
release in the lactating rabbit (Aulsbrook & Holland, 1969b). Because stimulation of similar sites in awake animals produces aversive or avoidance reactions (Spiegel et al., 1954; Olds & Olds,
1962) Aulsbrook & Holland suggest that this pathway may be part of
a nociceptive system that mediates the well known inhibitory effects
of painful and emotionally arousing stimuli on milk ejection (Cross,
1955a, 1955b).

Release of prolactin, as mentioned earlier, is under inhibitory
control by the brain. A prolactin inhibitory factor (PIF) has been
isolated from hypothalamic tissue and its inhibitory effects on pituitary secretion has been demonstrated in intact rats and in tissue cultures of anterior pituitary lobes (Meites, 1972). In the
lactating rat, suckling by the young results in a marked reduction
of hypothalamic PIF and rapid and abrupt increase in plasma prolactin as well as other hormones involved in lactation such as GH,
ACTH and thyrotropin releasing factor (Blake, 1974). The suppression of follicle stimulating hormone and lutenizing hormone, and

hence, the suppression of ovarian cycling during lactation are dependent on suckling induced release of prolactin.

Assay of prolactin or PIF, unlike that of oxytocin, is a time-
consuming and laborous process. As a result, there are fewer studies of the afferent pathway in the reflex release of prolactin. An
earlier hypothesis that oxytocin, released into the portal circulation, could stimulate the release of prolactin during suckling
(Benson & Folley, 1956) has not been supported (Meites, 1972). Instead, as in the case of oxytocin, sensory stimulation of suckling
appears to activate a neural afferent system that results in prolactin release. The brain stem pathway for prolactin was studied by Tindal & Knagg (1969) by determining the effects of daily
electrical brain stimulation on mammary secretion in pseudopregnant
rabbits. Analysis of positive stimulation sites indicated that the
ascending pathway follows the same course in the mesencephalon as
that found for oxytocin. The pathway appears to enter the posterior
hypothalamus dorsal to the mammillary bodies and extends rostrally
into the lateral hypothalamus. However, its exact course and termination within the hypothalamus has not yet been determined.

The use of hypothalamic lesions for identifying a "center"
for the control of prolactin has met with limited success. Experiments by Sawyer and co-workers (Haun & Sawyer, 1960, 1961; Kanematsu
et al., 1963; Sawyer et al., 1963) indicated that relatively discrete lesions of the posterior basal tuberal area result in the release of pituitary prolactin and lactogenesis in estrogen primed
rabbits. These results strongly suggest that the lesion interferes
with PIF release, although they do not prove that this posterior
basal tuberal region is the site for production of PIF. In related
studies it was found that estrogen implanted into this region increases prolactin content of the pituitary (Kanematsu & Sawyer, 1963).
As it has been demonstrated that estrogen can decrease hypothalamic
PIF (Ratner & Meites, 1964), it thus appears that PIF can be suppressed by both neurogenic and hormonal stimuli.

More rostral portions of the hypothalamus and forebrain may
also play a role in the control of prolactin. Grosz & Rothballer
(1961) reported that a transverse section through the tuber cinereum
at a point just behind the optic chiasma resulted in reactivation of
the partly involuted mammary glands of postpartum cats. Removal of
the entire telencephalon or more discrete lesions of the entorhinal
cortex and amygdala produce mammary growth and lactogenesis in ovariectomized, estrogen-primed rabbits (Beyer & Mena, 1965; Mena & Beyer,
1968).

Because prolactin is important not only in lactation but has
also been implicated in the initiation of maternal behavior (see
section on Hormonal induction of maternal behavior) it is unfortunate

that more information is not available concerning its neural control. Recently developed radioimmunoassays for prolactin (Niswender et al., 1969) may provide a more rapid and accurate method than the older bioassays for investigations of brain mechanisms controlling the synthesis and release of prolactin.

HORMONAL BASIS OF MATERNAL BEHAVIOR

Prematernal behaviors during pregnancy

Nest Building. Several behaviors during pregnancy may be considered maternal or prematernal. The best studied is nest building. During pregnancy rats and mice construct larger and more elaborate nests than do nonpregnant animals. In the mouse this increase occurs four or five days after mating, a time which coincides with the appearance of ovarian corpora lutea and the beginning of the progestational state of pregnancy (Koller, 1952, 1956). Exogenous progesterone given to virgin female mice causes an increase in nest building after two to three days (Koller, 1952, 1956; Lisk et al., 1969). Progesterone treatment is also effective in ovariectomized mice, but the greatest faciliation of nest building in castrates is obtained when small priming doses of estrogen are given before progesterone (Lisk, 1971); this is in accord with the known synergistic action of these two steroids.

The effect of progesterone on nest building in intact virgin female mice has recently been confirmed in our laboratory (Slotnick & Gelhard, unpublished observations). Two or three days after a 35mg pellet of progesterone was implanted subcutaneously in the nape of the neck, each mouse showed a dramatic and sustained increase in the amount of material used and each built a large nest with high walls and a partial ceiling.

In contrast to these results in mice, the construction of a maternal nest by rabbits and rats is inhibited by progesterone. The endocrine control of nest building in the rabbit has been reviewed (Zarrow et al., 1968, 1972). Construction of a maternal nest, during the last few days of the 31 to 32 day gestation period, is apparently stimulated by the decline in progesterone and increase in estrogen which occurs after day 27 of pregnancy (Challis et al., 1973). Removal of progesterone (by ovariectomy) after day 17 of gestation or injection of exogenous estrogen into the intact rabbit on days 20 to 22 induces maternal nest building. Exogenous progesterone given at the end of pregnancy delays the onset of maternal nest building and parturition.

In the rat, nesting activity increases slightly four to five days before parturition, and a maternal nest is made either the day before parturition or, in some cases just afterward (Rosenblatt & Lehrman, 1963). Denenberg et al. (1969) found a peak increase in nesting activity at 24 to 48 hours before parturition. This time course was confirmed in operant studies in which nesting material (paper strips) was obtained by bar pressing (Oley & Slotnick, 1970; Slotnick, unpublished observations).

The hormonal basis for this prepartum increase in nesting is not known, although it is presumably similar to that for the rabbit. In virtually the only hormonal study of nesting in this species, Denenberg et al. (1969) report that injections of progesterone on days 16 to 21 of pregnancy delayed the onset of peak nesting behavior (and parturition) and reduced the number of females that showed a prepartum increase in nest building. However, a variety of other endocrine manipulations that are effective in inducing maternal nest building in rabbits (including pseudopregnancy, treatment with estrogen in late pregnancy, and castration) had no clear effect on nesting in the rat. It is not clear whether these results reflect a difference between the hormonal control of nest building in rabbits and rats or are due to differences in testing procedures. However, other similarities between the rat and rabbit data suggest that, for both species, the construction of a maternal nest depends upon removal of the progesterone block at the end of pregnancy.

Self-licking. Pregnant rats show an increase in self-licking of the nipple line and genital region (Rosenblatt & Lehrman, 1963; Roth & Rosenblatt, 1967). Two to five days after the onset of pregnancy, there is a gradual and sustained increase in self-licking of these areas and a decrease in the amount of time spent licking other regions (head, forepaws, shoulder and upper back). The increased licking of the ventral body surface is probably stimulated by body growth during pregnancy and also perhaps by secretions from the vagina and the enlarged mammary glands. Roth & Rosenblatt (1968) demonstrated that increased self-licking of the ventral surface during pregnancy facilitates secretory activity of the mammary glands. By histological criteria, mammary development and secretory activity on day 22 of pregnancy were reduced to 50 percent of normal in animals prevented from licking "critical regions" by neck collars. Smaller deficits in mammary gland growth were seen in animals collared for only the first or second half of pregnancy. Roth & Rosenblatt suggest that the increased licking of the mammary glands is stimulated by enlargement of the gland; self-licking, in turn, provides a neurogenic stimulus that facilitates the release of galactogenic hormones and thus further augments mammary growth.

The relationship between self-licking during pregnancy and hormone-induced changes in the body surface provides an excellent example of a complex interaction between behavior and a neuroendocrine regulating mechanism. However, the functional role of self-

licking in the development of maternal behavior is unclear. Birch
(1956), in a widely quoted study, reported that female rats raised
with neck collars that were removed shortly before parturition tended to cannibalize their young or show inadequate maternal care;
quantitative data were not reported. Christophersen & Wagman (1965)
and Kirby & Horvath (1968) failed to replicate these findings, and
questioned the importance of preparturitive self-licking in the development of maternal behavior.

A nonhormonal basis for maternal behavior in virgin rats

Pregnancy, birth of young, and lactation are dependent upon
interactions among hormones and their target tissues. In contrast,
the expression of at least some aspects of maternal behavior may be
independent of hormonal stimulation in that they can occur in both
males and females at any stage of the reproductive cycle.

Retrieving young, licking them, adopting a nursing position,
and maternal nest building may all occur "spontaneously" in virgin
female rats upon their first adult encounter with young pups. Although 15 to 20 percent of animals show one or more components of
maternal behavior within minutes of the initial test, the full expression of maternal care generally requires continuous exposure to
pups for approximately five or six days (fresh litters are generally given each day). This procedure for inducing maternal behavior
by prolonged exposure to pups has frequently been referred to as sensitization and animals induced to become maternal are considered "sensitized." The factors leading to this induction of maternal behavior are not fully understood, and these terms should perhaps be replaced by more neutral or descriptive terms such as concaveation
(Wiesner & Sheard, 1933) or priming (Noirot, 1972a).

The duration of exposure required before virgin rats and mice
become maternally responsive is influenced by several environmental
variables (see review by Noirot, 1972a). For example, rats housed
with pups become maternal sooner if the cages are small (which increases the probability of contact with pups) than if cages are large
(Terkel & Rosenblatt, 1971). Pups one to two days old are more
readily accepted than older pups (Weisner & Sheard, 1933; Noirot,
1964). The presence of nearby cages with litters may also hasten
the onset of maternal responsiveness (Noirot, 1972a). Other variables
that affect the induction of maternal behavior include strain, age
at testing, and the health or vigor of the test pups (Noirot, 1972a).
Although some studies have indicated that males are less responsive
to the effects of pup exposure than are females, this may also depend upon the strain of animals used (Quadango & Rockwell, 1972).
These various factors, however, influence only the amount of time re-

quired before maternal behavior is expressed; eventually, almost all rats and mice allowed to live continuously with pups become maternally responsive.

The maternal behavior after pup exposure is similar in many respects to that seen in the postpartum animal. Fleming (1972) compared the behavior of primed virgin rats with that of primiparous rats living with their own litters. They were each given ten daily retrieving tests beginning on the first postpartum day (for dams) or the day after the first maternal responses (for virgins). Primiparous animals initially tended to retrieve pups faster, spent more time in the nest with pups, showed more nest building and spent more time in a nursing position over the pups. However, none of these differences was significant and over repeated tests behavior of the two groups was quite similar.

Nevertheless, important differences exist in both the range and quality of maternal behavior expressed by virgin and postpartum animals. The most obvious is the time required for maternal behavior to appear. In the parturient rat, maternal care activities begin with the birth of the first pup while virgin rats require days of continuous exposure to pups. Maternal activities such as aiding the young to emerge from the vaginal orifice, licking the afterbirth fluids, and eating the placenta cannot be adequately tested in the virgin. Preliminary data of Sachs et al. (1971) indicate that both maternally responsive and nonmaternal virgins eat the placenta and cannibalize the pups when presented with live Caesaren delivered fetuses with the placenta attached. Their results suggest that the inhibition of cannibalism of newborn pups may depend upon hormonal conditions at the end of pregnancy.

The use of more sensitive tests may further discriminate between the maternal behavior of primed virgin and lactating rats. For example, Bridges et al. (1972) reported that lactating rats show much more retrieving behavior than maternal virgins when the pups had been placed in a runway attached to the home cage. Similar results have been obtained for mice (Gandelman et al., 1970).

That maternal behavior induced in virgin rats is not dependent upon reproductive hormones has been clearly shown by Rosenblatt (1967). In his study no differences were found among intact, ovariectomized, or hypophysectomized virgin females for the duration of exposure to pups before retrieving, care of young, or nest building was first seen. Leblond & Nelson (1937a, 1937b) had obtained similar results for mice.

Pregnancy termination and initiation
of maternal behavior

The studies on the induction of maternal behavior, reviewed
above, suggest strongly that the neural substrate for this behavior
is present in both females and males, is independent of hormonal
control, and requires only appropriate stimulation from the young
before it is expressed. What role, then, do hormones play in the
expression of maternal care? One important difference between primiparous and virgin primed rats is the latency before maternal behaviors occur. It is not clear whether maternal behavior that
normally appears suddenly at birth of young depends on hormone
changes that occur at parturition, before parturition, or on parturitive experience ifself. Rosenblatt (1970) and Lott & Rosenblatt
(1969) found that nulliparous rats show no maternal interest when
tested with pups for one hour on days 12 to 22 of pregnancy. However, if rats are exposed continuously to pups in the latter half
of pregnancy, maternal behavior is elicited in only three to four
days -- a significant decrease from the five to six days of exposure required by virgin females.

This "pregnancy effect" is still quite different from the sudden appearance of the full complement of maternal behaviors shortly
after parturition. To examine the effect of terminating pregnancy
on the onset of maternal behavior, Lott & Rosenblatt (1969) removed
pups by Caesarean section or hysterectomy at different times during
gestation. (No differences were found between these two methods).
In addition, both hysterectomies and ovariectomies were performed on
some rats. Beginning 24 hours after surgery, the animals were allowed to live with five to ten day old pups and maternal behavior
was tested daily. The results (Table 2) demonstrate that when hysterectomy alone is performed on day 19 of pregnancy, rats require only
approximately 24 hours of exposure to pups before maternal behavior
appears. Terminating pregnancy at progressively earlier times resulted in a progressive increase in latency to maternal behavior.
However, this pregnancy termination effect was much reduced or abolished if both hysterectomies and ovariectomies were performed (Table
2, column 8). These results suggest that changes in ovarian hormones
that accompany termination of pregnancy may play a role in the facilitation of maternal behavior.

Recently Siegel (1974) repeated these experiments with similar
methods, except that he used younger test pups (three to five days
old) and began testing 48 hours rather than 24 hours after surgery.
The results described by Lott & Rosenblatt (1969) were confirmed:
rats subjected to hysterectomy in the latter half of pregnancy showed
a significant facilitation of maternal behavior as compared to normal
pregnant animals or those subjected to both hysterectomies and ovariectomies. However, Siegel found that even the latter group showed

Table II.

Latencies (days for the onset of retrieving in pregnant rats first exposed to pups 24 hours after various treatments. Latencies (mean + SD) are given from the day of operation or the equivalent day of pregnancy.

| (1) | (2) | (3) | Treatment | | | | | |
| | | | (4) | (5) | (6) | (7) | (8) | (9) |
Group	N	Day pups given	Hysterectomy[a]	N	Pregnant[b]	N	Hysterectomy + Ovariectomy	(4-8) p-value
19-days pregnant	8	20	2.25 ± 0.28					
16-days pregnant	16	17	2.31 ± 0.67	8	4.63 ± 0.99[c]	14	4.57 ± 2.02[d]	< .05
13-days pregnant	9	14	3.67 ± 1.35					
10-days pregnant	11	11	4.18 ± 2.01	9	7.33 ± 1.89	7	6.42 ± 3.02	< .005
8-days pregnant	8	9	6.37 ± 1.05					
Virgins	14	--	6.78 ± 2.80					
			$F = 14.23$					
			df = 5/60		$p < .005$		$p < .05$	
			$p < .01$					

[a] Some animals were hysterectomized and other had only their fetuses and the placentas removed by Caesarean-section. These procedures have given the same behavioral results.

[b] Comparison between means of columns 6 and 8 were not significant (t-test).

[c] Mean latency is significantly shorter than the latency of virgins at the .01 level of confidence.

[d] Mean latency is significantly shorter than the latency of virgins at the .02 to 0.5 levels of confidence.

(From Rosenblatt, 1970)

more rapid induction of maternal behavior than similarly operated
virgin controls; a result suggesting that a moderate effect of pregnancy termination may be present even if the ovaries are removed.

Moltz et al. (1966) extended these investigations by determining the effects of terminating pregnancy (by Caesarean section)
on the day of expected parturition (day 22). When tested 18 to 23
hours after surgery, the dams responded almost immediately (within
5 minutes) to foster pups. Furthermore, Caesarean-delivered rats
did not differ significantly from normal postpartum females on
measures of nest building, retrieving, or gain in pup weight over
a 21-day postpartum period. Fleischer & Slotnick (unpublished
observations) also found that nulliparous pregnant rats, delivered
by Caesarean section on the day of expected parturition and tested
24 hours later, responded toward foster pups as quickly and vigorously as did rats allowed to deliver normally.

Studies on artificial termination of pregnancy also bear on
the long-standing question of what role parturitive experience
plays in the development of the bond between the mother and her
young (Lehrman, 1961; Rosenblatt & Lehrman, 1963). The study of
Moltz et al. (1966) clearly indicates that parturitive experience
is not essential for the sudden onset of maternal behavior, or for
the continued care and maintenance of the litter. Rather, termination of pregnancy for the sudden appearance of maternal behavior
in the primiparous rat.

A recent report by Slotnick et al. (1973) provided evidence
that maternal responsiveness may, in fact, occur suddenly just before parturition and without artificial termination of pregnancy.
Nulliparous pregnant rats were given 6-minute tests during the latter half of pregnancy with pups one to four days old. On the afternoon of expected delivery, tests were given every three to six hours
until the onset of parturition. No maternal interest in pups was
observed until two to eleven hours before parturition. Then five
of eleven animals tested suddenly started retrieving, licking, and
crouching over the pups during the test, (see Fig. 6). The remaining six animals showed no maternal interest although they were
tested immediately before (and in some cases just after) the birth
of the first pup. When tested 12 to 18 hours after parturition,
all rats promptly retrieved test pups, and actively cared for them.
In a similar study, Sadowsky et al. (unpublished results, cited by
Siegel, 1974) also found a sudden increase in maternal responsiveness just before parturition in approximately 80 percent of animals
tested.

Thus it appears that the sudden onset of maternal behavior,
previously associated with the termination of pregnancy, may, occur
a few hours before parturition. Presumably, the appearance of ma-

ternal behavior at that time is due to the stimulation (or release
from inhibition) of appropriate parts of the brain by hormonal
changes near term. Why some of the animals in these studies did
not show a prepartum onset of maternal behavior is unclear. Hormonal events leading to parturition and those stimulating maternal
behavior may not be identical (although they may share common elements), and stimulation of maternal behavior may occur earlier in
regard to the onset of parturition in some animals then in others.

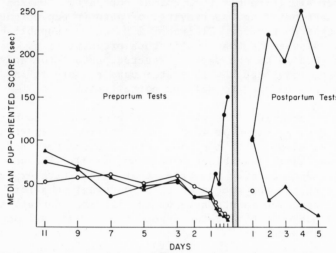

Fig. 6. Median time spent attending to pups during 6-min. tests
given prior to and following parturition. Litters were removed 12-
18 hrs. after parturition and dams were tested with foster pups.
(O) Nonpregnant controls, (●) pregnant animals which retrieved
pups prior to parturition, (▲) Pregnant animals which did not
retrieve pups prior to parturition. Note that rats which did not
retrieve pups prior to parturition show a rapid decline in postpartum
maternal behavior after being separated from their litters. (From
Slotnick et al., 1973).

Hormonal induction of maternal behavior

     The search for hormonal basis of maternal behavior in the rat
began 40 years ago with the studies of Riddle and associates (Riddle et al., 1935, 1942; Riddle, 1963). They tested the effects of
a wide variety of injections on initiation of pup retrieving in
normal, castrated, thyroidectomized, or hypophysecomized rats. Animals were usually injected daily for 10 days and then given a series
of daily 10-minute retrieving tests. Treatments with various substances, including prolactin, progesterone, luteinizing hormone,
phenol and thyroxin, appeared to stimulate pup retrieving. Unfortunately, methodological problems and inadequate statistical treat-

ment of data seriously compromised the usefulness of these studies,
and attempts to replicate some of them were not successful. Thus,
Beach & Wilson (1963) found no effects of prolactin or progesterone
and estrogen on the maternal behavior or virgin rats. Lott (1962)
and Lott & Fuchs (1962) also failed to induce maternal behavior
with prolactin or progesterone. More recently, however, some of
Riddle's early findings have been confirmed and advances have been
made in specifying the nature of hormonal changes at parturition.
An important factor in the success of these more recent studies has
been the use of the cohabitation or priming technique rather than
the brief daily pup retrieving tests used earlier. This allows
the substitution of an essentially all-or-none index for one which
yields a graded (latency) measure of maternal responsiveness for
each animal.

In 1968, Terkel & Rosenblatt reported that a single intravenous
injection of blood plasma from postpartum maternal rats given to
virgin females significantly reduced the amount of time required to
induce maternal behavior. Recipients showed the full complement of
maternal behaviors after approximately two days of cohabitation with
pups; in several animals maternal behavior appeared only four to
eight hours after the injection. Untreated control animals or those
injected with saline or blood from estrus-cycling rats in proestrus
or diestrus required approximately four to seven days before cohabitation with pups induced maternal responses. This study was
followed by an elegant series of experiments in which blood was continuously cross-transfused between two animals by means of implanted
heart catheters (Terkel, 1970; Terkel & Rosenblatt, 1972). The apparatus permitted reasonably unrestrained movement of both animals.
Seven of eight virgin females receiving blood by cross-transfusion
from a newly parturient rat showed maternal behavior within 48
hours; the mean latency was only 14.5 hours. Blood from newly parturient females was more effective than blood from females 24 hours
before or after parturition. However, blood from virgin animals
that spontaneously retrieved pups or had been primed by cohabitation
with pups failed to facilitate the onset of maternal responses in
naive virgins.

These results provided the first unequivocal evidence that
blood-borne factors from postpartum rats could induce maternal behavior in otherwise unresponsive recipient animals. Although the
active substance or substances have not been identified, techniques
for analyzing serum components are available and identification
should be possible.

One method for specifying hormonal changes essential for stimulating maternal behavior is to see whether disruption of hormonal
events at parturition produces a corresponding disruption in behavior. Moltz & Wiener (1966) and Moltz et al. (1969) determined
the effects of either ovariectomy performed shortly before term or

injections of 2 mg of progesterone on days 19 to 23 post coitum in
pregnant multiparous (maternally experienced) and nulliparous rats.
Because both treatments interfere with normal parturition, all
animals were delivered by Caesarean section. Twenty-four hours
after delivery, the animals were given newborn foster pups and
their maternal behavior was observed. After either treatment,
approximately 50 percent of the maternally inexperienced rats
failed to exhibit maternal behavior, and their litters died within 3 days. However, the remaining animals in this group and almost all of the treated multipara behaved maternally and raised
their litters to weaning. Moltz et al. (1969) suggest that ovariectomy or exogenous progesterone treatments in these studies interfered with maternal behavior because they prevented estrogen release
and the consequent rise in prolactin, both of which occur shortly
before term. Estrogen and prolactin, they suggest, act synergistically to stimulate or increase excitability of neural sites concerned
with maternal behavior. Furthermore, the effectiveness of estrogen
and prolactin in stimulating maternal behavior at parturition may
be increased by the "rebound from progesterone dominance" demonstrated electrophysiologically by Kawakami & Sawyer (1959). That
is, a sharp decline in progesterone concentration after a period
of progesterone dominance may increase neural sensitivity to estrogen and prolactin.

     If this hypothesis is correct, the failure of ovariectomy and
exogenous progesterone treatment to affect maternal behavior of
multiparous rats and 50 percent of primiparous rats in these studies is puzzling. Moltz & Wiener (1966) and Moltz (1971) proposed
that prior maternal experience of the multiparous rats may have
modified appropriate neural mediating systems to decrease their
threshhold for endocrine activation. In the case of inexperienced
animals, if there is variability in sensitivity to endocrine activation, those with lower threshholds (within the range of those of
multiparous rats) will not be adversely affected by the altered endocrine state. Presumably, animals with such low threshholds may
respond to circulating levels of estrogen still present after ovariectomy or progesterone treatment. This explanation is highly
speculative but could account for the failure of the hormonal treatments to affect multiparous and 50 percent of primiparous rats tested. It is true that experimentally altering hormonal balance may
produce considerable individual variability in response, particularly in male sexual behavior (see review by Davidson, 1972) and one
source of such variability may relate to prior experience. Rosenblatt & Aronson (1958) found that experienced male cats were sexually more responsive after castration than inexperienced castrates.
These results parallel those obtained by Moltz & Wiener for the effects of ovariectomy on maternal behavior of multiparous (experienced) and primiparous (inexperienced) rats. However, an ameliorating effect of experience on postcastration behavior has not been
found in all cases: studies in the rat (Block & Davidson, 1968)

and in the dog (Hart, 1968) failed to obtain differences between
experienced and inexperienced males in the rate of decline of sexual behavior after castration. Similarly, ovariectomy produces a
rapid and complete decline in sexual responsiveness in both experienced and inexperienced female rats (Davidson, 1972).

Another approach for studying the hormonal basis of maternal
behavior is to induce maternal behavior in virgin rats by stimulating the hormonal changes at the end of pregnancy. Moltz et al.
(1970) subjected ovariectomized virgin rats to the following series
of hormone injections: 12 mu of estrogen daily on days one to 11;
on days six to nine, 3 mg of progesterone twice daily and 50 IU of
prolactin on the evening of day nine and the morning of day 10.
On the afternoon of day 10, each animal was given six newborn pups
and observed for maternal behavior at periodic intervals. Control
groups were given two of the three hormones or vehicle only. Each
of ten females in the experimental group showed active maternal behavior 35 to 40 hours after introduction of pups. Control females
given only two of the three hormones showed marked variability in
latency to respond to pups: a moderate facilitation of maternal
responding was obtained in those given estrogen and progesterone
and, to a lesser extent, in those given estrogen and prolactin.
Most animals given vehicle only or progesterone and prolactin did
not show maternal behavior in seven days of testing. A summary of
these data is shown in Fig. 7.

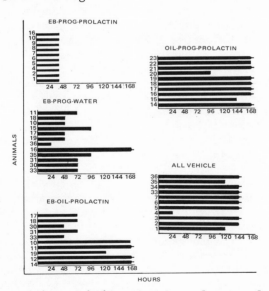

Fig. 7. Latency and variability in time of onset for the display of
maternal behavior in ovariectomized nulliparous rats after different
hormone and control treatments. See text for explanation. Broken
bar indicates that the animal had failed to act maternally at the conclusion of the observation period. (From Moltz et al., 1970)

Zarrow et al. (1971a) reported that a series of hormone injections designed to stimulate growth of the mammary gland and
lactation was also effective in inducing maternal behavior in castrated virgin rats. Two micrograms of estrogen and 4 mg of progesterone were given daily for 20 days, followed by 2 mg of cortisol acetate and 20 IU of prolactin daily. After four days of cortisol and prolactin treatment, the females were allowed to live
with pups and were tested each day. Of the 17 rats tested, 15 responded maternally within 24 hours after pups were offered, and
many retrieved within the first 15 minutes after initial exposure
to pups. Similar results were obtained if cortisol was not given.
Untreated control animals required four to five days of exposure
before maternal responses were observed.

These data lend additional support to the hypothesis that
estrogen and prolactin, acting after progesterone withdrawal, stimulate the onset of maternal behavior in the parturient animal.

Siegel (1974) attempted to replicate some of these findings
and to examine in detail the role of estrogen in stimulating maternal responsiveness. He confirmed the effectiveness of the hormone regimen used by Zarrow et al. (1971a), but obtained no reduction in latency with the treatment described by Moltz et al. (1970).
However, there was considerable variability in each group, and 10
of 25 animals showed spontaneous maternal behavior or cannibalized
pups. Siegel also found that a significant reduction in latency of
maternal behavior could be obtained with only 2.5 days of hormone
treatments. The most effective regimen was progesterone in decreasing dosages concurrent with estrogen in increasing dosages, followed by prolactin. Eight of ten animals tested showed maternal responses after three days of exposure to pups, whereas less than 40
percent of groups receiving only estrogen and prolactin or no hormones behaved maternally after five days of exposure. These results agree with the conclusion of Moltz (1971, 1974) that estrogen
and prolactin present after progesterone withdrawal effectively
stimulate maternal responsiveness.

In other experiments Siegel found that maternal behavior could
be stimulated by a single injection of a large amount of estrogen.
Immediately after ovaries and uterus were removed, virgin rats were
given 100 mu of estrogen and then offered pups 0.5, 24, or 48 hours
later. Most animals in each group showed maternal behavior after
only 24 to 48 hours of exposure to the pups. This facilitation was
not obtained if only 20 mu of estrogen was used or hysterectomies
were not performed. Siegel suggests that animals with the uterus
intact fail to respond to estrogen treatment because the uterus
competes with the brain in uptake of estrogen and thus reduces the
amount of hormone available for stimulating appropriate neural
structures. Klebanoff (1965) showed that uterine extracts from cy-

cling rats or from rats in early stages of pregnancy inactivate estrogen, whereas extracts from rats nearer term do not. This change in uterine function in late pregnancy could serve to make more estrogen available for stimulation of brain structures concerned with maternal behavior.

Maintenance of maternal behavior

For the first two to three weeks after birth, the dam exhibits a high degree of maternal responsiveness towards the pups. She provides them with warmth, maintains the maternal nest, licks, cleans, and nurses them. This is the "maintenance" period of maternal care. Later, beginning about the third week, as the sensory and motor capacities of the young develop rapidly and they become increasingly independent, there is a corresponding decline in maternal behavior. The synchrony between the behavioral development of the young and the maternal responses of the mother has been described by Rosenblatt (1970).

The effects of a brief separation from the pups on maternal responsiveness was examined by Rosenblatt & Lehrman (1963). When pups were removed at birth, less than 50 percent of the dams acted maternally three days later, and none were maternally responsive after four days. However, if a four day separation was imposed after the dams had been living with their pups for three or more days, most of the mothers were immediately responsive when tested five days after separation. Dams permanently separated from their pups at nine days postpartum and tested every other day showed a rapid decline in maternal behavior. These experiments clearly show that the maintenance of maternal behavior is strongly dependent upon the continued presence of the litter and that this dependence is greater at parturition than after several days of living with pups.

The normal decline in maternal behavior after two weeks of lactation can be prevented by replacing the growing pups with younger foster litters. Periodic replacement of the litter with young pups can greatly prolong the period of maternal care and lactation (Nicoll & Meites, 1959; Bruce, 1961).

Attempts to interfere with the maintenance of postpartum maternal behavior by altering hormonal balance have been singularly unsuccessful. Administration of 2 mg of progesterone daily for five days beginning 48 hours after birth (Moltz et al., 1969) or ovariectomy within 12 hours of parturition (Rosenblatt, 1970) had no detectable effect on maternal care. As described above, both of these treatments produced significant deficits in the initiation of maternal behavior when performed at term.

Interference with lactogenic hormones or oxytocin have also yielded negative results. Injections of ergocornine (an ergot derivative which inhibits prolactin release from the pituitary) beginning 12 hours postpartum (Numan et al., 1972), adrenalectomy (Thoman & Levine, 1970), and hypothalamic lesions that block the release of oxytocin (Yokoyama & Ota, 1959b) all failed to disturb maternal care, although these treatments significantly decrease or inhibit lactation. Obias (1957) found that the postpartum maternal behavior of females that were hypophysectomized on day 13 of pregnancy was similar to that of controls although the hypophysectomized dams did not lactate.

Perhaps the clearest evidence that neither mammary engorgement nor lactation is essential for the maintenance of maternal behavior in the postpartum rat is provided by a study of Moltz et al., (1967). All mammary glands, including nipples, were removed from 21 to 30 day old female rats. These animal were mated as adults, and after parturition they were tested with foster pups of increasing age for 20 days. The maternal behavior of these animals was comparable in all respects to that of sham-operated or normal controls. Interestingly, the presence of young inhibited the resumption of ovarian cycling in the mammectomized females. In the normal postpartum female, inhibition of ovarian cycling is assumed to result from the altered hormonal state during lactation (due particularly to increased levels of prolactin and inhibition of FSH release). In the postpartum mammectomized female, exteroceptive cues from the litter are apparently sufficient to inhibit ovarian cycling.

The available evidence indicates that continued responsiveness toward pups after parturition is relatively independent of hormonal stimulation. Apparently cohabitation with pups during this period is both a necessary and sufficient condition for the maintenance of maternal care. In this respect, the minimal conditions for the continued expression of maternal behavior in postpartum dams and in primed virgin females are identical.

Summary and comments

The studies reviewed above give us some indication of which hormones are involved in maternal behavior and how they may alter maternal responsiveness. In regard to the role of hormonal stimulation, the experiments on the induction of maternal behavior by cohabitation with pups are of fundamental importance because they demonstrate that almost all the appropriate maternal behaviors may be expressed by inexperienced male and female rats even in the absence of reproductive hormones. Clearly, activation of a neural substrate for maternal behavior does not require hormonal stimulation but, instead, depends primarily on stimuli provided by the young. Nevertheless, the experiments on pregnancy termination and effects of exogenous hormones indicate that endocrine changes during pregnancy and parturition significantly influence when maternal behavior will occur and, perhaps, the range and intensity of maternal care activities. These hormonal effects may be mediated partly by peripheral (somatic) changes during the course of pregnancy. Increase in body size, growth of mammary glands, and other changes all provide new afferent stimuli that may influence the behavior of the pregnant rat (Roth & Rosenblatt, 1967). Of course, the most obvious peripheral change resulting from pregnancy occurs at parturition. Termination of pregnancy and birth of the young represents a profound and sudden alteration in the state of the animal, and the appearance of pups at this time provides the adequate external stimuli for the expression of maternal care. Development of the mammary glands and lactogenesis is another hormonally dependent peripheral change, and the afferent stimuli provided during nursing may further enhance maternal responsiveness. However, the experimental elimination of self-licking during pregnancy (Christophersen & Wagman, 1965; Kirby & Horvath, 1968), parturitive experience (Moltz et al., 1966), and nursing (Moltz et al., 1967) have shown that behaviors associated with hormonally induced peripheral changes can be prevented without affecting either the initiation or maintenance of maternal behavior. Also, experiments on hormonal induction of maternal behavior in virgin male and female rats (Moltz et al., 1970; Zarrow et al., 1971a; Siegel, 1974) demonstrate that hormones may stimulate maternal behavior in the absence of the normal changes during pregnancy and parturition. Thus, while hormonally stimulated somatic changes and the afferent stimuli they provide may play a role in the development of maternal responsiveness, they are not essential for the hormonal stimulation of maternal behavior.

These results suggest that hormones stimulate maternal behavior by their action on the brain rather than by their peripheral effects. It is now well established that hormones may alter brain activity (see reviews by Vernikos-Danellis, 1972; Cross, 1973). Some reproductive hormones, notably progesterone and estrogen, are selectively concentrated in certain nuclei of the brain (Pfaff, 1968; Sar & Stumpf, 1973; review by McEwen & Pfaff, 1973). Although several investigators (such as Moltz, 1971; Fleming & Rosenblatt, 1974b) have postulated a neural substrate or center which is somehow responsible for the expression of maternal behavior and is sensitive to hormonal stimulation, little information is now available concerning the anatomical basis for such neuroendocrine effects. A recent study by Voci & Carlson (1973) indicates that hormones implanted in the brain may facilitate maternal care activities in mice. Brain implants of hormones have been used extensively in the study of sex behavior (Davidson, 1972), and these methods may also prove fruitful for studying the neuroendocrine basis of maternal behavior.

Estrogen and prolactin have been strongly implicated as the hormones that stimulate maternal behavior. Serum levels of both increase before parturition (Nagasawa & Yanai, 1972; Yoshinaga et al., 1969), and ovarian estrogen and estrogen-induced release of prolactin may be necessary for the facilitation of maternal behavior resulting from interruption of pregnancy near term (Moltz & Wiener, 1966; Rosenblatt, 1969). Also, when estrogen and prolactin are injected into virgin rats against a background of progesterone withdrawal (conditions that partly simulate the hormonal changes at the end of pregnancy), they significantly decrease the latency to maternal behavior (Moltz et al., 1970; Siegel, 1974). The two hormones may act synergistically to stimulate the neural substrate of maternal behavior. Estrogen enhances the effectiveness of progesterone by increasing its incorporation into target tissues, and similar synergistic mechanisms may be involved in estrogen and prolactin stimulation of appropriate brain areas. Evaluation of these two hormones separately and of their potential synergistic effects on maternal behavior should be possible in hypophysectomized rats or perhaps with the use of a prolactin inhibitor (Lu et al., 1971).

The role of progesterone is less clear. Because progesterone exerts an inhibitory effect on hypothalamic activity (Cross, 1973) and on the release of prolactin from the pituitary, the decline of progesterone near term is an important factor in determining the effectivenss of changes in estrogen and prolactin. Progesterone may simply play a permissive role, or, as suggested by Moltz et al., (1970), a "rebound" from progesterone dominance may act to decrease threshholds of appropriate neural structures to estrogen and prolactin. One test for the progesterone rebound hypothesis might be to determine if progesterone withdrawal would decrease the amount of estrogen and prolactin required to facilitate maternal behavior. Experiments by Siegel (1974) suggest this might be the case. A single large injection (100 mu) of estrogen facilitated the onset of maternal behavior in virgin rats but a smaller amount (20 ug) was ineffective. In another experiment, small daily doses of estrogen were effective when preceded by progesterone withdrawal. Because slightly different procedures were used in these experiments, the results are not conclusive. However they are consistent with the hypothesis that progesterone withdrawal may lower the threshhold for estrogen stimulation.

Are the changes in progesterone, estrogen and, prolactin at term and their presumed effects on the brain sufficient to account for the initiation of maternal behavior in the parturient rat? Although the "triad" hormone studies with virgin rats have demonstrated a significant decrease in latency to respond to pups, the induction of maternal behavior in these cases is only obtained after many hours of cohabitation with pups. Apparently, the immediate onset of maternal responsiveness, such as that observed after Caesarean section near term, has not been obtained by treatment with progesterone, estrogen, and prolactin. This failure, as Moltz et al., (1970) have suggested, may be because an optimal regimen of hormone treatment was not used, the dosages were too high or too low, or other hormones are involved in the stimulation of maternal behavior at parturition.

On the other hand, the delay of 24 to 48 hours before maternal behavior is observed in most of these studies may represent the time required for exogenous hormones to effectively stimulate the appropriate neural substrate; the presence of pups during this interval may be incidental to these physiological changes. In most studies, experimental animals were allowed to live with pups until maternal behavior occurred; because of this, it is unclear whether hormone treatments simply facilitated the induction of maternal behavior or produced endogenous changes in responsiveness independent of the presence of young. In one experiment by Siegel (1974), discussed above, pups were given to virgin rats -- either 0.5, 24, or 48 hours after combined ovariectomy-hysterectomy and injection of 100 mu of estrogen. Most animals showed maternal behavior only after 24 to 48 hours of exposure to pups, irrespective of the delay between treatment and presentation of pups. In this case, exposure to pups was apparently necessary to observe an effect of extrogen on maternal behavior. Certainly additional studies are needed to determine whether hormone treatments such as those used by Moltz et al., (1970) and Zarrow et al., (1971a) produce endogenous changes in maternal responsiveness (such as those which presummably occur as a function of pregnancy) or whether their effect is simply to facilitate induction of maternal behavior by cohabitation with pups.

SENSORY FACTORS CONTROLLING MATERNAL RESPONSIVENESS

Ultrasonic stimulation

A number of studies (reviewed by Noirot, 1972b), demonstrate that rat and mouse pups (as well as the young of other rodent species) emit ultrasonic cries or calls when isolated or handled roughly. In the rat, the call is very short in duration (about 90 ms) with a fundamental frequency of about 32 kHz. The frequency of the call lies close to the level of maximal auditory sensitivity of the adult rat (Gourevitch & Hack, 1966). The increase in calling during isolation is probably stimulated by a drop in body temperature of the nearly poikilothermic pup (Allin & Banks, 1971).

The function of these ultrasonics was investigated by Allin &

Banks (1972), who found that tape-recorded ultrasonics, projected
to a discrete portion of the cage, stimulated postpartum maternal
females (but not naive virgin controls) to leave their nest box and
search in the vicinity of the sound source. This finding and experiments cited by Noirot(1972b) indicate that cries by isolated
pups are effective stimuli for initiating retrieving behavior and
guide the female in locating a pup displaced from the nest. Also,
the cessation of retrieving by primiparous mice when the pups are
about 13 days old is correlated with a decline in the production
of ultrasonics by the pups at this age. (Noirot, 1972b)

Ultrasonic "distress" calls emitted when pups are roughly
handled by the dam tend to inhibit the mother's ongoing behavior.
Calls during retrieving may result in releasing the pup (or perhaps
grasping it more gently), and the call of pups in the nest may
inhibit pup licking or nest building. According to Noirot, when a
particular maternal activity is interrupted by ultrasonic cries,
another maternal activity usually takes its place. Thus, cries
during nest building may lead to pup licking or other pup-oriented
behaviors. Production of ultransonics may also be an important
factor in inhibiting the dam from stepping on or smothering pups
in the nest and may prevent pups from being bitten or otherwise
damaged during placentaphagia and cleaning of newborn at parturition.
Interestingly, a mutant strain of mouse ("fidgit") that is deaf and
cannot hear the cries of the young generally cannibalizes its litter at parturition (Noirot, 1972b).

Olfactory stimulation

The odor of pups appears to play an important role in maternal
responsiveness of rats and mice. When first exposed to pups, adult
virgin rats (Fleming, 1972) as well as pregnant rats (Slotnick et
al., 1973) hesitantly approach and invesigate them by sniffing
(rarely licking or manipulating them), and then withdraw and ignore
them.

Fleming (1972) and Fleming & Rosenblatt (1974a, 1974b) demonstrated that anosmia significantly facilitates the induction of
maternal behavior in virgin rats. After one-stage olfactory bulbectomy, 50 percent of virgin females tested became maternal in only
two to three days of exposure to pups (as compared to seven days
required by intact controls). However, the remaining bulbectomized
rats, but none of the controls, cannibalized their pups. Olfactory
bulbectomy increases some forms of aggressive behavior in rats
(Douglas et al., 1969; Karli et al., 1969), and Fleming & Rosenblatt showed that pup killing after bulbectomy was due to an increase in aggressiveness and not to anosmia per se. When the bulbs
were removed in two stages (one week between removals) or when "anos-

mia" was produced by intranasal syringing with zinc sulfate, cannibalism was eliminated and almost all experimental animals became maternal after only one to two days of testing. Alberts & Friedman (1972) have also shown that one-stage olfactory bulbectomy but not peripherally induced anosmia results in increased emotionality and muricidal behavior. Interference with olfaction by lesions of the lateral olfactory tract also reduced the latency to maternal behavior, although four of eleven animals with such lesions cannibalized pups in initial tests.

On the basis of their data and other studies on the nonhormonal basis for maternal behavior in the rat (Rosenblatt, 1967; Terkel & Rosenblatt, 1971) Fleming & Rosenblatt suggested that the prolonged exposure to pups does not "induce" maternal behavior in virgin rats but rather allows the animal to adapt to novel and presumably aversive stimuli provided by the pups. They assume that the neural substrate for maternal behavior is in a comparable state of activation or readiness in both virgin and parturient rats but that the former must first adapt to stimuli from the pup. Because pup odors are a significant part of this stimulus complex, rendering the animal anosmic results in a more rapid appearance of maternal behavior. The facilitation of maternal behavior produced by confining virgins and pups in small cages (Terkel & Rosenblatt, 1971) is interpreted along similar lines: in this situation the female cannot avoid the young, and the increased contact (including exposure to pup odors) more rapidly reduces fear and avoidance responses.

While this interpretation is generally consistent with their data, the experiments of Fleming & Rosenblatt were concerned with the effects of anosmia on maternal behavior and not specifically on the response of virgin rats to the odor of pups. Perhaps behavioral tests of preference (or aversion) to pup odors would provide additional information on the role of olfaction in the induction of maternal behavior. At present, it is not clear what adaptive value an initial fear or avoidance of pup odors would serve. Newly parturient rats or those delivered by Caesarean section at term and tested with cleaned pups do not display fear or avoidance of young, and one-stage bilateral bulbectomy has little or no effect on the postpartum expression of maternal behavior in the rat (Fleming & Rosenblatt, 1974a; Slotnick, 1969). Fleming & Rosenblatt (1974b) suggest hormonal changes during pregnancy may have a "calming" effect which overrides the female's potential fearfulness of the newborn pups; or the female may gain familiarity with odors from the genital region during pregnancy, which may reduce the novelty of similar odors from the pups at parturition. This latter suggestion, however, is unlikely because no deficits were found in postpartum maternal behavior in rats prevented from licking the genital region during pregnancy (Kirby & Horvath, 1968; Christophersen & Wagman, 1965). Furthermore, experiments by Charton et al.

(1971) indicate that adult rats may show a preference for the odor
of pups and that pup odors (particularly from the perineal regions)
may facilitate maternal activities of postpartum rats. Additional
evidence concerning the response of adult rats to the odors of pups
will be required to fully evaluate the mechanism by which anosmia
facilitates the onset of maternal behavior in the rat.

The effect of pup odors and of bilateral bulbectomy on maternal
behavior have also been investigated in the mouse. Although these
experiments are not directly comparable to those of Fleming & Rosenblatt, the results are, in several respects, contrary to those for
the rat. Noirot (1970) found that housing virgin female mice next
to cages with young or giving them a 5-minute exposure to young
presented in a perforated box strongly facilitated subsequent nest
building and retrieving. Such exposure to young provides both
auditory (distress call) and olfactory cues. By comparing the effects of exposing virgin mice to either a perforated box containing
a nest which had housed pups (mainly olfactory stimuli) or to a
nonperforated box containing young (mainly auditory stimuli),
Noirot partly separated the effects of olfactory and auditory priming. As compared to controls exposed only to an empty box, females
exposed to nest odors showed more intensive pup-oriented activities
in a later test, while females exposed to ultrasonic cries of pups
showed more nest building.

Other studies also point to a critical role for olfaction in
the expression of mouse maternal behavior. Gandleman and coworkers
demonstrated that olfactory bulbectomy results in a dramatic and
virtually complete elimination of nest building and maternal behavior (Gandleman et al., 1971, 1972; Gandleman, 1973; Zarrow et
al., 1971b). After removal of the olfactory bulbs, both multiparous
and primiparous mice failed to build nests and either cannibalized
their litters after parturition (the majority of cases) or ignored
the pups. Similar results were obtained with bulbectomized virgin
mice; in only a few cases, in which autopsy revealed an incomplete
bulbectomy, did experimental mice show maternal responses.

The factors underlying these bulbectomy-induced deficits in
maternal behavior have not been elucidated and, unfortunately, the
behavior of experimental animals was not described in detail. The
disruption of maternal behavior was probably not due to a hormonal
imbalance produced by bulbectomy: similar effects were obtained
in virgin and postpartum mice, and pregnant experimental and control mice did not differ in regard to duration of pregnancy or
mammary development (Gandleman et al., 1971). The deficits in
nest building also appear to be quite general. Exposure to cold
(7°C) did not stimulate bulbectomized mice to build nests, and ex-
ogeneous progesterone had only a small effect in stimulating col-
lection of nesting material (Zarrow et al., 1971b).

The absence of maternal behavior and the presence of cannibalism were probably not secondary to an increase in aggressiveness in bulbectomized mice. In contrast to findings with rats (as reported above) Zarrow, et al., (1971b) reported that bulbectomized mice were no more irritable than controls when handled. Ropartz (1968) and Slotnick & McMullen (unpublished observations) found that bulbectomy reduces or eliminates intraspecific aggression in male mice. Perhaps olfactory cues (together with distress cries) play a critical role in inhibiting attack on the young and cannibalism in virgin animals or cannibalism after placentophagia in the postpartum mouse. However, this hypothesis would not bear on the absence of nest building in bulbectomized mice. At present, no single explanation for these dramatic effects of olfactory bulbectomy is available. There is evidence that mouse sexual (Rowe & Edwards, 1972) and aggressive (Ropartz, 1968, Rowe & Edwards, 1971) behavior may be highly or totally dependent upon olfaction.

The contrasting effects of olfactory bulbectomy and evidence for the role of olfaction in maternal behavior of rats and mice may now be summarized. The studies of Fleming & Rosenblatt (1974a, 1974b) indicate that elimination of olfactory cues facilitates the onset of maternal behavior in the rat. In the mouse, however, olfactory stimulation increases maternal behavior and bulbectomy eliminates it. By interfering with olfaction at the receptor level or by lesions of the lateral olfactory tract, Fleming & Rosenblatt showed that the bulbectomy-induced facilitation of rat maternal behavior was due to interference with olfaction and not to a nonspecific "nonolfactory" function of the bulbs. Although a similar analysis has not been made for the mouse, the available evidence strongly suggests that rats and mice differ in regard to the role of olfaction in maternal behavior. Other differences between rats and mice in neural control of maternal behavior have been demonstrated and are discussed below.

Evidence for a maternal pheromone

In addition to a role for odor of pups on the initiation of maternal behavior, odors from the female attract pups and may have an important role in the maintenance of mother-young interactions. Leon & Moltz (1971, 1972) tested preference of pups for the odor of the mother over that of nulliparous females in an olfactory apparatus consisting of a start box and small open area connected to two goal boxes that contained the stimulus females or their bedding. Odors from the goal boxes were carried by an air stream across the open area to the start box. A test consisted of placing a pup in the start box and allowing it to crawl to one of the goal boxes. When pups at different ages were tested, a strong preference for the odor of the mother was seen at 14 to 21 days (Fig. 6).

This preference was not shown by pups one and ten days old but began to emerge at 12 days and rapidly declined by 27 days of age, when the young become completely independent of the mother.

The odor preference on the part of the pups was not specific to the mother, but was exhibited to other lactating females. Moreover, a striking synchrony was found between the age at which the preference emerged and the number of days the female was lactating: 16-day-old pups were most strongly attracted to females that had been lactating for 16 to 21 days. Pups exhibited no preference between females that had been lactating 16 and 21 days but preferred the former to those of other lactational ages or to virgin rats. Thus it appears that the time at which the female emits this (as yet undefined) odor corresponds closely to the age at which the pups are maximally attracted to the odor.

Leon & Moltz (1971) have suggested that the odor from the lactating female to which the pups are attracted may be considered a pheromone, that is, an odor that is released into the environment by one individual (sender) and produces a specific reaction in another individual (receiver) of the same species (Butler, 1970). As yet, the source of the odor is unknown, and additional information concerning the nature of the chemical cue and a more detailed analysis of how it affects the behavior of the pups would be highly desirable.

Although these experiments by Leon and coworkers were limited to testing of pups in a maze for preference behavior with odors of different females, their results suggest a functional role for the development of an odor bond (Leon & Moltz, 1972; Moltz et al., 1974). The age at which the odor bond is first seen in the pup (12 to 14 days) corresponds to a time when the young, having developed considerable motor and sensory capacities, begin to leave the nest and explore the surrounding environment. The dam also begins to show a decline in pup retrieving at this lactational age. However, the young continue to nurse until about 27 days of age; during this initial stage of independence, the odor bond may serve to reunite the mother and young for periodic maternal care.

Conditioned release of oxytocin and prolactin

The possiblity that sensory factors other than suckling may influence the release of oxytocin was suggested by early reports of dairy farmers that milk letdown occurs in cows in response to preparations for milking (Ely & Peterson, 1941). Recent studies have experimentally demonstrated that stimuli associated with milking or nursing may cause release of oxytocin. For example, Peeters et al. (1960) recorded an increase in intramammary pres-

sure in the lactating cow when the calf was shown to the mother;
and Cleverley (1968) found that when cows were accustomed to a
strict milking routine, entrance of the milker alone caused an increase in plasma oxytocin. Release of oxytocin in lactating goats
was demonstrated after presentation of the kid (McNeilly, unpublished results cited by Cowie & Tindal, 1971, p. 209), and in
studies summarized by Caldeyro-Barcia (1969), mammary pressure in
lactating women was shown to increase in response to the cries
or presentation of their babies.

Although it has been suggested that this release of oxytocin
is a result of conditioning (for instance, Cowie & Tindal, 1971),
only an early Russian study by Grachev (cited by Lehrman, 1961,
p. 1343) appears to have demonstrated acquisition of a conditioned milk ejection response. Using a lactating goat, Grachev found
that after 18 pairings of a ringing bell and hand milking, sound
of the bell alone caused an ejection of milk from a catheterized
mammary gland.

"Conditioned" release of oxytocin in the rat has been studied
by Deis (1968). On alternate days, lactating rats were separated
from their litters for nine hours, then caged next to an actively
nursing rat for 30 minutes before being allowed to nurse their
pups. This prior exposure to the nursing animal resulted in increased release of milk (determined by weight gain of the litter)
as compared to nonexposed controls. Rats made deaf by injections
of alcohol into the middle ear did not show this effect. Deis
concluded that auditory stimuli during the exposure period mediated
a conditioned release of oxytocin, which increased the amount of
milk available to the suckling young.

In carefully controlled studies, Grosvenor and associates
(Grosvenor, 1965; Grosvenor et al., 1965; Grosvenor et al., 1970)
demonstrated that stimuli other than suckling may cause the release
of pituitary prolactin. Rats that had been lactating for 7 to 14
days were separated from their pups for 7 to 10 hours (a time sufficient for accumulation of pituitary prolactin) and were then allowed to nurse their litter or were exposed to their pups but not
allowed to make contact with them. The exposure consisted of sus-
pending pups in a basket under the wire mesh cage floor. After
30 minutes of nursing or exposure, the mothers were killed and the
concentration of pituitary prolactin was determined by the pigeon
crop assay of Nicoll (1967). As expected, suckling stimulation resulted in a significant drop in pituitary prolactin. Exposure to
pups produced an equivalent decrease in primiparous rats lactating
for 14 days but not in those lactating for only 7 days. However,
exposure was effective in multiparous rats lactating for seven
days.

These results indicate that suckling stimuli normally cause a release of prolactin but that this release becomes conditioned to other stimuli from the pups somewhere between days seven and fourteen of laction. Since multiparous rats show the exposure effect on day seven (the earliest postpartum day tested), it appears that the effects of prior nursing experience are retained through a second pregnancy.

The stimuli involved in mediating this exposure-induced release of prolactin were examined by Mena & Grosvenor (1971). A significant reduction in pituitary prolactin still occurred when auditory and visual stimuli from the pups were removed, but there was no reduction if odor cues from the pups were blocked. In a second experiment, lactating animals were tested after being made deaf and anosmic, blind and anosomic, or blind and deaf. Surgical procedures were performed on days 14 to 16 of pregnancy, and animals were tested on postpartum day 14. Only the anosmic-blind group failed to show a significant reduction in pituitary prolactin when exposed to pups. In addtion, the anosmic-deaf and the deaf-blind rats exhibited strong interest toward the inaccessible pups, but the anosomic-blind rats took little notice of them, and, 18 of the 30 anosmic-deaf and anosmic-blind rats cannibablized their litters in the first 13 days after parturition.

These results clearly implicate pup odors in maternal care and in the exposure-induced release of prolactin. Because blocking odor cues from the pups was sufficient to eliminate prolactin release in the intact animal but release occurred in anosmic-deaf animals, Mena & Grosvenor suggest that visual cues may become important for this response in the anosmic animal. Auditory stimuli were ineffective in both experiments. However, it was not reported whether pups vocalized during these tests or how effectively auditory cues were eliminated.

BRAIN MECHANISMS AND MATERNAL BEHAVIOR

The cerebral cortex

The earliest systematic study of brain mechanisms in maternal behavior (Beach, 1937) was addressed to the basic question of whether an innately determined activity was dependent upon the cerebral cortex. Theories then current suggested that learned behaviors were mediated by the cortex but that unlearned ("native") behaviors were dependent only on more primitive or subcortical parts of the brain. In Beach's study, cortical lesions varying in size and location were made in virgin rats; after recovery from surgery the animals were mated and tested for maternal behavior after parturition.

On the first four days after delivery, nest building, retrieving of pups, and reactions to air and heat blasts directed at the nest site were assessed. Animals with small lesions involving less than 20 percent of the cortex showed few deficits, but animals with larger lesions had deficits in nesting, retrieving, and care of the young. No one cortical region appeared to be critical, and the extent of maternal deficits was closely related to the amount of cortex removed and not to the locus of the lesions. Rats with greater than 40 percent destruction of the cortex were severely impaired and in many cases failed to build a nest, did not clean pups during parturition, and showed little or no postpartum responsiveness toward pups. These animals occasionally carried their pups in an aimless manner, they did not nurse them or show any well-coordinated pattern of maternal care. Beach suggested that the deficits did not result from motor or sensory disorders (although these may have been present) but rather from a loss of an integrative activity normally provided by the cortex. Lesions produced in infancy were not as detrimental for maternal behavior as lesions of equal size made in adulthood (Beach, 1938). Studies of Stone (1938) and Davis (1939) on the effects of cortical lesions on maternal behavior were in agreement with Beach's findings.

The limbic system

No further analysis of brain mechanisms in maternal behavior appeared until 1955 with the publication of a study by Stamm on the medial cerebral cortex. During the intervening years, the concept of how the nervous system functions in regard to species-typical behaviors had changed considerably. Experiments of Kluver & Bucy (1939), Rosvold et al. (1954), and others had indicated that a group of cortical and subcortical structures known as the limbic system (MacLean, 1952) probably played an important role in species-typical behavior. The report by Stamm (1955) was the first to implicate part of this system, the cingulate cortex, in the control of maternal behavior.

Maternally experienced rats were subjected to lesions of the medial cerebral cortex (which included the cingulate cortex) or to more laterally placed neocortical lesions; after parturition maternal behavior was assessed with tests similar to those used by Beach (1937). Although the medial lesions involved only about 16 percent of the cortical mantle, animals in this group showed severe impairment of nest building and retrieving and did not nurse their litters. When subjected to blasts of heat or air, these rats ran aimlessly about the cage, picking up and dropping pups but not gathering them together in a protected corner. Eighty percent of their pups died within 48 hours of parturition.

Despite these deficits, parturitional behavior was apparently normal, and maternal behavior improved when dead young were replaced with healthy older pups. Rats with lateral lesions of equivalent size showed few or no maternal deficits, in agreement with Beach's finding that more than 20 percent of the neocortex had to be removed before significant deficits occurred. However, Stamm's study indicated that a specific cortical region (the cingulate cortex) may be critical for the normal expression of maternal care. A report by Wilsoncroft (1963) indicated that the anterior but not the posterior portion of the cingulate cortex was essential for normal maternal behavior.

A more detailed study of the cingulate cortex and maternal behavior was conducted later by Slotnick (1967b). Maternally experienced rats were subjected to partial or complete lesions of the cingulate cortex, mated, and tested for maternal behavior, which was assessed by detailed observations during retrieving tests. In general, the results reported by Stamm were confirmed: animals with cingulate lesions did not construct maternal nests and pup retrieving behavior was erratic and confused. Pups would be carried into the nest and then out of the nest again and deposited randomly about the cage. Although animals often retrieved material and piled it together, they would frequently scatter it again over the cage floor; a nest was seldom constructed. Most animals with cingulate lesions kept their litters alive during the 5-day postpartum test period, but weight gain of pups was only about half that of controls. As in Stamm's study, maternal behavior of experimental animals improved with time. However, this improvement did not require stimulation by more vigorous foster pups, but apparently resulted from continued exposure to the same pups or to the test procedures, or both. Histological analysis revealed that most lesions were almost entirely confined to the interhemispheric (cingulate) cortex and probably involved less than 10 percent of the cerebrum. As shown in Table III, the extent of maternal deficits was significantly related to the severity of retrograde degeneration of the thalamic nuclei that project to this limbic cortical region. In contrast to Wilsoncroft's (1963) findings, the greatest deficits were obtained when the entire cingulate cortex was destroyed; lesions limited to either the anterior or posterior portions resulted in less severe maternal impairments.

Experiments on mice with cingulate cortical lesions have not fully confirmed the effects found in rats. Carlson & Thomas (1968) found that cingulate cortical lesions in hybrid mice resulted in only a moderate deficit in retrieving behavior, no greater than that shown by animals with neocortical lesions of similar size. Slotnick & Nigrosh (1974) also found that albino mice with cingulate cortical lesions retrieved pups more slowly than controls but had no

Table III. Mean ratings of degeneration in each of the anterior thalamic nuclei, mean 5-day gain in weight of litters, and mean score for all retrieving tests on postpartum days 1-4 for animals with partial cingulate (PC) and full cingulate (FC) lesions.

Rat No.	AM Right	AM Left	AV Right	AV Left	AD Right	AD Left	Average Degeneration	5-Day Gain in Litter Weight	Average Retrieving Score Postpartum Test Days
Group PC. Animals with lesions limited to the anterior cingulate cortex.									
20	2.7	4.0					3.3*	3.05**	363***
22	3.2	1.0					2.1	5.12	124
53	3.6	2.4					3.0	4.79	209
61	3.5	3.3					3.4	4.18	341
Group PC. Animals with lesions limited to the posterior cingulate cortex.									
15			4.0	4.0	3.0	3.8	3.7	3.70	133
29			4.0	3.6	3.0	2.4	3.2	3.25	312
46			3.6	4.0	2.8	2.8	3.3	3.30	183
Group FC. Animals with full cingulate lesions.									
1	3.2	3.2	3.6	2.4	3.0	2.0	2.9	2.85	480
6	2.7	2.0	2.0	1.1	1.0	0.0	1.5	4.61	461
14	3.1	3.7	2.8	2.5	1.8	1.6	2.6	4.00	376
18	4.0	4.0	4.0	4.0	3.0	3.2	3.7	-1.00	1200
25	3.6	3.2	4.0	4.0	3.2	3.6	3.5	0.00	619
32	3.5	2.7	2.9	4.0	1.6	3.5	3.0	2.45	622
42	4.0	3.2	3.8	3.2	2.0	2.5	3.1	1.92	825
B9	2.5	3.5	3.1	4.0	1.5	3.5	3.0	3.01	274
B24	4.0	3.8	4.0	4.0	4.0	4.0	3.9	2.06	914

* Average degeneration is based only on the anterior nuclei that were affected by the lesion.

** Pup weight in grams.

*** Retrieving time in seconds.

(From Slotnick, 1967b)

deficits in nesting or other aspects of maternal care. Although
the amount of damage to the cingulate cortex (as determined by the
extent of retrograde degeneration in the anterior thalamic nuclei)
was significantly correlated with retrieving deficits, even mice
with nearly complete lesions did not differ greatly from controls.

These results indicate that rats and mice differ in regard to
limbic cortical control of maternal responsiveness. Unfortunately,
the effect of cingulate cortical lesions on maternal behavior has
not been examined in other species.

Additional studies have implicated subcortical components of
the limbic system in maternal behavior. Kimble, et al. (1967) found
that primiparous rats with large dorsal hippocampal lesions tended
to cannibalize their pups, spent little time nursing surviving pups,
did not build maternal nests, and were generally unresponsive to
pups. The lesions, produced by aspiration, necessitated removal of
the overlying neocortex. To evaluate this damage, other rats with
large neocortical lesions were studied as controls. Surprisingly,
these rats showed no maternal deficits even though 40 to 50 percent
of the neocortex was destroyed. These results stand in sharp contrast to the severe deficits in maternal behavior reported by
Beach (1937, 1938), Stone (1938), and Davis (1939) after cortical
lesions of similar size. Kimble et al. (1967) suggested that in
these earlier studies, the deficits in maternal behavior resulted
not from cortical damage but rather from inadvertent damage to the
underlying hippocampus. Beach did report that lesions in about
half of his animals extended into the dorsal convexity of the hippocampus, but he described this hippocampal damage as "always super-
ficial and rarely affect[ing] both sides of the brain" (Beach,
1937). He did not compare the behavior of rats with and without
hippocampal damage. If the suggestions of Kimble et al. are correct, it will be necessary to re-evaluate the role of the neocortex
in expression of maternal behavior.

However, the failure to find an effect of cortical lesions
may be partly related to the testing procedures used by Kimble et
al. In their study, animals were not disturbed for testing until
six days after delivery whereas Beach's daily tests of maternal behavior started the first postpartum day (Beach, 1937). Tests that
disburb the dam and litter may reveal lesion effects that may otherwise not be apparent (Slotnick, 1963). Also, the efficiency of
maternal behavior tends to improve during the first few postpartum
days in normal as well as brain-damaged rats (Stamm, 1955; Slotnick,
1967b). Thus, the test procedures used by Kimble et al. may not
have been sensitive enough to detect certain lesion effects. The
degree to which brain-damaged animals are able to care for their
litters when left undisturbed is also an important question and has
been largely ignored in most lesion studies. Perhaps some of the

differences in behavior between rats with cortical lesions studied
by Beach and by Kimble et al. may reflect an inability of the brain-
damaged animals to respond appropriately to disturbances of the nest
and young during the initial postpartum period.

The effects of other limbic lesions on maternal behavior were
evaluated in an extensive study (Slotnick, 1969, in preparation).
In separate groups of virgin rats the olfactory bulbs were removed
or lesions were produced in the septum, amygdala, mammillary bodies,
or interpeduncular nucleus. Normal animals and those with sham
lesions served as controls. Tests of nesting, retrieving, and pup
care during the first three to four postpartum days revealed that
some lesions selectively interfered with maternal care whereas
others were without effect. Extensive damage or removal of the
olfactory bulbs and large lesions of the amygdala resulted in little or no disturbance of maternal behavior. Lesions of the interpeduncular nucleus resulted in a transitory deficit in retrieving
behavior; performance was confused on the first retrieving test
but indistinguishable from that of controls thereafter.

Most animals with mammillary body lesions showed no deficits
in retrieving, but nursing and nesting behaviors were disturbed.
Each animal in this group either failed to adopt the nursing position over retrieved pups or did so only briefly and did not nurse
the litter (see sequential analysis in Fig. 8). These rats licked
retrieved pups and kept them piled together in one corner of the
nest, but they generally rested in another part and pushed away
pups that crawled toward them. These animals did not construct a
typical maternal nest but simply gathered paper strips into a compact flat pile.

Rats with septal lesions showed the most severe deficits in
maternal behavior (see Fig. 8). These rats showed normal parturitional activities but did not clean all of their pups. None of the
animals built a nest or even gathered all of the paper strips together. They frequently carried pups about the cage, sometimes
bringing them into the nest site (defined as the corner of the cage
where some paper strips were gathered and where the dam usually
rested) and then carried them out again. Bouts of such "retrieving"
activity lasted many minutes and were greatly augmented whenever
the animal was disturbed for testing. Few of these rats nursed
their young or even adopted a nursing position over them, and none
of the pups survived longer than 48 hours. In contrast to rats with
cingulate cortical lesions (reported above) the animals were unable
to maintain alive healthy foster pups and showed little or no improvement in behavior over repeated tests.

Fig. 8. (Opposite page). Sequential analysis
of maternal behavior during a pup retrieval
test on postpartum day 1 for two rats with
septal lesions (panels A and B) and one rat
with destruction of the mammillary bodies
(panel C). Maternal behavior was recorded
by an observer using a panel of switches
connected to a multiple-pen event recorder.
Compare with the sequential analysis of
normal maternal behavior presented in Fig.
1. See text for explanation.

Fleischer (1973) confirmed these findings for rats with
septal lesions. Even relatively small lesions well within the
septal area resulted in a similar pattern of disorganized pup
care and failure to construct a nest. Fleischer also found
that virgin rats with septal lesions could be induced to show
maternal responses after four to six days of cohibitation with
pups. However, like their primiparous counterparts the virgin
rats did not construct nests and repeatedly manipulated and
carried pups about the cage.

Both Slotnick (1969) and Fleischer (1973) found that septal
lesions in virgin female rats resulted in a syndrome of hyperemotionality similar to that reported for male rats with septal
lesions (Brady & Nauta, 1953). This hyperemotionality generally
decreased in the first week after surgery and had completely disappeared by the postpartum tests (about 35 to 45 days after surgery). This immediate consequence of septal lesions may account
for the observation that normal maternally responsive rats given
septal lesions two or three days after parturition showed no maternal interest when replaced with their pups but instead attacked
and killed them (Fleischer, 1973).

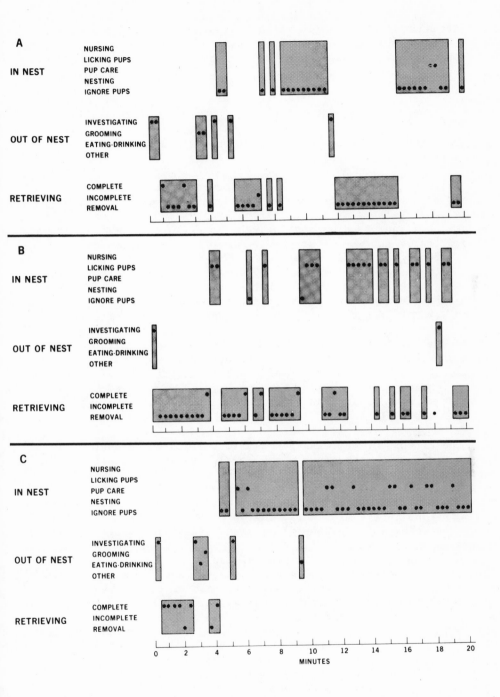

Hypothalamic lesions

Although the effects of various hypothalamic lesions on reproductive endocrinology have been examined in many studies, few
have specifically dealt with maternal behavior. The hypophysotro-
pic portion of the hypothalamus is directly concerned with regulation of reproductive hormones, and a systematic study might provide information concerning the hypothalamic sites at which hormones
act to affect maternal responsiveness. While it is generally assumed that the neural substrate for the initiation of maternal behavior in the parturient animal involves the hypothalamus, unequivocal evidence is not available.

Halloway & Stevenson (1967) investigated the effects of a
variety of medial hypothalamic lesions on the course of pregnancy
in the rat. Relatively small lesions were placed in the posterior
preoptic area and the supraoptic, ventromedial, dorsomedial, arcuate,
premammillary, and mammillary nuclei in different groups of rats on
day 10 of pregnancy. As compared to pair-fed controls, animals
with lesions showed little or no abnormality in duration of pregnancy or number of pups born. (Pair-fed controls were used because some lesions resulted in an altered weight gain during the
latter half of gestation.) Litter weights of animals with lesions
of the supraoptic, arcuate, or premammillary nuclei were significantly smaller than control. Although animals were killed within
two hours after the birth of the last pup, Halloway and Stevenson
noted that rats with ventromedial hypothalamic lesions were vicious,
did not build nests, and ate the pups as they were born. Animals
in the remaining groups had built nests and apparently showed normal
parturient behavior.

The effects of medial hypothalamic lesions on lactation have
been described by Yokoyama & Ota (1959a). Relatively small lesions
were made seven days after delivery, and litter weight was used
to assess lactational performance. Lesions in the vicinity of the
supraoptic nuclei, unilateral lesions of the arcuate nucleus, or
small lesions in the midtuberal region of the hypothalamus did not
block lactation or (apparently) maternal behavior. Lesions that
destroyed the paraventricular nuclei or the paraventricular hypophyseal tract interfered with the release of milk during nursing.
Some of these animals became savage, cannibalized pups, or showed
no maternal interest in them. However, five of the ten animals in
this subgroup recovered after a few days and again were maternal
but could not nurse their young. Lesions located more posteriorly
and involving the dorsomedial and ventromedial hypothalamic nuclei
also interfered with lactation but apparently did not affect other
aspects of maternal behavior. Because the mammary glands of all
of these animals were well developed and milk could be expressed
by palpation, the lesions probably interfered with lactation by

blocking oxytocin release (either by destruction of the paraventricular nuclei or tract or by severing afferent input to the nucleus) rather than by suppressing the release of galactopoietic hormones. In a second study, Yokoyama & Ota (1959b) demonstrated that after similar hypothalamic lesions, pups were able to obtain milk if exogenous oxytocin was given to the dam.

These studies indicate that destruction of pathways involved with the release of oxytocin may be without effect on the maintenance of maternal responsiveness. Herrenkohl & Rosenberg (1974) clearly demonstrated the independence of these two factors. When the medial basal portion of the hypothalamus was deafferented during the latter half of pregnancy by use of the Halasz knife (Halasz & Pupp, 1965), the young of experimental animals gradually lost weight and died. However, in behavioral tests with foster pups, the experimental animals did not differ from controls in retrieving or in the amount of time spent in a nursing position over the pups. Moreover, when the experimental animals were given exogenous oxytocin, the pups obtained milk. A selective impairment in oxytocin release by partial isolation of the medial basal hypothalamus has also been reported by Yokoyama et al. (1967).

The effects of medial hypothalamic lesions was also studied by Kurcz (1965). Although Kurcz provided little information concerning maternal behavior, the results are in general accord with the studies of Yokohoma & Ota (1959b) and Herrenkohl & Rosenberg (1974), which indicate that medial hypothalamic lesions may selectively impair lactational performance but not maternal behavior. No histological analysis was given, but the lesions apparently involved the ventromedial hypothalamic nuclei. Rats given lesions several months before mating became strongly hyperphagic and only 14 of 44 became pregnant. These obese animals had a long (up to 48 hours) and difficult delivery, and many of the pups were born dead. When tested several hours later with normal pups, Kurcz reported that their maternal behavior was normal. However, the pups were not able to obtain sufficient milk from these mothers and most died after three to five days. Animals given lesions during pregnancy did not become markedly obese and apparently delivered live litters. These rats were also reported to show good maternal behavior, but their pups and additional foster pups died of starvation.

In contrast to medial hypothalamic lesions which have minimal effects, discrete lesions of the midlateral hypothalamus causes a profound disruption of maternal behavior in the postpartum rat (Avar & Monos, 1964, 1966, 1967, 1969a, 1969b). Lesions were produced on day 16 or 17 or pregnancy and were located either just lateral or ventrolateral to the fornix at the level of the ventro-

medial nuclei (Avar & Monos, 1966). Rats with lesions were hypo-
phagic and hypodipsic for the remainder of pregnancy, gave birth
to significantly more dead young (29 percent) than did controls
(8 percent), and tended to cannibalize pups, nearly all of which
died within three days of parturition. Newborn foster pups offered
to operated animals also died within two to three days, and the
death rate was similar to that of healthy pups isolated from maternal care. When pups were isolated from maternal care, those born
to operated animals died at a faster rate than did those from normal
dams, and normal postpartum rats showed little or no maternal interest in pups from experimental animals. Apparently, pups from
experimental rats were less viable than those of controls and did
not provide adequate stimuli for maternal care. This effect on
viability was probably due to inadequate parturitional activities
of the experimental rats; experimental rats licked the young and
ate the placenta at parturition but also "nibbled" the pups as
well. Also, even before parturition, operated animals did not build
maternal nests and after parturition they ". . . did not collect
the young into nests but left them scattered about on the floor of
the cage and instead of avoiding them, they trod them down. When
the young were placed into the upper compartment they did not fetch
them and showed no interest in them when they had been returned to
the lower compartment" (Avar & Monos, 1967).

Because experimental and control animals did not differ in regard to duration of pregnancy, number of pups born, development of
the mammary glands, or later ovarian cycling, Avar & Monos (1967,
1969a) suggested that the lesions specifically interfered with
maternal responsiveness rather than with neuroendocrine mechanisms
of pregnancy or lactation. The transient decrease of food and water
intake may have contributed to these behavioral effects; however a
pair-fed control group showed normal maternal behavior except four
of sixteen rats which cannibalized their pups.

The results of these studies are difficult to evaluate because
there is little information concerning the nature of the lesions
and only brief descriptions of maternal behavior. Lateral hypothalamic lesions involving the medial forebrain bundle produce severe
deficits in a wide variety of motivated behaviors (Epstein, 1971;
Hitt et al., 1970) as well as sensory "neglect" (Marshall et al.,
1971). Additional studies will be required to determine if the deficits described by Avar and Monos are specific to maternal responsiveness or are a result of a more general loss in motivated behaviors
usually associated with damage to the lateral hypothalamus.

Summary and Comments

In comparison to the endocrinological factors in maternal behavior, the neural basis of such behavior has received relatively
little systematic study. Nonetheless, it is evident that destruction of specific parts of the brain may result in quite severe deficits in maternal care. The once widely accepted conclusions of
Beach (1937) that neocortical lesions result in maternal deficits
and that the extent of such deficits depends upon the amount of
cortex removed has been challenged recently by Kimble et al. (1967).
Whether the failure of Kimble et al. to replicate Beach's findings
is due to differences in lesion size or test procedures has not
been determined.

Lesions confined to the limbic system, particuarly the cingulate
cortex, hippocampus, septal area and the related mammillary nuclei
of the hypothalamus cause severe disturbances in maternal behavior of
rats (Stamm, 1955; Kimble et al., 1967; Slotnick, 1967b, 1969). A
variety of factors might be postulated to account for these maternal
deficits. For example, such brain lesions might interrrupt endocrine balance or neuroendocrine mechanisms underlying maternal behavior, or interfere with motor or sensory processes necessary for
the normal expression of maternal care. Another possibility is
that a "motivational center" might exist in the brain, destruction
of which would result in an absence of maternal behavior.

Because hormones have their primary behavioral effect on the
initiation of maternal behavior (see section on Hormonal induction
of maternal behavior) interference with hormonal balance by brain
lesions might be expected to affect the initiation of maternal behavior at parturition. Any severe disturbance of endocrine or
neuroendocrine regulation by brain lesions would also be reflected
in reproductive capacity. However, several lines of evidence suggest that the behavioral deficits produced by limbic lesions do
not stem from an interference with endocrine factors. No differences between normal and limbic damaged animals have been reported
in parturitional activities, "interest" in pups immediately following parturition, nor in length of gestation, litter size or weight
of the litter at birth. Although maternal care in these studies
was generally inadequate to insure survival of the young, in almost all cases the dams appeared to be motivated to express maternal behavior and responded quickly to young during retrieving tests.
Poor retrieving performance and inadequate care of the litter were
frequently related to excess carrying of pups about the cage, extended periods spent in caring for one or two isolated pups and
an apparent inability to maintain a nest and gather the young together. As none of the groups with limbic lesions described by
Stamm (1955), Kimble et al. (1967), Slotnick (1967b, 1969), or
Fleischer (1973) appeared disinterested in the pups, it is unlike-

ly that these lesions disrupted a "motivational center" for Maternal behavior.

Additional studies have, in fact, provided strong evidence
that these maternal deficits did not stem from an interruption of
neuroendocrine reflexes or hormonal balance. Maternally responsive
male rats given cingulate cortical lesions showed the same aberrant
pattern of retrieving as experimental postpartum females (Slotnick,
1967b) and virgin females with septal lesions became maternal as
quickly as controls when exposed to pups but showed the same disruption of maternal responding as did their postpartum counterparts
(Fleischer, 1973).

These results indicate that brain lesions may affect maternal
behavior of the postpartum animal without interfering with hormonal
factors underlying the initiation or maintenance of maternal care.
Deficits due to limbic lesions appear to stem from a disruption of
sequential activities involved in maternal behavior. Such lesions
may alter the animal's perception of otherwise appropriate stimuli
or may disrupt pathways essential for integration of sequentially
organized behaviors.

Only studies of rats with lateral hypothalamic lesions (Avar
& Monos, 1967, 1969b) have reported a complete absence of postpartum maternal behavior. Experimental animals in these studies
partly cannabalized or simple ignored their young at parturition
and showed no further maternal interest in them. In this case,
the possibility exists that the lesions destroyed a center for the
initiation of maternal care or perhaps a neural area which is responsive to the hormonal changes that stimulate the onset of maternal behavior at parturition. However, as mentioned above (section
on The hypothalamus) lateral hypothalamic lesions are known to interfere with a variety of motivated behaviors and additional studies are needed to assess the specificty of these effects in regard
to maternal care and the neuroendocrine mechanisms underlying the
onset of maternal behavior. In particular, it would be of considerable interest to determine the effects of similar lesions on
the induction of maternal behavior of virgin rats by hormones and
by cohabitation with pups. Such studies might help clarify the
mechanisms underlying the absence of maternal behavior resulting
from lateral hypothalamic lesions.

Studies in which oxytocin release is interrupted by medial
hypothalamic lesions have clearly demonstrated a neuroendocrine related interference with care of the young (Yokoyama & Ota, 1959b;
Herrenkohl & Rosenberg, 1974). Such lesions interrupt lactational
performance and ability to maintain the litter. However, behavioral tests indicate that animals with these lesions are maternally
responsive and still attempt to nurse their young. While the occur-

rence of milk release (and its conditioning to exteroceptive cues from the young) may influence maternal behavior, this has not been demonstrated experimentally and the available evidence indicates a considerable degree of independence of these factors.

In summary, the available studies have demonstrated that brain lesions may interfere with maternal care but they have provided little information as to where in the nervous system hormones or experiential factors act to stimulate the onset of maternal behavior. It seems reasonable to assume that a neural substrate exists which is responsive to appropriate environmental and hormonal stimulation and, in turn, mediates the display of nesting, retrieving, nursing and other activities involved in maternal behavior. Of course, this area of experimentation is still in its infancy and much work remains to be done before we can gain a full understanding of the sensory and neuroendocrine factors underlying maternal behavior.

ACKNOWLEDGEMENTS

My most sincere thanks are due to Patricia Goldman and Paul D. MacLean for critically reviewing the manuscript and for their many helpful suggestions. Work of the author's laboratory presented in this paper was supported in part by USPHS Grant HD 03131.

REFERENCES

ADER, R. & GROTA, L. J., 1970, Rythmicits in the maternal behavior of Rattus Norvegicus, Anim. Behav. 18:144.

ALBERTS, J. & FRIEDMAN, M., 1972, Olfactory bulb removal but not anosmia increases emotionality and mousekilling. Nature 238: 454.

ALLIN, J. T. & BANKS, E. M., 1971, Effects of temperature on ultrasound production by infant albino rats, Dev. Psychobiol. 4:149.

ALLIN, J. T. & BANKS, E. M., 1972, Functional aspects of ultrasound production by infant albino rats (Rattus Norvegicus), Anim. Behav. 20:175.

AULSBROOK, L H. & HOLLAND, R. C., 1969a, Central regulation of oxytocin release with and without vasopressin release, Amer. J. Physiol. 216:830.

AULSBROOK, L. H., & HOLLAND, R. C., 1969b, Central inhibition of oxytocin release, Amer. J. Physiol. 216:830.

AVAR, Z. & MONOS, E., 1964, The effect of hypothalamic lesion on
     the time of onset and course of labour, and on the develop-
     ment of the foetus, Acta Med. Acad. Scient. Hung. 20:395.

AVAR, Z. & MONOS, E., 1966, Effect of lateral hypothalamic lesions
     on pregnant rats and foetal mortality, Acta Med. Acad. Scient.
     Hung. 22:259.

AVAR, Z. & MONOS, E., 1967, Effect of lateral hypothalamic lesion
     on maternal behaviour and foetal vitality in the rat, Acta
     Med. Acad. Scient. Hung. 23:255.

AVAR, Z. & MONOS, E., 1969a, Biological role of lateral hypothalamic
     structures participating in the control of maternal behaviour
     in the rat. Motility, explorative behaviour, lactation, and
     the effects of reduced food intake, Acta Physiol. Acad. Scient.
     Hung. 35:285.

AVAR, Z. & MONOS, E., 1969b, Behavioural changes in pregnant rats fol-
     lowing far-lateral hypothalamic lesions, Acta Physiol. Acad.
     Scient. Hung. 35:295.

BEACH, F. A., 1937, The neural basis of innate behavior. I.   Ef-
     fects of cortical lesions upon the maternal behavior pattern
     in the rat, J. Comp. Psychol. 24:393.

BEACH, F. A., 1938, The neural basis of innate behavior: II. Rel-
     ative effects of partial decortication in adulthood and in-
     fancy upon the maternal behavior of the primiparous rat, J.
     Genet. Psychol. 53:109.

BEACH, F. A. & WILSON, J. R., 1963, Effects of prolactin, progester-
     one and estrogen on reactions of non-pregnant rats to foster
     young, Psych. Rep. 13:231.

BENSON, G. K. & FOLLEY, S. J., 1956, Oxytocin as stimulator for the
     release of prolactin from the anterior pituitary, Nature 177:
     700.

BEYER. C., ANGUIANO, L. G. & MENA, F., 1961, Oxytocin release in
     response to stimulation of cingulate gyrus, Amer. J. Physiol.
     200:625.

BEYER, C. & MENA, F., 1969, Neural factors in lactation, in: Physi-
     ology and pathology of adaptation mechanisms, (P. Alexander,
     and Bacq, Z. M., eds.) p. 310-344.

BEYER, C. & MENA, F., 1965, Induction of milk secretion in the rab-
     bit by removal of the telencephalon, Amer. J. Physiol. 208:585.

BIRCH, H. G., 1956, Sources of order in the maternal behavior of animals, Amer. J. Orthopsychiat. 26:279.

BLAKE, C. A., 1974, Stimulation of pituitary prolactin and TSH release in lactating and proestrous rats, Endocrinology, 94:503

BLOCH, G. J. & DAVIDSON, J. M., 1968, Effects of adrenalectomy and experience on postcastration sex behavior in the male rat, Physiol. Behav. 3:461.

BOICE, R., 1973, Domestication, Psych. Bull. 80:215.

BRADY, J. V. & NAUTA, W. J. H., 1953, Subcortical mechanisms in emotional behavior, J. Comp. Physiol. Psychol. 46:339.

BRIDGES, R., ZARROW, M. X., GANDELMAN, R., & DENENBERG, V. H., 1972, Differences in maternal responsiveness between lactating and sensitized rats, Dev. Psychobiol. 5:123.

BRUCE, H. M., 1961, Observations on the suckling stimulus and lactation in the rat, J. Reprod. Fert. 2:17.

BUTLER, C. G., 1970, Chemical communication in insects: Behavioral and ecological aspects, in "Advances in chemoreception. Vol. I. Communication by Chemical signals, (J. W. Johnston, Jr., Moulton, D. G., & Turk, A. eds.) pp. 35-78, Appleton-Century-Crofts, New York.

CALDEYRO-BARCIA, R., 1969, Milk ejection in women, in "Lactogenesis: The initiation of milk secretion at parturition (M. Reynolds, & Folley, S. J., eds.) pp. 229-243, University of Pennsylvania Press, Philadelphia.

CALHOUN, J. B., 1962, "The ecology and sociology of the Norway rat," pp. 1-288, U. S. Department of Health, Education and Welfare, Bethesda.

CARLSON, N. R. & THOMAS, G. J., 1968, Maternal behavior of mice with limbic lesions, J. Comp. Physiol. Psychol. 66:731.

CATCHPOLE, H. R., 1969, Hormonal mechanisms during pregnancy and parturition, in "Reproduction of domestic animals," (H. H. Cole & Cupps, P. T. eds.), pp. 415-440, Academic Press, New York.

CHALLIS, J. R. G., DAVIES, I. J., & RYAN, K. J., 1973, The concentrations of progesterone, estrone and estradiol-17 in the plasma of pregnant rabbits, Endocrinology 93:971.

CHARTON, D., ADRIEN, J. & COSNIER, J., 1971, Déclencheurs chimiques
  due comportement de léchage despetites par la Ratte parturiente,
  Rev. Comp. Anim. 5:89.

CHRISTOPHERSEN, E. R. & WAGMAN, W., 1965, Maternal behavior in the
  albino rat as a function of self-licking deprivation, J. Comp.
  Physiol. Psychol. 60:142.

CLEVERLEY, J. D., 1968, The detection of oxytocin release in response to conditioned stimuli associated with machine milking
  in the cow, J. Endocrin. 40:ii.

COWIE, A. T., 1972, Lactation and its hormonal control, in: Reproduction in mammals. Vol. 3. Hormones in reproduction (ed.
  by C. R. Austin & R. V. Short). Cambridge University Press,
  Cambridge. pp. 106-143.

COWIE, A. T. & TINDAL, J. S., 1971, "The physiology of lactation,"
  pp. 1-392, Arnold, London.

CROSS, B. A., 1955a, The hypothalamus and the mechanism of sym-
  pathetico-adrenal inhibition of milk ejection, J. Endocrin.
  12:15.

CROSS, B. A., 1955b, Neurohormonal mechanisms in emotional inhibition of milk ejection, J. Endocrin. 12:29.

CROSS, B. A., 1961, Neural control of oxytocin secretion, in "Oxytocin, (R. Caldeyro-Barcia, H. Heller, eds.), pp. 24-47,
  Pergamon Press, Oxford.

CROSS, B. A., 1973, Unit responses in the hypothalamus, in "Frontiers in Neuroendocrinology, (W. F. Ganong & L. Martini, eds.)
  pp. 133-171, Oxford University Press, New York.

DAVIDSON, J. M., 1972, Hormones and reproductive behavior, in
  "Hormones and Behavior," (S. Levine, ed.), pp. 63-103, Academic
  Press, New York.

DAVIS, C. D., 1938, The effect of ablations of neocrotex on mating,
  maternal behavior and the production of pseudopregnancy in
  the female rat and on copulatory activity in the male, Amer.
  J. Physiol. 127:374.

DEIS, R. P., 1968, The effect of an exteroceptive stimulus on milk
  ejection in lactating rats, J. Physiol. 197:37.

DENENBERG, V. H., TAYLOR, R. E. & ZARROW, M. X., 1969, Maternal behavior in the rat: An investigation and quantification of nest

building, Behaviour 34:1.

DOUGLAS, R., ISAACSON, R. & MOSS, R., 1969, Olfactory lesions, emotionality and activity, Physiol. Behav. 4:379.

ELY, F. & PETERSEN, W. E., 1941, Factors involved in the ejection of milk, J. Dairy Sci. 24:211.

EPSTEIN, A., 1971, The lateral hypothalamic syndrome: Its implications for the physiological psychology of hunger and thirst, in "Progress in physiological psychology Vol. 4 (E. Stellar & J. M. Sprague, eds.), pp. 263-317. Academic Press, New York.

EVERETT, J. W., 1964, Central neural control of reproductive functions of the adenohypophysis, Physiol. Rev. 44:373.

FLEMING, A. S., 1972, Olfactory and experiential factors underlying maternal behavior in the lactating and cycling female rat, Doctoral dissertation, Rutgers University.

FLEMING, A. S. & ROSENBLATT, J. S., 1974a, Olfactory regulation of maternal behavior in rats: I. Effects of olfactory bulb removal in experienced and inexperienced lactating and cycling females, J. Comp. Physiol. Psychol. 86:221.

FLEMING, A. S. & ROSENBLATT, J. S., 1974b, Olfactory regulation of maternal behavior in rats: II. Effects of peripherally induced anosmia and lesions of the lateral olfactory tract in pup-induced virgins, J. Comp. Physiol. Psychol. 86:233.

FLEISCHER, S. F., 1973, Deficits in maternal behavior of rats with lesions of the septal area, Unpublished doctoral dissertation, Columbia University.

FLINT, A. P. F. & ARMSTRONG, D. T., 1973, The appearance of an endometrial 20-hydroxysteroid dehydrogenase towards the end of pregnancy in the rat, Endocrinology 92:624.

FUCHS, A. R. & SAITO, S., 1971, Pituitary oxytocin and vasopressin content of pregnant rats before, during and after parturition, Endocrinology 88:574.

GANDELMAN, R., 1973, The development of cannibalism in male Rockland-Swiss mice and the influence of olfactory bulb removal, Develop. Psychobiol. 6:159.

GANDELMAN, R., ZARROW, M. X. & DENENBERG, V. H., 1970, Maternal behavior: Differences between mother and virgin mice as a function of the testing procedure, Develop. Psychobiol. 3:207.

GANDELMAN, R., ZARROW, M. X. & DENENBERG, V. H., 1972, Reproductive and maternal performance in the mouse following removal of the olfactory bulbs, J. Reprod. Fert. 28:453.

GAMDELMAN, R., ZARROW, M. X., DENENBERG, V. H. & MYERS, M., 1971, Olfactory bulb removal eliminates maternal behavior in the mouse, Science 171:210.

GOUREVITCH, G. & HACK, M. H., 1966, Audibility in the rat, J. Comp. Physiol. Psychol. 62:289.

GROSVENOR, C. E., 1965, Evidence that exteroceptive stimuli can release prolactin from the pituitary gland of the lactating rat, Endocrinology 77:1037.

GROSVENOR, C. E., MAIWEG, H. & MENA, F., 1970, A study of factors involved in the development of the exteroceptive release of prolactin in the lactating rat, Horm. Behav. 1:111.

GROSVENOR, C. E., MENA, F., DHARIWAL, A. P. S. & MCCANN, S. M., 1965, Reduction of milk secretion by prolactin-inhibiting factor: Further evidence that exteroceptive stimuli can release pituitary prolactin in rats, Endocrinology 81:1921.

GROSZ, H. J. & ROTHBALLER, A. B., 1961, Mypothalamic control of lactogenic function in the cat, Nature 190:349.

GROTA, L. J., 1973, Effects of litter size, age of young, and parity on foster mother behavior in Rattus Norvegicus. Anim. Behav. 21:78.

HALASZ, B. & PUPP, L., 1965, Hormone secretion of the anterior pituitary gland after physical interruption of all nervous pathways in the hypophysiotrophic area, Endocrinology, 77:553.

HART, B. L., 1968, Role of prior experience in the effects of castration on sexual behavior of male dogs, J. Comp. Physiol. Psychol. 66:719.

HAUN, C. K. & SAWYER, C. H., 1960, Initiation of lactation in rabbits following placement of hypothalamic lesions, Endocrinology 67:270.

HAUN, C. K. & SAWYER, C. H., 1961, The role of the hypothalamus in initiation of milk secretion, Acta Endocrin. 38:99.

HERRENKOHL, L. R. & ROSENBERG, P. A., 1974, Effects of hypothalamic deafferentation late in gestation on lactation and nursing behavior in the rat, Hormon. Behav. 5:33.

HITT, J. C., HENDRICKS, S. E., GINSBERG, S. I. & LEWIS, J. H., 1970, Disruption of male, but not female, sexual behavior in rats by medial forebrain bundle lesions, J. Comp. Physiol. Psychol. 73: 377.

HOLLOWAY, S. A. & STEVENSON, J., 1967, Effect of various ablations in the hypothalamus on established pregnancy in the rat, Canad. J. Physiol. Pharm. 45:1081.

INNES, W. T., 1964, "Exotic Aquarium Fishes," pp. 1-541. Metaframe, Maywood.

KANEMATSU, S., HILLIARD, J. & SAWYER, C. H., 1963, Effect of hypothalamic lesions on pituitary prolactin content in the rabbit, Endocrinology 73:345.

KANEMATSU, S. & SAWYER, C. H., 1963, Effects of intrahypothalamic and intraphypophyseal estrogen implants on pituitary prolactin and lactation in the rabbit, Endocrinology 72:243.

KARLI, P., VERGNES, M. & DIDIERGEORGES, R., 1969, Rat-mouse interspecific aggressive behavior and its manipulation by brain ablation and by brain stimulation, in "Aggressive Behavior," (S. Garattini & E. B. Sand, eds.), Wiley, New York, pp. 47-55.

KAWAKAMI, M. & SAWYER, C. H., 1959, Neuroendocrine correlates of changes in brain activity threshholds by sex steroids and pituitary hormones, Endocrinology 65:652.

KIRBY, H. W. & HORVATH, T., 1968, Self-licking deprivation and maternal behaviour in the primiparous rat, Canad. J. Psychol. 22:369.

KIMBLE, D. P., ROGERS, L. & HENDRICKSON, C. W., 1967, Hippocampal lesions disrupt maternal, not sexual behavior in the albino rat, J. Comp. Physiol. Psychol. 63:401.

KLEBANOFF, S. J., 1965, Inactivation of estrogen by rat uterine preparations, Endocrinology 76:301.

KLUVER, H. & BUCY, P. C., 1939, Preliminary analysis of functions of the temporal lobes in monkeys, Arch. Neurol. Psychiat. 42: 979.

KNAGGS, G. S., TINDAL, J. S. & TURVEY, A., 1971, Paraventricular-hypophyseal neurosecretory pathways in the guinea-pig, J. Endocrin. 50:153.

KOLLER, G., 1952, Der Nestbau der weissen Maus und seine hormonale

Auslosung, Verh. dtsch. zool. Ges., Freiburg, pp. 160-168.

KOLLER, G., 1956, Hormonale und psychische Steuerung beim Nestbau weiser Mause, Zool. Anz (Suppl.) Verh. dtsch. zool. Ges. 19:125.

KURCZ, M., 1965, A terhesség, a szülés és a laktáció zavara a kisérleti "hypothalamikus" elhizás esetében (Disorders of pregnancy, birth and lactation in experimental hypothalamic obesity) Kiser. Orvostu. 17:471.

LEBLOND, C. P. & NELSON, W. O., 1937a, Maternal behavior in hypophysectomized male and female mice, Amer. J. Physiol. 120:167.

LEBLOND, C. P. & NELSON, W. O., 1937b, Presence d'instinct maternal sans stimulation hormonale. C. R. Soc. Biol. 124:1064.

LEHRMAN, D. S., 1961, Hormonal regulation of parental behavior in birds and infrahuman mammals, in "Sex and Internal Secretions, Vol. II, 3rd. Ed. (W. C. Young, ed.) Williams & Wilkins, Baltimore, pp. 1268-1382.

LEON, M. & MOTZ, H., 1971, Maternal pheromone: discrimination by pre-weaning albino rats, Physiol. Behav. 7:265.

LEON, M. & MOLTZ, H., 1972, The development of the pheromonal bond in the albino rat, Physiol. Behav. 8:683.

LINKIE, D. M. & NISWENDER, G. D., 1972, Serum levels of prolactin, luteinizing hormone, and follicle stimulating hormone during pregnancy in the rat, Endocrinology 90:632.

LISK, R. D., 1971, Oestrogen and progesterone synergism and elicitation of maternal nest-building in the mouse (Mus Musculus), Anim. Behav. 19:606.

LISK, R. D., PRETLOW, R. A. & REIEDMAN, S. M., 1969, Hormonal stimulation necessary for elicitation of maternal nest-building in the mouse (Mus. Musculus), Anim. Behav. 17:730.

LIU, T. M. Y. & DAVIS, J. W., 1967, Induction of lactation by ovariectomy of pregnant rats, Endocrinology 80:1043.

LOCKARD, R. B., 1968, The albino rat: A defensible choice or a bad habit?, Amer. Psychol. 23:734.

LOTT, D. F., 1962, The role of progesterone in the maternal behavior of rodents, J. Comp. Physiol. Psychol. 55:610.

LOTT, D. F. & FUCHS, S. S., 1962, Failure to induce retrieving by sensitization or the injection of prolactin, J. Comp. Physiol.

Psychol. 55:1111.

LOTT, D. F. & ROSENBLATT, J. S., 1969, Development of maternal
    responsiveness during pregnancy in the rat, in "Determinants
    of infant behaviour," Vol. IV. (B. M. Foss, ed.) Methuen,
    London pp. 61-67.

LU, K., KOCH, Y. & MEITES, J., 1971, Direct inhibition by ergocornine
    of pituitary prolactin release, Endocrinology 89:229.

LYONS, W. R., 1958, Hormonal synergism in mammary growth,
    Proc. Roy. Soc. (London) Series B, 149:303.

MACLEAN, P. D., 1952, Some psychiatric implications of physiologi-
    cal studies of frontotemporal portion of limbic system (visceral
    brain), Electroenceph. Clin. Neurophysiol. 4:407.

MCCANN, S. M. & DHARIWAL, A. P. S., 1966, Hypothalamic releasing
    factors and the neurovascular link between the brain and the
    anterior pituitary, in "Neuroendocrinology" Vol. I. (L. Martini
    & W. F. Ganong, eds.), pp. 261-296, Academic Press, New York.

MCCANN, S. M., DHARIWAL, A. P. S., & PORTER, J., 1967, Regulation
    of the adenohypophysis, Ann. Rev. Physiol. 30:589.

MCEWEN, B. S. & PFAFF, D. W., 1973, Chemical and physiological
    approaches to neuroendocrine mechanisms: Attempts at inte-
    gration, in "Frontiers in Neuroendocrinology," (W. F. Ganong,
    & L. Martini eds.) pp. 267-355, Oxford University Press, New
    York.

MARSHALL, J. F., TURNER, B. H. & TEITELBAUM, P., 1971, Sensory ne-
    glect produced by lateral hypothalamic damage, Science 174:
    523.

MEITES, J., 1972, Hypothalamic control of prolactin secretion, in
    "Lactogenic Hormones", (G. E. W. Wolstenholme & J. Knight eds.)
    pp. 325-350, Churchill Livingstone, London.

MENA, F. & BEYER, C., 1968, Induction of milk secretion in the rab-
    bit by lesions in the temporal lobe, Endocrinology 83:618.

MENA, F. & GROSVENOR, C. E., 1971, Release of prolactin in rats by
    exteroceptive stimulation: Sensory stimuli involved, Horm.
    Behav. 2:107.

MOLTZ, H., 1971, The ontogeny of maternal behavior in some selected
    mammalian species, in "The Ontogeny of Vertebrate Behavior,"
    (H. Moltz, ed.), pp. 263-313, Academic Press, New York.

MOLTZ, H., GELLER, D. & LEVIN, R., 1967, Maternal behavior in the
totally mammectomized rat, J. Comp. Physiol. Psychol. 64:225.

MOLTZ, H., LEIDAHL, L., & ROWLAND, D., 1974, Prolongation of pheromonal emission in the maternal rat, Physiology and Behavior
(In press) Vol. 12 #3 March, 1974 p. 409-412.

MOLTZ, H., LEVIN. R. & LEON, M., 1969, Differential effects of progesterone on the maternal behavior of primiparous and multiparous rats, J. Comp. Physiol. Psychol. 67:36.

MOLTZ, H., LUBIN, M. & NUMAN, M., 1970, Hormonal induction of maternal behavior in the ovariectomized nulliparous rat, Physiol.
Behav. 5:1373.

MOLTZ, H., ROBBINS, D. & PARKS, M., 1966, Caesarean delivery and
the maternal behavior of primiparous and multiparous rats,
J. Comp. Physiol. Psychol. 61:455.

MOLTZ, H. & WIENER, H., 1966, Effects of ovariectomy on maternal
behavior of primiparous and multiparous rats, J. Comp. Physiol.
Psychol. 62:382.

MORISHIGE, W. K., PEPE, G. J., & ROTHCHILD, I., 1973, Serum luteinizing hormone, prolactin and progesterone levels during pregnancy in the rat, Endocrinology 92:1527.

NAGASAWA, H. & YANAI, R., 1972, Changes in serum prolactin levels
shortly before and after parturition in rats, Endocrin. Japon.
19:139.

NALBANDOV. A. V., 1973, Control of luteal function in mammals, in
"Handbook of Physiology," Section 7, Vol. 2, American Physiological Society, Washington, D. C. pp. 153-167.

NICOLL, C. S., 1967, Bioassay of prolactin: analysis of the pigeon
crop-sac response to local prolactin injection by an objective
and quantitative method, Endocrinology 80:641.

NICOLL, C. S. & MEITES, J., 1959, Prolongation of lactation in the
rat by litter replacement, Proc. Soc. Exp. Biol. Med. 101:81.

NISWENDER, G. D., CHEN, C. L., MIDGLEY, A. R., MEITES, J., & ELLIS,
S., 1969, Radioimmunoassay for rat prolactin, Proc. Soc. Exp.
Biol. Med. 130:793.

NOBLE, G. K. & CURTIS, B., 1939, The social behavior of the jewel
fish, Hemichromis bimaculatus Gill., Bull. Amer. Mus. Nat. Hist.
76:1.

NOBLE, G. K. & MASON, E. R., 1933, Experiments on the brooding
    habits of the lizards, Eumeces and Ophisauras, Amer. Mus.
    Novit. No. 619:1.

NOIROT, E., 1964, Changes in responsiveness to young in the adult
    mouse: II. The effect of external stimuli, J. Comp. Physiol.
    Psychol. 57:97.

NOIROT, E., 1970, Selective priming of maternal responses by audi-
    tory and olfactory cues from mouse pups, Develop. Psychobiol.
    2:273.

NOIROT, E., 1972a, The onset of maternal behavior in rats, hamsters,
    and mice: A selective review, in "Advances in the Study of
    Behavior," Vol. 4 (D. S. Lehrman, R. A. Hind & E. Shaw, eds.)
    pp. 107-145, Academic Press, New York.

NOIROT, E., 1972b, Ultrasounds and maternal behavior in small ro-
    dents, Develop. Psychobiol. 5:371.

NUMAN, M., LEON, M. & MOLTZ, H., 1972, Interference with prolactin
    release and the maternal behavior of female rats, Horm. Behav.
    3:29.

OBIAS, M. D., 1957, Maternal behavior of hypophysectomized gravid
    albino rats and development and performance of their progeny,
    J. Comp. Physiol. Psychol. 50:120

OLDS, M. E. & OLDS, J., 1962, Approach-escape interactions in rat
    brain, Amer. J. Physiol. 203:808.

OLEY, N. N. & SLOTNICK, B. M., 1970, Nesting material as a rein-
    forcement for operant behavior in the rat, Psychon. Sci. 21:
    41.

PEPE, G. J. & ROTHCHILD, I., 1973, Serum progesterone levels in
    ovariectomized rats injected with progesterone and estrone:
    Relation to pregnancy maintenance and growth of decidual
    tissue, Endocrinology 93:1193.

PEETERS, G., STORMORKEN, H., & VANSCHOUBROEK, F., 1960, The effect
    of different stimuli on milk ejection and diuresis in the
    lactating cow, J. Endocrin. 20:163.

PFAFF, D. W., 1968, Autoradiographic localization of radioactivity
    in the rat brain after injection of tritiated sex hormones,
    Science 161:1355.

PSYCHOYOS, A., 1967, The hormonal interplay controlling egg-implanta-
    tion in the rat, in "Advances in Reproductive Physiology," Vol.

2, (A. McLaren ed.), Academic Press, New York, pp. 257-277.

QUADAGNO, D. M. & ROCKWELL, J., 1972, The effect of gonadal hormones in infancy on maternal behavior in the adult rat, Horm.
Behav. 3:55.

RAJ, H. G. M. & MOUDGAL, N. R., 1970, Hormonal control of gestation
in the intact rat, Endocrinology 86:874.

RATNER, A. & MEITES, J., 1964, Depletion of prolactin-inhibiting
activity of rat hypothalamus by estradiol or suckling stimulus,
Endocrinology 75:377.

REICHLIN, S., 1963, Medical Progress, Neuroendocrinology. New Eng.
J. Med. 269:1182.

RICHTER, C. P., 1955, Self-regulatory functions during gestation
and lactation, in "Gestation: Transactions of the second
conference, March 8, 9, and 10 (G. B. Wislocki, Chm) Princeton University Press, Princeton, pp. 11-89.

RIDDLE, O., 1963, Prolactin or progesterone as the key to parental
behaviour: A review, Anim. Behav. 11:419.

RIDDLE, O., LAHR, E. L. & BATES, R. W., 1935, Maternal behavior induced in virgin rats by prolactin, Proc. Soc. Biol., 32:730.

RIDDLE, O., LAHR, E. L. & BATES, R. W., 1942, The role of hormones
in the initiation of maternal behavior in rats, Amer. J.
Physiol.137:299.

ROPARTZ, P., 1968, The relation between olfactory stimulation and
aggressive behaviours in mice, Anim. Behav. 16:97.

ROSENBLATT, J. S., 1967, Nonhormonal basis of maternal behavior
in the rat, Science 156:1512.

ROSENBLATT, J. S., 1969, The development of maternal responsiveness
in the rat, Amer. J. Orthopsychiat. 39:36.

ROSENBLATT, J. S., 1970, Views on the onset and maintenance of ma-
ternal behavior in the rat, in "Development and Evolution of
Behavior," (L. R. Aronson, E., Tobach, D. S. Lehrman, & J. S.
Rosenblatt, eds.), pp. 489-515, Freeman, San Francisco.

ROSENBLATT, J. S. & ARONSON, L. R., 1958, The decline of sexual behavior in male cats after castration with special reference to
the role of prior sexual experience, Behaviour 12:285.

ROSENBLATT, J. S. & LEHRMAN, D. S., 1963, Maternal behavior of the laboratory rat, in "Maternal Behavior of Mammals," (H. S. Rheingold ed.) Wiley, New York.

ROSVOLD, H. E., MIRSKY, A. F. & PRIBRAM, K. H., 1954, Influence of amygdalectomy on social behavior in monkeys, J. Comp. Physiol. Psychol. 47:173.

ROTH, L. L. & ROSENBLATT, J. S., 1967, Changes in self-licking during pregnancy in the rat, J. Comp. Physiol. Psychol. 63:397.

ROTH, L. L. & ROSENBLATT, J. S., 1968, Self-licking and mammary development during pregnancy in the rat, J. Endocrin. 42:363.

ROWE, F. A. & EDWARDS, D. A., 1971, Olfactory bulb removal: Influences on the aggressive behaviors of male mice, Physiol. Behav. 7:889.

ROWE, F. A. & EDWARDS, D. A., 1972, Olfactory bulb removal: Influences on the mating behavior of male mice, Physiol. Behav. 8:37.

SACHS, B. D., WARDEN, A. F. & POLLAK, E., 1971, Studies on postpartum estrus in rats, Paper presented at the Eastern Regional Conference on Reproductive Behavior, Haverford, Pennsylvania.

SAR, M. & STUMPF, W. E., 1973, Neurons of the hypothalamus concentrate [^{3}H] progesterone or its metabolites, Science 182:1266.

SAWYER, C. H., HAUN, C. K., HILLIARD, J., RADFORD, H. M., NANEMATSU, S., 1963, Further evidence for the identity of hypothalamic areas controlling ovulation and lactation in the rabbit, Endocrinology 73:338.

SCHALLY, A. V., ARIMURA, A. & KASTIN, A. J., 1973, Hypothalamic regulatory hormones, Science 179:341.

SCHARRER, E. & SCHARRER, B., 1963, "Neuroendocrinology," pp. viii-289, Columbia University Press, New York.

SIEGEL, H. I., 1974, Hormonal basis of the onset of maternal behavior in the laboratory rat, Unpublished doctoral dissertation, Rutgers University.

SLOTNICK, B. M., 1963, Disturbances of maternal behavior in rats following lesions of the dorsal limbic cortex, Doctoral dissertation, University of Illinois, Urbana.

SLOTNICK, B. M., 1967a, Intercorrelations of maternal activities in the rat, _Anim. Behav._ 15:267.

SLOTNICK, B. M., 1967b, Disturbances of maternal behavior in the
rat following lesions of the cingulate cortex, _Behaviour_,
29:204.

SLOTNICK, B. M., 1969, Maternal behavior deficits following forebrain lesions in the rat, _Amer. Zool._ 9:4.

SLOTNICK, B. M., CARPENTER, M. L. & FUSCO, R., 1973, Initiation of
maternal behavior in pregnant nulliparous rats, _Horm. Behav._
4:53.

SLOTNICK, B. M. & NIGROSH, B. J., 1974, Maternal behavior of mice
with cingulate cortical, amygdala or septal lesions,
J. Comp. Physiol. Psychol. (In press).

SPIEGEL, E. A., KLETZKIN, M. & SZEKELY, E. G., 1954, Pain reactions on stimulation of the tectum mesencephali, _J. Neuropath._
13:212.

SPIES, H. G. & NISWENDER, G. D., 1971, Levels of prolactin, LH and
FSH in the serum of intact and pelvic-neurectomized rats,
Endocrinology 88:937.

STAMM, J. S., 1955, The function of the median cerebral cortex
in maternal behavior in rats, _J. Comp. Physiol. Psychol._ 48:
347.

STONE, C. P., 1938, Effects of cortical destruction on reproductive
behavior and maze learning in albino rats, _J. Comp. Psychol._
26:217.

TERKEL, J., 1970, Some aspects of maternal behavior in the rat with
special reference to humoral factors at the time of parturition,
Doctoral dissertation, Rutgers University.

TERKEL, J. & ROSENBLATT, J. S., 1968, Maternal behavior induced by
maternal blood plasma injected into virgin rats, _J. Comp.
Physiol. Psychol._ 65:479.

TERKEL, J. & ROSENBLATT, J. S., 1971, Aspects of nonhormonal maternal behavior in the rat, _Horm. Behav._ 2:161.

TERKEL, J. & ROSENBLATT, J. S., 1972, Humoral factors underlying
maternal behavior at parturition: Cross transfusion between
freely moving rats, _J. Comp. Physiol. Psychol._ 80:365.

THOMAN, E. B. & LEVINE, S., 1970, Effects of adrenalectomy on maternal behavior in rats, Develop. Psycho. Biol. 3:237.

TINDAL, J. S. & KNAGGS, G. S., 1969, An ascending pathway for release of prolactin in the brain of the rabbit, J. Endocrin. 45:111.

TINDAL, J. S. & KNAGGS, G. S., 1971, Determination of the detailed hypothalamic route of the milk-ejection reflex in the guinea-pig, J. Endocrin. 50:135.

TINDAL, J. S., KNAGGS, G. S., & TURVEY, A., 1967, The afferent path of the milk-ejection reflex in the brain of the guinea-pig, J. Endocrin. 38:337.

TINDAL, J. S., KNAGGS, G. S., & TURVEY, A., 1969, The afferent path of the milk-ejection reflex in the brain of the rabbit, J. Endocrin. 43:663.

VERNIKOS-DANELLIS, J., 1972, Effects of hormones on the central nervous system, in "Hormones and Behavior" (S. Levine, ed.), pp. 11-62, Academic Press, New York.

VOCI, V. E. & CARLSON, N. R., 1973, Enhancement of maternal behavior and nest building following systemic and diencephalic administration of prolactin and progesterone in the mouse, J. Comp. Physiol. Psychol. 83:388.

WIESNER, B. P. & SHEARD, N. M., 1933, "Maternal Behavior in the Rat," Edinburgh, Oliver and Boyd.

WILSONCROFT, W. E., 1963, Effects of median cortex lesions on the maternal behavior of the rat, Psych. Rep. 13:835.

WOODS, W. H., HOLLAND, R. C. & POWELL, E. W., 1969, Connections of cerebral structures functioning in neurohypophyseal hormone release, Brain Res. 12:26.

YOKOYAMA, A., HALASZ, B., & SAWYER, C. H., 1967, Effect of hypothalamic deafferentation on lactation in rats, Proc. Soc. Exp. Biol. Med. 125:623.

YOKOYAMA, A. & OTA, K., 1959a, The effect of hypothalamic lesions on litter growth in rats, Endocrin. Japon 6:14.

YOKOYAMA, A. & OTA, K., 1959b, Effect of oxytocin replacement on lactation in rats bearing hypothalamic lesions, Endocrin. Japon. 6:268.

YOSHINAGA, K., HAWKINS, R. A. & STOCKER, J. F., 1969, Estrogen
    secretion by the rat ovary in vivo during the estrus cycle
    and pregnancy, Endocrinology 85:103.

ZARROW, M. X., BRODY, P. N., & DENENBERG, V. H., 1968, The role
    of progesterone in behavior, in "Perspectives in Reproduction
    and Sexual Behavior (M. Diamond, ed.) pp. 363-389, Indiana
    University Press, Bloomington.

ZARROW, M. X., DENENBERG, V. H. & SACHS, B. D., 1972, Hormones
    and maternal behavior in mammals, in "Hormones and Behavior,"
    (S. Levine ed.), Acadmenic Press, New York.

ZARROW, M. X., GANDELMAN, R. & DENENBERG, V. H., 1971a, Prolactin:
    Is it an essential hormone for maternal behavior in the mam-
    mal? Horm. Behav. 2:343.

ZARROW, M. X., GANDELMAN, R., & DENENBERG, V. H., 1971b, Lack of
    nest building and maternal behavior in the mouse following
    olfactory bulb removal, Horm. Behav. 2:227.

CHAPTER 16

HORMONAL CONTROL OF FEEDING BEHAVIOR AND ENERGY BALANCE

Jack Panksepp, Ph.D.

Department of Psychology
Bowling Green State University
Bowling Green, Ohio   43403

CONTENTS

INTRODUCTION

Life ultimately depends on an organism's capacity to sustain
the flame of intracellular metabolism. Hence all living animals store
fuel within their bodies, and they possess many behavioral and physiological processes to insure the relative stability of these stores.
While eating and related instrumental behaviors oversee the maintenance of adequate energy intake, hormones and ancillary patterns of
enzyme induction establish a balance between the storage and usage
of the ingested nutrients.

To understand the relationship between hormones and feeding behavior, we would have to specify in detail the regulatory machinery
which permits maintenance of stable body fuel reserves. Unfortunately, the precise nature of the biochemical process which subserves
body energy regulation remains unidentified. In general terms, however, it is clear that the metabolically useful energy content of food
determines how much an animal eats. Though a multitude of short-term
influences such as bulk, taste and tonicity of food often obscure this
fact, the central role of energy has been adequately demonstrated by
methods such as diluting the energy density of food with metabolically
inert materials (Adolph, 1947) or by force feeding animals with nutrients (Cohn & Joseph, 1962; Panksepp, 1971). In all such experiments, animals voluntarily modify food consumption so that daily energy
intake remains stable. Though precise caloric compensation may not be
apparent in each meal an animal eats, the imprecision of individual
meals is eventually corrected by changes in the satiating capacity of
future meals and the hunger-inducing capacity of intermeal intervals
(Panksepp, 1973; 1974).

Maintenance of relatively constant energy intake under constant

environmental conditions must reflect surveillance of certain body
energy transactions by metabolic or hormonal detectors somewhere in
the body. Whether this detection process applies to a circumscribed
body nutrient compartment or to some more inclusive measure of body
nutrient levels is not known. For instance, regulation may specifically reflect the state of fat stores, glycogen stores, lean body mass,
specialized cells within the central nervous system, or a general
body energy monitor which measures the integral of all metabolic fuels
which have appeared in the bloodstream during certain spans of time.
In fact, so many factors influence feeding behavior, that it is often
assumed that a very complex multifactor system must be the ultimate
basis for the capacity to regulate fuel reserves. But existing evidence does not preclude a more optimistic possibility. A single process, such as fat metabolism, may be pivotal in overall regulation
and other control mechanisms may remain subservient to that central
process (Panksepp, 1974).

Whatever the mechanism, information concerning the state of body
nutrition is eventually encoded in the neural activity of primitive
vegatative centers of the brain, especially the hypothalamus. Extremes of obesity and self-starvation and related hormone imbalances
result from damage of specific sub-areas of the hypothalamus. Damage
to ventromedial sectors leads to overeating and the development of
grotesque obesity in both animals and men. Damage to ventrolateral
sectors leads to severe loss of appetite, loss of weight, and with
extensive damage, loss of life. However, the possibility has arisen
recently that the apparent preeminence of the hypothalamus in energy
regulation may be due to its anatomical location rather than to unique
intrinsic functions. Many neural systems which mediate motivated behaviors arise from cell bodies in the brainstem and ascend through
the narrow hypothalamic corridor known as the medial forebrain bundle (Fuxe et al., 1970). These extra-hypothalamic circuits clearly
do participate in feeding (Ahlskog & Hoebel, 1973; Grossman, 1972;
Ungerstedt, 1971), but at the present time, it remains very likely
that the brain collects a significant portion of metabolic information from the body directly through the auspices of hypothalamic
transducer mechanisms (Debons et al., 1970; Oomura, 1973; Panksepp,
1972), and as far as anyone knows, it is primarily through these systems that hormones modulate feeding behavior.

ON THE GENERAL NATURE OF HORMONAL CONTROL
OF FEEDING AND WEIGHT REGULATION

Hormones may modify feeding in three general ways: 1) The central nervous system may sense hormone levels directly, and variations
in levels may be utilized as error signals by neural comparators which
control feeding. Indeed, some hormones clearly modify neural activity rapidly (Foote et al., 1972), but there is presently no clear evidence that any such mechanisms participates in ongoing regulation of

energy balance. 2) Hormones may indirectly modify the excitability
of feeding systems by activating genetic mechanisms which control the
manufacture of enzymes necessary for synthesis of neurotransmitters
and other substances which convey the flow of information from neuron
to neuron. For example, glucocorticoids supposedly can increase levels of the putative synaptic-transmitter serotonin by increasing levels of tryptophan hydroxylase (Azmitia & McEwen, 1971). 3) Finally,
and probably most significantly, hormones participate in regulation
of feeding and body weight by modulating the rates and types of energy transactions within the body. This is probably the main way hormones do modify feeding. Still, no mechanism of action has been
conclusively identified, and the study of relationships between hormones and feeding remains largely an empirical matter.

HORMONES AND BODY ENERGY METABOLISM

Since the role of hormones in the organization of feeding and
energy balance will probably be understood in terms of metabolic processes which are promoted and hindered, some major interactions between hormones and metabolism will be briefly reviewed. Specific
citations and more elaborate treatment of the research literature
may be found in endocrinology texts such as that edited by Williams
(1968).

Although all hormones modify carbohydrate, fat and protein metabolism to some extent, most body nutrient transfers during basal environmental conditions are controlled by three hormones--insulin,
glucocorticoids and growth hormone. Moreover, thyroxine exerts a
major steady-state influence which becomes a major variable with environmental temperature fluctuations; adrenaline and glucagon are
important in the momentary control of blood glucose, and gonadal
hormones mediate sexually dimorphic dispositions in feeding and metabolism.

Insulin has long been known to be unique among hormones in its
cardinal role of organizing anabolic (growth) processes within the
body. It promotes glycogen, lipid, protein and RNA synthesis, while
concurrently inhibiting release of stored nutrients from adipose
tissue (i.e., the antilipolytic effect of insulin). Moreover, insulin is the only hormone which can lower blood sugar directly. In
the absence of insulin, blood sugar rises beyond levels which the
kidney can reabsorb, and the classical diabetic symptom of glucose
loss in urine appears. In general, the action of insulin is opposed
by glucocorticoids, growth hormone, glucagon, adrenaline and thyroxine.
This is not to say that all these latter hormones act synergistically.
Some act like insulin in certain ways (for example, growth hormone
also promotes protein synthesis), but in most instances their action
is contrary to that of insulin.

Glucocorticoids (cortisol, corticosterone, etc.) promote the breakdown of fat and muscle, and antagonize the blood glucose lowering action of insulin. By preventing phosphorylation of glucose, glucocorticoids may also decrease intracellular glucose catabolism. Concurrently, these steroids increase synthesis of glucose and glycogen in the liver. In general, glucocorticoids promote rapid utilization of body energy and thus tend to exacerbate any existing diabetic symptoms.

In many important ways growth hormone acts like a glucocorticoid. It promotes the breakdown of fat and antagonizes the hypoglycemic effects of insulin. It inhibits glucose catabolism, but increases the uptake and oxidation of fatty acids in muscle. However, unlike the glucocorticoids, it promotes positive nitrogen balance (protein synthesis) with the assistance of insulin. Concurrent uptake of amino acids by the liver leads to increased synthesis of glucose. Thus, unlike glucocorticoids, growth hormone promotes the deposition of lean body mass, but like glucocorticoids, it promotes breakdown of fat, decreases glucose utilization and promotes glucose synthesis.

Thyroxine stimulates catabolism of body tissues generally-oxygen consumption and heat production of all but a few tissues, such as brain and heart, are markedly increased. To this end, thyroxine increases fat, protein and glycogen breakdown and also increases synthesis of glucose. The main stimulus leading to increased thyroxin secretion is a decrease in environmental temperature.

Adrenaline and glucagon have actions very similar to thyroxin in that both stimulate breakdown of fat, glycogen and protein and increase synthesis of glucose in the liver. It is thought that adrenaline is released primarily in response to emergency situations which demand extra energy expenditure, while glucagon is secreted primarily in response to acute decreases in blood sugar. Both are closely involved in maintaining the stability of blood glucose levels from moment to moment.

Of course the metabolic actions of the various hormones are interrelated in a complex fashion. Not only are there normally occurring sequences of hormone release--for instance, feeding is followed by insulin release, and several hours later when insulin activity wanes, growth hormone is released--but the action of one hormone may enhance or block the action of another. For instance, the lipolytic effect of epinephrine depends on the presence of glucocorticoids (Skidmore et al., 1972) and insulin stimulated glucose metabolism in adipose tissue is increased by pretreatment with growth hormone (Batchelor & Mahler, 1972). Furthermore, metabolic effects of hormone may vary with the age of an animal (Miller & Allen, 1973). Eventually the analysis of hormonal modulation of feeding behavior will have to face such complexities.

EFFECTS OF HORMONES ON FEEDING

For a long time it has been recognized that endocrine disorders are accompanied by marked changes in appetite, body weight and the distribution of body nutrients. For example, juvenile-onset diabetes, maturity-onset diabetes, Graves' disease, myxoedema, acromegaly, Cushing's disease and various gonadal disorders are all characterized by relatively consistent changes in feeding behavior and body composition (Williams 1968; Zoudek, 1944). However, since most of the clinical literature concerning endocrine disorders and appetite changes is anecdotal, that material will not be discussed in detail. The following literature survey will deal primarily with systematic experimtental studies of hormone manipulations, feeding behavior and weight regulation of common laboratory animals. It is assumed that such basic physiological findings will often translate to the human condition quite straightforwardly.

Insulin and insulin deficiency. Since insulin is the prime controler of fat deposition and glucose utilization in the body, it is reasonable that it would also control feeding behavior. In rats, food intake increases approximately thirty minutes after injection of fast forms of insulin, at about the time blood glucose reaches asymptotically low levels (Booth & Brookover, 1968; Booth & pitt, 1968). Glucose administered in conjunction with insulin reduces the feeding effect, but nonmetabolizable sugars do not (Booth & Pitt, 1968). The most likely cause of insulin induced feeding is reduced intracellular energy production resulting from the precipitous fall in blood glucose. However, at the onset of insulin action, when blood metabolites are entering cells rapidly, intracellular metabolism should be increased, and it might be expected that animals would exhibit increased satiety. Indeed, a marginal augmentation of satiety has been observed in well fed animals during the initial half hour after insulin administration (Lovett & Booth, 1970). Insulin-induced feeding may thus result from "the hastening of the end of satiety, rather than the stimulation of a distinctive hunger signal" (Lovett & Booth, 1970). It should be emphasized that insulin-induced feeding may be unique to omnivorous animals, for insulin does not increase feeding in herbivorous creatures such as goats and sheep (Baile & Mayer, 1968; Baile & Martin, 1971).

Slower acting forms of insulin (such as protamine zinc insulin) have been used to make rats overeat for prolonged periods and become obese (McKay et al., 1940, Panksepp, 1973). In fact, long-term insulin administration is the easiest way to induce normal animals to voluntarily gain considerable extra weight. With the proper dose schedule, laboratory rats will gain up to 100 grams, primarily as fat, during a two week period. After termination of insulin treatment, these overweight animals reduce their weight to normal by voluntarily reducing food intake (Fig. 1.).

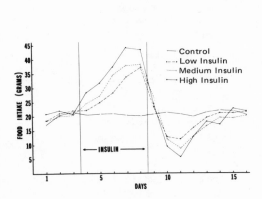

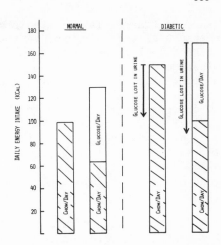

Fig. 1. Food intakes of rats in response to daily injections of the following dose schedules of Protamine Zinc Insulin: Low--2, 4,6,8,8 Units on successive days; Medium--4,8,12,14,7 Units; High--6,12,18,20,10 Units. During the five days of insulin administration controls gained 5 grams; low, 18 grams; medium, 48 grams; high, 64 grams (Panksepp, Unpublished data).

Fig. 2. Daily caloric intakes of normal and diabetic rats during access to just chow or chow + 5 and 35% glucose solutions. Each bar represents mean data for two day periods (Unpublished data, Panksepp & Meeker).

It is not yet clear whether the brief hyperphagia following fast acting insulin and the sustained overeating during prolonged treatment with slower acting forms of insulin are caused by the same physiological changes. Several lines of evidence suggest that different mechanisms may be involved. For instance, the facilitation of feeding by fast acting insulin declines markedly with repeated daily injections (Booth & Brookover, 1968), apparently because of depletion of adrenalin (Booth, 1970). Slower acting forms of insulin, however, can maintain overeating for weeks. While the mild hyperphagic effects of fast acting insulin are mediated primarily by a reduction of intracellular glucose metabolism, the prolonged effect of slower acting forms may be mediated by the profound shift of metabolism toward anabolic processes such as fat deposition and inhibition of fat utilization. In any case, it would be useful if future studies employed both short and long term insulin treatments to see if two modes of action could be dissociated.

Normally, insulin secretion occurs just after feeding (Fajan & Floyd, 1972; Steffens, 1970). Since insulin permits nutrients access to intracellular metabolic machinery, a normal role of insulin in controlling feeding may be the initiation of satiety after eating. This possibility has been tested several times with conflicting results. No decrease in the satiating effects of glucose, or the hunger inducing effects of 2-deoxy-D-glucose is observed in rats made diabetic temporarily with mannoheptulose (Panksepp et al., 1972). To the contrary, chronic streptozotozin diabetes reduces the capacity of small glucose loads to inhibit feeding (Booth, 1972), and alloxan diabetes prevents feeding normally elicited by injections of 2-deoxy-D-glucose in rats (Nance & Gorski, 1973). Although the effects of insulin on short term satiety remain ambiguous, diabetic animals clearly compensate for ingested glucose calories on a long-term basis (Fig. 2.).

Insulin may also prime feeding control systems in anticipation of a meal. Not only can sweet taste elicit the reflexive release of insulin (Valenstein et al., 1969), but the secretion of insulin can probably be conditioned to neutral stimuli associated with meals (Balugara, 1968; Woods & Shogren, 1972). Anticipatory insulin secretion may be the physiological basis for appetite wheting effects of cocktails and appetizers. Such early warning systems may not only prepare the body for forthcoming food, but also advise the regulatory system of amounts eaten prior to full digestion and assimilation of nutrients (LeMagnen, 1969; Nicholaidis, 1969).

Paradoxically, both states of high and low systemic insulin produce hyperphagia--like insulin treated animals, diabetic animals also overeat (Kumaresan & Turner, 1965). Of course, due to lack of insulin, they are unable to gain weight. It is unlikely that this overeating is due merely to the lack of insulin, for acute reductions of insulin with mannoheptulose and anti-insulin serum do not increase appetite, and may in fact reduce feeding (Anderson et al., 1963; Panksepp et al., 1972). Similarly, feeding is markedly reduced during the first few days after production of diabetes with alloxan (Kumaresan & Turner, 1965). Thus, it seems likely that diabetic hyperphagia reflects a compensatory response of the regulatory system to depletion of body nutrient stores (Panksepp & Nance, 1972) and energy loss in the urine (Fig. 2). As would be expected, diabetic hyperphagia is reduced by insulin therapy (Young & Liu, 1965).

Insulin and brain mechanisms. Insulin induced feeding probably reflects metabolic changes in hypothalamic receptors. Administration of glucose into the lateral hypothalamus of intact animals suppresses insulin induced feeding (Booth, 1968), and lateral hypothalamic lesions abolish the capacity of animals to overeat to peripheral injections of insulin (Epstein & Teitelbaum, 1967). Ventromedial hypothalamic (VMH) lesions do not impair feeding in response to a single injection of insulin (Epstein & Teitelbaum, 1967), but repeated daily injections are not as effective in producing overfeeding as in normal animals (Panksepp & Nance, 1972).

In general, the brain does not require insulin for transmembrane transport of nutrients. However, during the past decade it has become very clear, that discrete parts of the brain are insulin sensitive (Debons et al., 1970; Szabo & Szabo, 1972), and it appears that these areas of the brain participate in the control of feeding. For instance, gold-thioglucose has long been known to damage certain parts of the brain associated with weaknesses of the blood brain barrier such as found in the medial hypothalamus (Liebelt & Perry, 1967), and insulin appears to mediate the effect. Diabetic animals are relatively insensitive to the neurotoxic effects of gold-thioglucose (Debons et al., 1968), but sensitivity can be reinstated by injections of insulin either into the body or directly into the medial hypothalamus (Debons et al., 1970). However, several other hormonal manipulations (adrenalin, thyroxine, hydrocortisone) can also reinstate sensitivity in diabetics (Baile et al., 1971). Though this may indicate that insulin is not of unique significance to the function of medial hypothalamic metabolic detectors, it may also indicate how a variety of hormonal influences converge to modulate activity of feeding control networks.

Although it has traditionally been thought that medial hypothalamic glucoreceptors mediate short-term satiety by rapid oxidation of glucose (Mayer, 1955), it now seems more likely that this part of the brain mediates long-term regulation of energy balance (Panksepp, 1971). Thus, the insulin sensitive cells in the medial hypothalamus may provide a local brain storage depot for nutrients by which the brain takes account of deviations of body nutrient stores (probably fat) from a reference set-point level (Panksepp, 1972; Panksepp & Pilcher, 1973). In fact, it appears likely that the hypothalamus contains two glucose sensitive systems--an insulin sensitive one in the medial hypothalamus and an insulin independent one in the lateral hypothalamus (Smith, 1972). Of course, the lateral hypothalamic receptors could be indirectly affected by insulin when blood glucose levels are precipitously decreased.

Althought the normal function of medial hypothalamic glucoreceptors appears to depend on insulin, there has been little success in modifying feeding by direct administration of insulin into any part of the brain. Many have tried, but because of the general lack of positive results, detailed reports have not appeared in the literature. From the vantage that these receptors participate in long-term regulation of feeding rather than short-term satiety, we have injected insulin into the medial hypothalamus of rats repeatedly during the course of the day and measured overall daily food intake. The results have been mixed. In some experiments, feeding has been reliably suppressed after insulin injections into the medial hypothalamus, but in other experiments, no effect has been observed. We have been unable to identify the critical variables. They may be anatomical, temporal or artifactual. Hopefully, future research will resolve the issue.

Insulin and hypothalamic obesity. Until recently, it was generally believed that the VMH participates in the inhibition of feeding by sensing a satiety factor which builds up in the bloodstream
after feeding. But when Hales & Kennedy (1964) demonstrated that
hypothalamic obesity is accompanied by oversecretion of insulin, the
possibility arose that hypothalamic hyperphagia is merely a secondary consequence of hyperinsulinemia (Hustvedt & Løvø, 1972; York &
Bray, 1972). Indeed, ventromedial hypothalamic lesions do not produce any additional hyperphagia in diabetic animals (Goldman et al.,
1972, Panksepp & Nance, 1972; Young & Liu, 1965) this may only be
because diabetics already eat much more than normal animals. The
best way to assess the role of insulin secretion in the genesis of
hyperphagia would be to use neurologically intact diabetics, reduce
their hyperphagia with insulin therapy, and then inflict ventromedial hypothalamic damage to see if overeating still occurs. In
such animals, the lesions should evoke no excess insulin secretion.
Such experiments have yielded conflicting results. York & Bray
(1972) report that food intake of diabetic animals with medial hypothalamic lesions is directly proportional to the amount of exogenous insulin administered. It should, however, be noted that this
conclusion is inconsistent with some data presented in that article.
For example, it was also reported that lesioned diabetics receiving
either 2 or 4 units of insulin, eat reliably more than unlesioned
diabetics receiving identical insulin therapy (29.5gm vs. 20.6gm).
Friedman reports similar findings (Friedman, 1972). Furthermore,
by using a high fat diet to reduce the overeating of diabetes, Friedman also demonstrated hyperphagia in VMH lesioned diabetics receiving no insulin therapy. In general then, these data indicate that
VMH lesions can increase feeding without hyperinsulinemia.

It has been reported that vagotomy also eliminates hypothalamic
hyperphagia and obesity (Brooks et al., 1946; Powley & Opsahl, 1974).
Since the vagus mediates neural control of insulin secretion, those
results revive the spectre of hyperinsulinemia in the genesis of hypothalamic hyperphagia. It has to be remembered, however, that vagotomy produces extremely severe gastrointestinal disturbances (Alvarez,
1948). Here is one description of the "recovery" of 10 hypothalamic
hyperphagic rats after vagal transections (Brooks et al., 1946):
"Four of these animals died within two to three weeks. . . All of the
rats were ill for many days and lost much weight. They would endeav-
or to eat but the food would be partially regurgitated. In those
animals which died, the oesophagus was enormously distended with fluid and food and the stomach was flaccid and enlarged." Since VMH
lesioned animals are very prone to emotional disturbances (Wheatley,
1944), reductions in feeding after vagotomy may be the consequence
of many nonspecific mechanisms.

In summary, although hypothalamic obesity depends on availability of insulin, as do all other obesities, it is very unlikely that
hypothalamic hyperphagia can be explained merely in terms of a primary hyperinsulinemia. Possibly the most compelling evidence against

that explanation is the difficulty entailed in inducing normal rats
to gain much more than 150 grams with most diligent daily administration of insulin. It would be very unlikely that weight gains reported for hypothalamic obesity (up to 600 grams) could ever be achieved
by administration of exogenous insulin. Add to this the relative insensitivity of VMH lesioned animals to the appetite inducing effects
of long-term insulin administration (Panksepp & Nance, 1972), and
the probability that hypothalamic hyperphagia is merely the result
of a primary hyperinsulinemia becomes very small.

Glucocorticoids. In both normal and adrenalectomized rats, low
doses of glucocorticoids stimulate food intake and increase body
weight (Grossie & Turner, 1965; Hausberger & Hausberger, 1960; Hollifield, 1968), while high doses reduce food intake and lead to a precipitous loss of weight (Stevenson & Franklin, 1970). Thus, we
have a seemingly paradoxical situation where the body is depleted of
nutrient reserves but there is no compensatory increase in feeding.
In fact, high doses of the potent synthetic glucocorticoid, dexamethasone, prevent the elicitation of feeding and weight gain with
insulin (Fig. 3.). Possibly the extreme catabolic effect of dexamethasone produces such high levels of circulating nutrients that
regulatory centers controlling feeding mistakenly interpret the state
to represent recent consumption of large amounts of food.

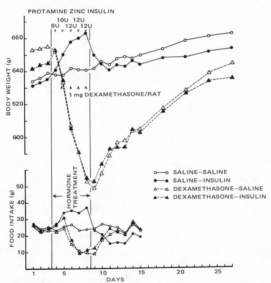

Fig. 3. Food intakes and body weights of rats receiving daily injections of insulin and dexamethasone (Panksepp, Unpublished data).

Why low levels of adrenal glucocorticoids increase feeding is
not clear. Possibly a low catabolic effect is translated accurately
as depletion of body nutrients, and feeding behavior is adjusted upward appropriately. Possibly the insulin resistance produced by glu-

cocorticoids leads to such vigorous compensatory release of insulin that insulin induced feeding occurs (Åkerblom et al., 1973, Hausberger, 1960). In any case, the normal daily release of glucocorticoids may facilitate feeding. In rats maximal corticosterone secretion occurs during early evening when feeding is highest (Galicich et al., 1963), and in animals allowed food or water only once a day, maximal secretion of corticosterone shifts so as to just precede the feeding period (Johnson & Levine, 1973). Both adrenalectomized animals (Grossie & Turner, 1965) and hypoadrenal humans (Williams, 1968) exhibit a decrease in appetite.

Adrenalin. Adrenalin injections can reduce appetite in many species (Russek et al., 1967). It is unlikely that this merely reflects the autonomic changes and weakness which adrenalin also produces, for doses which reliably reduce food motivation have little effect on behavior maintained by rewarding electrical stimulation of the lateral hypothalamus (Mogenson et al., 1969). Furthermore, it appears unlikely that the effects are directly due to calorigenic effects since noradrenalin increases body temperature and oxygen consumption as vigorously as adrenalin, but fails to reduce feeding (Russek et al., 1967). The effect may be due to increased intracellular glucose in liver (Russek et al., 1967).

Thyroxin. Prolonged administration of thyroxin markedly reduces body weight gain in rats, and the effect is larger in males than females (Grossie & Turner, 1961). In conjunction with the reduced weight, the hyperthyroid animals exhibit increased food intakes. This probably reflects a regulatory attempt to compensate for the extreme energy expenditure provoked by intensified body metabolism. Conversely, because of decreased metabolic demands, thyroidectomized animals can maintain relatively normal growth with reduced food intake (Grossie & Turner, 1965).

Growth hormone and hypophysectomy. In hypophysectomized rats, growth hormone increases food intake and body weight (Andik et al., 1966; Goldman et al., 1970; Pfaff, 1969). A similar pattern, though of smaller magnitude occurs in intact rats. However, because of the rapid growth during treatment, food intake with respect to body weight may actually decrease (Grossie & Turner, 1965). Animals with growth hormone secreting tumors also gain weight more rapidly than normal animals (Åkerblom et al., 1972). Of course, these changes probably reflect bone and muscle growth, for growth hormone treatment is a very effective way of reducing body fat (Goldman, 1973).

Growth hormone is usually released several hours after meals (Hunter et al., 1966) and during the first period of slow wave sleep each night (Parker et al., 1972). It normally makes fat available as a source of energy when other more temporary nutrient stores have been utilized. Accordingly, a hunger signal associated with lipolysis may be mediated by growth hormone (Kennedy, 1966), possibly via direct inhibition of the ventromedial hypothalamic "satiety" mechanism (Kennedy, 1966; Kurtz et al., 1972). Similarly, the avid eating of young animals may reflect chronic inhibition of the medial hypothalamus by growth hormone (Kennedy, 1957).

Glucagon. Glucagon can diminish sensations of hunger, gastric contractions, food intake and body weight gain in man (Mayer, 1960; Schulman et al., 1957). These findings are in accord with the function of glucagon which is to increase availability of glucose for metabolic purposes. Lesions of the ventromedial hypothalamus markedly reduce the capacity of glucagon to inhibit hunger contractions (Mayer, 1960). Whether the medial hypothalamic system which mediates glucagon effects on gastric activity is the same as that damaged by gold-thioglucose is not known.

Gonadal hormones. Mature female animals usually maintain lower body weights than males. In rats, this difference remains even when males and females are pair-fed with identical amounts of food (Kim et al., 1952). Although part of the sex difference seems due to intrinsic genetic factors, a considerable part of the difference can be explained by effects of neonatal androgen on brain organization and the activational effects of gonadal hormones on adult behaviors (Wade, 1972). Male body weight is decreased by neonatal castration and female weight is increased by administration of masculinizing doses of testosterone soon after birth (Bell & Zucker, 1971). Similarly, in adult rats, castration decreases and ovariectomy increases food intake and body weight (Kakolewski, 1968). These effects can be reversed by administration of testosterone and estrogen (Bell & Zucker, 1971; Mook et al., 1972). Similarly, treatment of normal female rats with testosterone induces weight gain and treatment of males with estrogen produces weight loss (Bell & Zucker, 1971).

Male and female rats also exhibit marked differences in taste reactivity. For instance, when allowed to choose between water and a concentrated (.75%) saccharin solution, normal female rats, but not those which have been masculinized at birth, exhibit a greater preference for saccharin than males (Wade & Zucker, 1969). However, this effect should not be interpreted to mean that females prefer sweets more than males. In reality, females may be less sensitive to the aversive aspects of the .75% saccharin solution.

It is possible that both the organizational effects of neonatal androgens and the changes which follow adult gonadectomy are ultimately mediated by biasing ventromedial hypothalamic energy regulatory mechanisms. Three lines of evidence support that conclusion. First, sex differences in food intake and body weight can be eliminated by ventromedial hypothalamic lesions (Valenstein et al., 1969). Second, after peripheral injections of labeled estrogen and testosterone, radioactivity is concentrated among other places in the arcuate nucleus of the ventromedial hypothalamus (Stumpf, 1970). Third, direct implantation of estrogen into the medial hypothalamus depresses food intake in a manner analagous to peripheral injections (Wade & Zucker, 1970). Although it has been reported that ventromedial hypothalamic lesions do not abolish the appetite depressant effects of estrogen (King & Cox, 1973), this failure may be due to placement of lesions so as to spare the periventricular zone where estrogen concentrates.

Progesterone and prolactin also participate in the regulation of body weight and food intake especially during the time of pregnancy and lactation when feeding is much higher than normal (Kennedy, 1953). Injections of both progesterone and prolactin into intact non-pregnant female rats increases feeding (Hervey & Hervey, 1967; Pfaff, 1969). No such effect is observed in males, though castrated males with ovarian transplants do become sensitive to the weight promoting effects of progesterone (Hervey & Hervey, 1965). In females the progesterone effect also seems to depend on the presence of ovarian estrogen since it can be eliminated by ovariectomy and reinstated with estrogen therapy (Roberts et al., 1972). Still, there is some doubt as to the absolute necessity of estrogen, since adrenalectomy can also restore progesterone sensitivity in ovariectomized animals (Roberts et al., 1972). This, however, may merely reflect improvement in the general health of the adrenalectomized animals (Ross & Zucker, 1974).

The mechanisms by which gonadal hormones come to modify feeding are not known. Although it is possible that these hormones directly modify activity of neural systems, it might be that their effects are mediated secondarily via changes in energy metabolism. For instance testosterone is known to promote fat deposition, while estrogen can inhibit the process (Cook, 1964). Oxidative metabolism in the limbic system is modulated by ovarian hormones (Martin et al., 1972). During the estrous cycle, changes in food intake parallel cyclic changes in glucose tolerance and plasma insulin. On the day of estrous, food intake is low while glucose tolerance is good; on the day of diestrus, food intake is high and glucose tolerance is impaired (Bailey & Matty, 1972; Taittelin & Gorski, 1973).

Gastric hormones. During and after feeding, release of local gastric hormones may modulate the decline of appetite. Enterogastrone, a duodenal hormone which normally slows passage of food through the gastrointestinal tract, has been reported to markedly reduce food intake of hungry mice (Schally et al., 1967), but this effect may have been due to the presence of polypeptide impuritites in enterogastrone extracts (Glick et al., 1971). More recently, cholecystokinin, another duodenal hormone released when food enters the small intestine, has been found to inhibit feeding in rats (Smith et al., 1974). Such local gastric factors probably control feeding on a short term basis, and it is likely that the regulatory system could perform quite adequately without them. They do, however, provide another early warning system by which animals can gauge energy intake prior to absorption and metabolism of ingested food.

FEEDING AND PUTATIVE NEUROTRANSMITTERS

In the brain, feeding is controlled by neural systems which employ biogenic amines such as norepinephrine, dopamine and serotonin as transmitters. This has been appreciated since the demonstration that feeding can be elicited in sated rats by microapplication of norepinephrine into the lateral hypothalamus (Grossman, 1962). That such systems actually participate in normal feeding is affirmed by the capacity of perfusates collected by push-pull techniques from the hypothalamus of hungry donor monkeys to elicit feeding when infused into the hypothalamus of satiated recipients (Yaksh & Myers, 1972).

Although it is likely that all of the aforementioned amine systems participate in the regulation of feeding and energy balance in some manner, adrenergic systems may be of cardinal importance in both hunger and satiety. In rats, feeding appears to be controlled by alpha-adrenergic "hunger" synapses in the medial hypothalamus, and beta-adrenergic "satiety" synapses in the lateral hypothalamus (Liebowitz, 1972). The appetite reducing effect of adrenergic stimulants such as amphetamine is now understood in terms of predominant activation of the beta-adrenergic "satiety" system. It is possible that the alpha-adrenergic feeding system arises from norepinephrine containing cell bodies in the periventricular zone of the third ventricle (Liebowitz, 1972) while the beta-adrenergic satiety system arises from brain stem neurons which contribute to the ventral noradrenergic pathway defined by histochemical techniques (Ahlskog & Hoebel, 1973). Overeating and obesity can be produced by destruction of this latter system. Still, this scheme may not generalize simply across species. Feeding can be elicited by activation of both alpha- and beta- adrenergic systems in sheep (Baile, 1974), while no evidence for an adrenergic feeding system has been obtained in cats (Myers, 1964).

Dopaminergic neural systems also participate in the control of feeding. Destruction of the ascending nigro-striatal dopamine system produces extremely severe anorexia (Ungerstedt, 1971). Since this neural system ascends through the far lateral hypothalamus, it seems certain that the loss of appetite after lateral hypothalamic lesions is at least partially due to destruction of ascending dopamine fibers. That dopamine concentrations in the hypothalamus increase following food deprivation, may indicate that increased activity in this system normally accompanies hunger (Friedman et al., 1973). Conversely, dopamine systems may also participate in the elaboration of satiety (Krug, 1973).

It is generally believed that serotonin systems exert little control over feeding. Still, several reports have found that injections of serotonin into the hypothalamus can increase (Jinger & Kelly, 1972) or decrease (Booth, 1968) feeding. Furthermore, as depicted in Fig. 4, inhibition of serotonin synthesis by daily administration of parachlorophenylalanine, reduces body weight of rats to a stable level about 25% below control levels (Panksepp & Nance, 1974). This weight reduction is similar to that following lateral hypothalamic lesions placed in the trajectory of ascending serotonergic fiber systems (Powley & Keesey, 1970). Accordingly, a serotonergic system may modulate the set-point at which body weight is regulated.

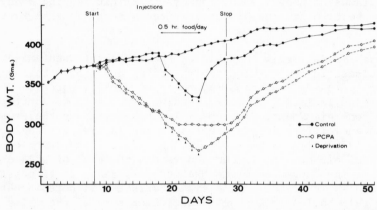

Fig. 4. Body weight changes during daily administration of PCPA. On the first day of treatment experimental subjects received 200 mg/kg PCPA intragastrically, and on each successive drug day they received 50 mg/kg. During days 19-24 half the animals were allowed food for only one hour a day. [Data from Panksepp & Nance, (1974). Reprinted by permission].

The analysis of how neurotransmitters and hormones come to modify neural activity is receiving a noticeable impetus from the discovery that many of these substances operate via activation of the intracellular second messenger cyclic adenosine-3' -5' - monophosphate (cyclic AMP). Cyclic AMP administered into various parts of the hypothalamus can both increase and decrease feeding (Booth, 1972; Montemurro, 1971). It is noteworthy that insulin is one of the few hormones that does not activate the intracellular cyclic-AMP mechanism, in fact it tends to reduce cyclic-AMP while promoting activation of the sister nucleotide cyclic-GMP (Illiano et al.,

1973). In general, cyclic-AMP is thought to antagonize the invigoration of metabolism which cyclic-AMP promotes (Goldberg et al., 1973) Thus, both in terms of behavioral action, as well as in terms of the intracellular second-messenger system, insulin has an action which is opposite to that of most other hormones.

HORMONES AND THE RECOVERY OF FEEDING AFTER BRAIN DAMAGE

Recently, it has been demonstrated that recovery of function after brain damage can be hastened by several hormone treatments. Nerve growth factor, which is structurally similar to insulin, reduces the duration and severity of anorexigenic lateral hypothalamic lesions (Berger et al., 1973). Similarly, pretreatment of animals with insulin prior to lateral lesions promotes recovery of feeding; while pretreatment with glucagon delays recovery (Balagura et al., 1973). In general, these findings support the idea that insulin, in addition to its well known metabolic effects, also enhances the differentiation and growth of cells (Krug et al., 1972). Further, other hormones which are capable of increasing intracellular levels of cyclic-AMP may speed repair to damaged neural tissue (Hier et al., 1973; Pichichero et al., 1973).

HORMONES AND THE GENESIS OF OBESITY

All known forms of obesity are accompanied by endocrine imbalances. The most frequently encountered changes are increased secretion of insulin (Albrink, 1968, Stein & Hirsch, 1972) and glucocorticoids (Coppinschi et al., 1966; Hausberger & Hausberger, 1960), and decreased secretion of thyroxine (Hinman & Griffith, 1973; Williams, 1968; York et al., 1972) and growth hormone (Miller et al., 1971; Woods et al., 1974) (Fig. 5.). Considerable controversy exists as to which of these changes are causes and which are consequences of obesity. Of the above changes, only experimentally induced increases of insulin (McKay et al., 1940) and glucocorticoids (Mayer et al., 1956) can produce obesity in animals. However, Glucocorticoids may provoke obesity secondarily by increasing insulin secretion. If a general hormonal cause of obesity is to be found it will certainly be closely related to deranged pancreatic function. The only hormonal change which is present in every known form of obesity is excess insulin secretion.

Of course, excess insulin secretion in obesity may merely be secondary to overeating. Normal weight people also develop high insulin levels when forced to gain weight (Sims et al., 1973). Furthermore, insulin levels decrease markedly in pathologically obese animals and men when food is restricted (Karam et al., 1965; Stern & Hirsch, 1972).

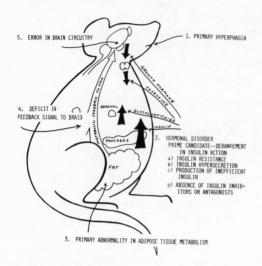

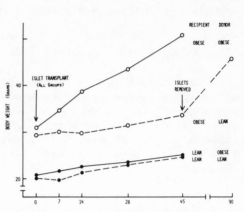

Fig. 5. A summary of the main possible causes of obesity. The most commonly encountered hormone changes which accompany obesity are indicated.

Fig. 6. Body weights of lean and genetically obese mice (ob/ob) as a function of days after transplantation of pancreatic tissue from normal and lean animals. [Data from Strautz, (1970). Reprinted by permission].

Still, it is generally believed that the high insulin levels of obesity reflects a basic biological dysfunction. One possibility is that certain target tissues are insensitive to the action of insulin and thereby hypersecretion occurs in a regulatory endeavor to stimulate cellular functions controlled by insulin. Such insulin-resistance may reflect a decrease of insulin receptors on cell membranes of obese individuals (Goldfine et al., 1973), and this may itself be a secondary consequence of derangements of other hormone systems. For instance, glucocorticoids (Goldfine et al., 1973), growth hormone (Emmer et al., 1971) and free fatty acids (Randle et al., 1966) all tend to decrease tissue sensitivity to insulin.

That many obese individuals exhibit normal glucose-tolerance curves (Albrink, 1968; Stunkard & Blumenthal, 1972) does not neccessarily mean their insulin sensitivity is normal. A deficit in insulin action may coexist with normal glucose tolerance. For instance, in large fat cells insulin binds adequately to cell membranes and allows glucose entry, but it fails to properly promote oxidation of the glucose which has entered (Livingston et al., 1972). This insulin-resistant state may reflect faulty transmission of the insulin

receptor signal to intracellular metabolic control mechanisms. The
ultimate cause of insulin resistance which so commonly occurs in o-
besity remains unknown, but it may well be that this is one of the
main sites of pathology which eventually precipitates overeating
and obesity.

The hypersecretion of insulin in some forms of diabetes may also
reflect the absence of systemic factors which normally restrain pancreatic insulin production or release (Young et al., 1969). The
normal pancreas may itself contain such inhibitory factors, for the
mere transplantation of normal pancreatic islets into genetically
obese mice (ob/ob) inhibits development of obesity (Fig. 6.), and
reduces the abnormally high glucose and insulin levels to normal
(Strautz, 1970). When the pancreatic transplant is removed, obesity returns. Unfortunately, these lucrative findings are yet to be
replicated.

HORMONES AND THE TREATMENT OF OBESITY

Clearly, obesity is not a single disease. There may be many
causes (Fig. 5.). It is unlikely that a single effective tretment
for all obesities will ever exist. Probably the only manipulation
which could conceivably reduce all forms of obesity is elimination
of circulating insulin. Without insulin, nutrients will not be
stored in adipose tissue effectively. Diabetic animals eat great
quantitites of food but lose weight. Unfortunately, the diabetic
"cure" of obesity is not compatible with good health. A more be-
nign method for restraining abnormal insulin secretion may, however,
prove extremely effective in controlling obesity.

A variety of other hormone manipulations lead to weight loss in
laboratory animals, but their effectiveness only in certain syndromes
highlights the existence of distinct pathogenic processes in different obesities. Adiposity in genetically obese mice of several strains
(NH, NZO, A^y/a) can be greatly reduced or eliminated by bilateral
adrenalectomy and hypothysectomy (Bray & York, 1971). Hypophysectomy is also effective in ob/ob mice (Roberts et al., 1972) but adrenalectomy is of little help (Naeser, 1973). Neither of these manipulations prevents hypothalamic obesity produced with electrolytic
lesions (Cox et al., 1968; York & Bray, 1972), but hypophysectomy
does markedly reduce obesity in gold-thioglucose treated mice (Herbai, 1970; Redding et al., 1966). A common feature of these manipulations, which may be the basis of the observed therapeutic effects,
is removal of adrenal and pituitary diabetogenic factors such as glucocorticoids and growth hormone which may be antagonizing some normal
metabolic effects of insulin.

Several exogenous hormone manipulations can also reduce obes-

ity. Administration of high doses of the synthetic estrogen, dieth-
ylstylbesterol (Montemurro, 1971), androgens (Kandutsch et al., 1972)
or growth hormone (York & Bray, 1972) markedly reduces hypothalamic
obesity in rats. Although low doses of cortisol do not reliably decrease rate of weight gain in adrenalectomized rats with medial hypothalamic lesions (York & Bray, 1972), it is likely that more potent synthetic glucocorticoids, such as dexamethasone, would reduce
weight in all kinds of obesity as readily as they reduce weight of
normal animals (Fig. 3).

Two kinds of hormone therapy--thyroxin and human chorionic
gonadotrophin--have been used widely in human obesities. Considerable controversy exists as to whether either is really effective.
Thyroid preparations have been used for fifty years as an aid to
weight reduction, because they increase metabolic rate and accordingly draw heavily on stored nutrients. The main drawback to thyroid therapy seems to be the sizeable loss of weight which is attributable to breakdown of muscle rather than fat (Bray et al.,
1973), but this shortcoming may be due to the exact manner the
therapy is employed (Lamki et al., 1973). Chorionic gonadotrophin,
a fetal hormone which supposedly permits the unborn child easier
access to the mother's stored nutrients, has been reported to be
effective in reducing weight in conjunction with a low calorie
diet. Supposedly the treatment promotes the ease and comfort with
which a low calorie diet can be followed, rather than directly enhancing weight loss (Gusman, 1969).

The future should hold more effective hormonal aids for weight
reduction. For example, during the past decade reports concerning
the possible existence of a specific "fat-mobilizing" hormone have
appeared in the literature with tantalizing persistence (Curtis-
Prior & Hanley, 1973), and if such a factor is distinct from known
lipolytic substances in the body, a very specific fat reducing
therapy may be developed. Likewise, with the advent of synthetic
growth-hormone production, the lipolytic property of that hormone
may be harnessed in such a way that undesirable diabetogenic side
effects are minimized. Further, hormone cocktails should come into wider use. For instance, fat mobilizing substances may be used
in conjunction with catabolic hormones such as thyroxine or phospho-
diesterase inhibitors such as theophylline which increase cyclic-
AMP in tissues. It is unlikely that a useful role for potent catabolic hormones such as glucocorticoids will ever be found. Adrenal
steroids have the undesirable tendency to precipitate psychological
depressions (Glasser, 1953), and their diabetogenic and anti-inflam-
matory effects would surely cause more ailments in the obese than
they would cure.

Presently, judicious exercise in combination with a controlled
diet remains the most effective form of weight reduction. In fact,
exercise may contribute to weight reduction by more than the mere

increase of energy expenditure. It is a common human experience
that moderate exercise can reduce hunger (Mayer et al., 1954).
Similarly, a well known laboratory curiosity is a reliable reduction in food consumption and body weight when rats are given access to exercise wheels (Stevenson et al., 1966). In addition to
direct thermal effects, it is possible that the reduced appetite
after exercise is also mediated by hormonal changes. Physical
training reduces levels of circulating insulin in both obese and
lean humans (Fahlén et al., 1972). This may be a secondary consequence of increased production of an insulin-like substance in
muscles. After exercise, blood nutrients appear to have readier
access to intracellular metabolic machinery. This insulin-like
effect is so potent that the ventromedial hypothalamus of diabetic
mice recovers sensitivity to the toxic effects of gold-thioglucose
after exercise (Baile et al., 1971). Unfortunately, exercise does
not reinstate sensitivity to gold-thioglucose in genetically obese
mice (McLaughlin et al., 1973). In fact, sensitivity is decreased.
This may indicate that exercise may be relatively ineffective as
an aid for appetite control in some forms of obesity.

ON THE BASIC NATURE OF FEEDING CONTROL SYSTEMS

    Although no definitive proof has been obtained, it appears
likely that the parameter ultimately regulated in energy balance
is the level of adiposity in the body, and that the control of
food intake is subservient to a process related to adipose tissue
metabolism. The most compelling lines of evidence for lipostatic
control is the consistent finding that fattening of normal animals,
whether accomplished by forced feeding (Cohn & Joseph, 1962), insulin injections (Panksepp, 1973) or electrical stimulation of the
lateral hypothalamus (Steinbaum & Miller, 1965), is followed by
compensatory reduction in feeding until the increased weight (primarily fat) is lost. The brain thus appears to be monitoring the
total amount of body fat or some correlate thereof. A striking
demonstration of this proposition is apparent in the parabiosis experiments of Hervey (1959), relevant data from which are summarized
in Fig. 7. When two normal animals are joined together, their body
fat gradually decreases to half the normal level during a 5-9 month
period. Further, if normal animals are confronted by the grotesque
fat stores (approximately 50% of body weight) of partners with ventromedial hypothalamic lesions, their fat contents dwindle to neg-
ligable levels, and most animals eventually die from apparent starvation. Although some more recent work has failed to observe the trans-
fer of any powerful "satiety" factor across the parabiotic union of
normal and VMH rats (Fleming, 1969; Han et al., 1963), it is quite
possible that the failure reflects major procedural differences. In
the unsuccessful "replications," animals were allowed food for only
10-15 hours each day rather than continuously, and the weight gains
of lesioned animals were markedly lower than those observed by Her-

vey (1959). More recent work confirms Hervey's findings. Parabiotic
union of two normal mice, or two genetically obese mice, suppresses
the normal weight gains of the individual animals (Chlouverakis,
1972) (Fig. 8).

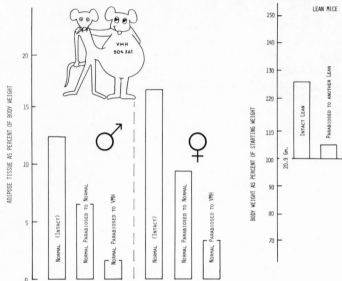

Fig. 7. Body fat of normal males   Fig. 8. Body weight changes of
and females parabiosed to either   genetically obese mice (ob/ob)
normal or hypothalamic hyperphagic   and lean littermates parabiosed
rats. [Data from Hervey, (1959).   to each other in all combinations.
Reprinted by permission].   [Data according to Chlouverakis,
                                     (1972). Reprinted by permission].

     That the intact organism monitors total body fat is further sug-
gested by findings that adipose tissue stores enlarge to compensate
for surgical removal of body fat (Chlouverakis & Hojnicki, 1974;
Liebelt et al., 1965; Schemmel et al., 1971). In some cases, though
not all, this recovery has been reported to be accompanied by increased food intakes. Recent work employing the parabiotic union
of genetically obese animals with lean littermates has clarified
the kinds of deficits which may characterize various forms of o-
besity. Pairing of genetically obese (ob/ob) mice with lean littermates reduces the weight gains of both animals, though the obese
animals are affected more (Chlouverakis, 1972). Again, it seems
that normal mice are affected by an abundance of a "satiety" signal
from obese animals, but the obese mice also receive some kind of
normalizing influence from the lean animals. As in Strautz's studies (Fig. 6), the normalizing influence may be related to pancreatic
mechanisms since insulin levels and sensitivity were markedly improved in obese animals joined to normals (Chlouverakis, 1972).

Apparently a different or more severe metabolic defect causes the obesity of genetically diabetic mice (db/db). The regulatory systems of both normal and obese (ob/ob) mice are savagely attacked when conjoined to that of a diabetic animal (Fig. 9). A potent "satiety" factor which diabetics produce, but to which they are not themselves sensitive appears to cross the parabiotic bridge to quell the appetite of the partners (Coleman, 1973; Coleman & Hummel, 1969). However, there also appears to be another "satiety" influence emanating from normals and ob/ob's which reduces the food intake and weight gain of the diabetics. Clearly then, both diabetic (db/db) and obese (ob/ob) mice are capable of responding to a normalizing regulatory influence which they supposedly do not produce within their own bodies. Conversely, both kinds of obese animals produce a "satiety" signal which is very effective in suppressing the feeding behavior of a normal animal, but which has less effect on their own regulatory systems.

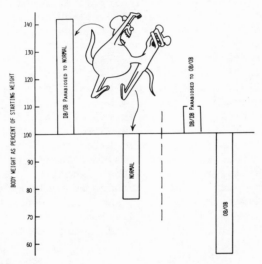

Fig. 9. Body weight changes of genetically obese mice (db/db) and lean littermates parabiosed to each other. [Data from Coleman, (1973) and Coleman & Hummel, (1969). Reprinted by permission].

Still, the nature of the regulatory signal which allows a normal animal to maintain a relatively stable body weight has eluded identification. It is generally thought to emanate directly from the adipose tissue mass of the body. Free-fatty acids may participate as a "hunger" or nutrient depletion signal since levels increase with food deprivation (Gordon, 1960; Walker & Remley, 1970). Hervey (1969) has proposed the the size of fat depots may be measured by a tracer dilution method involving steroid hormones. A constant amount of steroid, which is soluble in plasma and fat, would be partitioned in a fixed ratio between these two body compartments. Accordingly, the amount of hormone tracer in plasma would vary inversely with the amount of fat present. With food deprivation there would be a decrease in body fat, leading to an increase in the plasma concentration of the tracer and concurrent activation of hypothalamic feeding circuits. In addition to steroids, prostaglandins from fat stores (Baile et al., 1973) and the ratio between basal insulin and growth hormone levels (Woods et al., 1974) have been proposed as signals by which adiposity and feeding is regulated. Unfortunately, there is little direct evidence that any of these mechanisms actually mediates the regulatory impulse.

However, there are some logical guidelines as to what the general nature of the signal might be. As described by Hervey, a normal animal connected to another normal reduces its body fat to half the level it would maintain alone. It thus follows that in parabiosis, one brain is looking at the total amount of fat to which the bloodstream is exposed--viewing it as a unit though half of it belongs to another animal. This straightforward finding has one profound consequence: Whatever the regulatory lipostatic signal is, it is unlikely to be the concentration of a substance released continuously from the fat mass. Were it released continuously, the total signal strength after parabiosis would not be modified in either animal, for a constant signal from each animal would be diluted in the blood of the other. Even with complete mixing, this would still leave each animal with a normal concentration of the "signal" in its own bloodstream. In order for each animal in parabiotic union to perceive twice the signal it normally would, the "signal" must be released asynchronously in each animal. Thus when one animal is transmitting the signal, the other animal is probably not, and vice versa. Further, it would have to be assumed that the dose-response curve of the signal would be relatively flat so dilution between two bloodstreams would have little effect on effective signal intensity. Each animal could thus be exposed to its own lipostatic signal as well as to that of its partner. Such a pulsatile signal may be derived from the adipose tissue mass, for instance, as free-fatty acids or from a variety of correlated hormonal processes. For instance, the signal may merely be insulin which is secreted in response to the feeding of each animal. Conversely, it may be that there is no lipostatic signal at all, and the reason a parabiosed animal loses half of its body fat is because it is being stimulated more frequently by catabolic influences such as growth hormone which recruit body fat. But this specific possibility is unlikely because the "satiety" is transmitted from hypothalamic obese animals to normals and it is known that VMH lesioned animals have a severe growth hormone deficit (Bernardis & Frohman, 1970). In any case, Hervey's data which so elegantly speaks for regulation of body fat, does not neccessitate the conclusion that fat stores are in themselves regulated very precisely. Rather, the observed stability of the stores may be the consequence of a correlated process.

The reason identification of the regulatory signal which conveys information concerning body energy balance has remained so elusive may be because in reality no direct regulatory information about body fat stores is conveyed to the central nervous system. The regulatory signal may be elaborated entirely in the brain itself, and it may only be in dynamic nutritional balance with energy stores of the body. In other words, the hypothalamus, possibly ventromedial sectors, may keep a running tabulation of body nutrient transactions by local storage of nutrients and thereby modulate feeding behavior directly as a consequence of fluctuations of its own local metabolic processes. Accordingly, contrary to popular opinion, feeding would be the regulated process, and the stability of body nutrient stores would be a secondary correlate thereof.

There is evidence that just such a system may exist within the ventromedial hypothalamus. After administration of ^{14}C labeled glucose loads into rats, radioactivity lingers for a longer time in the medial hypothalamus than other parts of the brain (Panksepp, 1972). Furthermore, the retention of the label in the VMH relative to the rest of the brain is highest in a lipid subfraction, possibly indicating that hypothalamic cells are keeping a biochemical ledger of systemic nutrients transactions related to body fat (Panksepp & Pilcher, 1973). In any case, it is quite likely that the capacity of VMH cells to store nutrients reflects the same process which makes this part of the brain so sensitive to the cytotoxic effects of gold-thioglucose. Not only are both effects related to availability of insulin, but both are diminished by pretreatment of animals, with 2-deoxy-D-glucose (Likuski et al., 1967, Panksepp & Nance, 1974). Indeed, this medial hypothalamic nutrient uptake mechanism seems to be deficient in some forms of obesity. Gold-thioglucose produces smaller lesions in genetically obese mice than in lean littermates (Baile et al., 1970). This apparently reflects the presence of a functional lesion of the VMH since addition of a real electrolytic lesion has little additional effect on weight gain of ob/ob mice (Chlouverakis et al., 1973).

CONCLUDING REMARKS

Behind almost every basic scientific search lies a human problem --behind feeding research lie the riddles of obesity and anorexia nervosa. So far science has brought little substantial help to those who suffer from appetite disorders. However, the past few years have been full of promise. The solution to energy balance regulation seems within our reach. In fact, all the needed information to solve the puzzle may already be scattered in the scientific journals waiting to be gathered, milled, and leavened into understanding.

An appreciation of the relationships between hormones, feeding and metabolism will surely be central to such understanding. At a very general level, we can presently conclude that most hormones influence feeding by modulating intracellular energy metabolism, but the specific transducer linkages by which metabolic information is translated into neural activity remain unknown. Fortunately, we do know where to seek the answers. It is fairly certain that the cardinal interface between long-term body metabolism and brain activity resides with the medial hypothalamus.

On a conceptual level there is also reason for optimism. For a long time body energy regulation was thought to be a linear system whereby body nutrient stores transmitted a message of bodily nutrition to the brain. However, it is now possible that long-term body energy balance is organized in terms of a parallel circuit --ingested nutrients going independently to the body fat stores and to regulatory centers of the brain. If so, the development of effective therapies for obesity may be simpler than if regulation operated according to linear principles. Parallel systems can be manipulated independently more easily than serial systems. It would indeed be fortunate if changes in body weight could be dissociated from the regulatory distress of hunger. If and when that time comes, hormones will surely be among the medicines which make it possible.

ACKNOWLEDGEMENTS

Preparation of this chapter was partially supported by NSF grant GB-40150. I wish to thank Drs. Robert Conner and John Jalowiec for valuable criticisms of the manuscript.

REFERENCES

ADOLPH, E. F., 1947, Urges to eat and drink in rats. Am. J. Physiol. 151:110.

AHLSKOG, J. E. & HOEBEL, B. G., 1973, Overeating and obesity from damage to a noradrenergic system in the brain. Science 182:166.

ÅKERBLOM, H. K., MARTIN, J. M., GARY, G. L. & MOSCARELLO, M., 1972, Experimental hypersomatotropism II Metabolic effects in rats bearing the MtT-W15 tumor, Horm. Metab. Res. 4:15.

ÅKERBLOM, H. K., MARTIN, J. M. & GARY, G. L., 1973, Relative role of cortisone and growth hormone on glucose intolerance and insulin secretion in rat, Horm. Metab. Res. 5:34.

ALBRINK, M. J. (ed.), 1968, Endocrine Aspects of Obesity, Am. J. Clin. Nutr. 21:1395-1485.

ALVAREZ, W. C., 1948, Sixty years of vagotomy; A review of some 200 articles, Gastroenterology 10:413.

ANDERSON, J. W., KILBOURN, K. C., ROBINSON, J. & WRIGHT, P. H., 1963, Diabetic acidosis in rats treated with anti-insulin serum, Clin. Sci. 24:417.

ANDIK, I., SARDI, F. & SCHMIDT, P., 1968, The effect of growth hormone on feed intake and food selection, Acta Physiol. Acad. Sci. Hung. Tom. 29:177.

AZMITIA, E. C. & MCEWEN, B. S., 1969, Corticosterone regulation of tryptophan hydroxylase in midbrain of the rat, Science 166:1274.

BAILE, C. A., 1974, Putative neurotransmitters in the hypothalamus and feeding, Fed. Proc. 33:1166.

BAILE, C. A., HERRERA, M. G. & MAYER, J., 1970, Ventromedial hypothalamus and hyperphagia in hyperglycemic obese mice, Am. J. Physiol. 218:857.

BAILE, C. A. & MAYER, J., 1968, Effects of insulin-induced hypoglycemia and hypoacetoemia on eating behavior in goats, J. Dairy Sci. 51:1495.

BAILE, C. A. & MARTIN, F. H., 1971, Hormones and amino acids as possible factors in the control of hunger and satiety in sheep, J. Dairy Sci. 54:897.

BAILE, C. A. & MCLAUGHLIN, C. L., ZINN, W. & MAYER, J., 1971, Exercise, lactate, hormones and gold-thioglucose lesions of the hypothalamus of diabetic mice, Am. J. Physiol. 221:150.

BAILE, C. A., SIMPSON, C. W., BEAN, S. M., MCLAUGHLIN, C. L. & JACOBS, H. L., 1973, Prostaglandins and food intake of rats: a component of energy balance regulation? Physiol. Behav. 10:1077.

BAILEY, C. J. & MATTY, A. J., 1972, Glucose tolerance and plasma insulin of the rat in relation to the oestrus cycle and sex hormones, Horm. Metab. Res. 4:266.

BALAGURA, S. J., 1968, Conditioned glycemia responses in the control of food intake, J. Comp. Physiol. Psych. 65:30.

BALAGURA, S., HARRELL, L. & RALPH, T., 1973, Glucodynamic hormones modify the recovery period after lateral hypothalamic lesions, Science 182:59.

BATCHELOR, B. R. & MAHLER, R. J., 1972, Growth hormone induced enhancement of insulin sensitivity in adipose tissue, Horm. Metabl. Res. 4:87.

BELL, D. D. & ZUCKER, I., 1971, Sex differences in body weight and eating: Organization and activation by gonodal hormones in the rat. Physiol. Behav. 7:21.

BERGER, B. D., WISE, C. D. & STEIN, L. 1973, Nerve growth factor: enhanced recovery of feeding after hypothalamic damage, Science 180:506.

BERNARDIS, L. L. & FROHMAN, L. A., 1970, Effect of lesion size in the ventromedial hypothalamus on growth hormone and insulin levels in weanling rats, Neuroendorinol. 6:319.

BOOTH, D. A., 1968, Mechanism of action of norepinephrine in eliciting an eating response on injection into the rat hypothalamus, J. Pharm. Exp. Therap. 160:336.

BOOTH, D. A., 1972, Unlearned and learned effects of intrahypothalamic cycle AMP injection on feeding, Nature (New Biology). 237:222.

BOOTH, D. A., 1970, Effects of insulin on feeding in hypophysectomized and adrenal-demedullated rats, Horm. Behav. 1:305.

BOOTH, D. A., 1968, Effects of intrapothalamic glucose injections on eating and drinking elicited by insulin, J. Comp. Physiol. Psych. 65:13.

BOOTH, D. A., 1972, Feeding inhibition by glucose loads, compared between normal and diabetic rats, Physiol. Behav. 8:801.

BOOTH, D. A. & BROOKOVER, T., 1968, Hunger elicited in the rat by a single injection of bovine crystalline insulin, Physiol. Behav. 3:439.

BOOTH, D. A. & PITT, M. E., 1968, The role of glucose in insulin-induced feeding and drinking, Physiol. Behav. 3:447.

BRAY, G. A., MELVIN, K. E. W. & CHOPRA, I. J., 1973, Effect of triiodothyronine on some metabolic responses of obese patients, Am. J. Clin. Nutr. 26:715.

BRAY, G. A. & YORK, D. A., 1971, Genetically transmitted obesity in rodents, Physiol. Rev. 51:593.

BROOKS, C. M., LOCKWOOD, R. A. & WIGGINS, M. L., 1946, A study of the effect of hypothalamic lesions on the eating habits of the albino rat, Am. J. Physiol. 147:735.

CHLOUVERAKIS, C., 1972, Insulin resistance of parabiotic obese-hyperglycemic mice, Horm. Metab. Res. 4:143.

CHLOUVERAKIS, C., BERNARDIS, L. L. & HOJNICKI, D., 1973, Ventromedial hypothalamic lesions in obese-hyperglycaemic mice, Diabetologia 9:391.

CHLOUVERAKIS, C. & HOJNICKI, D., 1974, Lipectomy in obese hyperglycemic mice, Metabolism 23:133.

COHN, C. & JOSEPH, D., 1962, Influence of body weight and body fat on appetite of "normal" lean and obese rats, Yale J. Biol. Med. 34:598.

COLEMAN, D. L., 1973, Effects of parabiosis of obese with diabetes and normal mice, Diabetologia. 9:294.

COLEMAN, D. L. & HUMMEL, K. P., 1969, Effects of parabiosis of normal with genetically diabetic mice, Am. J. Physiol. 217:1298.

COOK, D. L., 1964, Steroids and lipid metabolism, Academic Press, New York.

COPINSCHI, G., CORNIL, A., LECLERCQ, R. & FRANCKSON, J. R. M., 1966, Cortisol secretion rate and urinary corticoid excretion in normal and obese subjects, Acta Endocrinol. 51:186.

COX, V. C., KAKOLEWSKI, J. W. & VALENSTEIN, E. S., 1968, Effect of ventromedial hypothalamic damage in hypophysectomized rats, J. Comp. Physiol. Psych. 65:145.

CURTIS-PRIOR, P. B. & HANLEY, T., 1973, A fat-mobilizing factor in rat serum, Acta Endocrinol. 74:409.

DEBONS, A. F., KRIMSKY, I., LIKUSKI, H. J., FROM, A. & CLOUTIER, R. J., 1968, Gold-thioglucose damage to the satiety center: inhibition in diabetes, Am. J. Physiol. 214:652.

DEBONS, A. G., KRIMSKY, I. & FROM, A., 1970, A direct action of insulin on the hypothalamic satiety center, Am. J. Physiol. 219:938.

EMMER, M., GORDEN, P. & RO, J., 1971. Diabetes in association with other endocrine disorders, Med. Clin. N. Amer. 55:1057.

EPSTEIN, A. N., TEITELBAUM, P., 1967, Specific loss of the hypothalamic control of feeding in recovered lateral rats. Am. J.

Physiol. 213:1159

FAHLÉN, M., STENBERG, J. & BJÖRNTORP, P., 1972, Insulin secretion in obesity after exercise, Diabetologia. 8:141.

FAJAN, S. S. & FLOYD, J. C., JR., 1972, Stimulation of islet cell secretion by nutrient and by gastrointestinal hormones released during digestion, Handbook of Physiology, Section 7: Vol. 1 Endocrine Pancreas. pp. 473-494, Am. Physiol. Soc. Washington, D. C.

FLEMING, D. G., 1969, Food intake studies in parabiotic rats, Ann. N. Y. Acad. Sci. 157:985.

FOOTE, W. E., LIEB, J. P., MARTZ, R. L. & GORDON, M. W., 1972, Effect of hydrocortisone on single unit activity in midbrain raphe, Brain Res. 41:242.

FRIEDMAN, E., STARR, N. & GERSHON, S., 1973, Catecholamine synthesis and the regulation of food intake in the rat, Life Sci. 12:317.

FRIEDMAN, M. I., 1972, Effects of alloxan diabetes on hypothalamic hyperphagia and obesity, Am. J. Physiol. 222:174.

FUXE, K., HÖKFELT, T., UNGERSTEDT, U., 1970, Morphological and functional aspects of central monoamine neurons, Int. Rev. Neurobiol. 13:93.

GALICICH, J. H., HALBERG, F. & FRENCH, L. A., 1963, Circadian adrenal cycle in C mice kept without food and water for a day and a half, Nature. 197:811.

GLASSER, G. H., 1953, Psychiatric reactions induced by corticotropin (ACTH) and cortisone, Psychosom. Med. 15:280.

GLICK, Z. D., THOMAS, D. W. & MAYER, J., 1971, Absence of effect of injections of the intestinal hormones secretin and cholecystokinin-pancreozymin upon feeding behavior, Physiol. Behav. 6:5.

GOLDFINE, I. D., KAHN, C. R., NEVILLE, D. M., JR., ROTH, J., GARRISON, M. M. & BATES, R. W., 1973, Decreased binding of induced insulin resistance, Biochem. Biophys. Res. Comm. 53:852.

GOLDBERG, N., HADDOX, M. K., HARTLE, D. K. & HADDON, J. W., 1973, In Proceedings of the Fifth International Congress of Pharmacology, pp. 146-169, Karger, Basel.

GOLDMAN, J. K., 1973, In vivo effects of growth hormone on in vitro adipose tissue metabolism, Hormone Res. 4:207.

GOLDMAN, J. K., SCHNATZ, J. D., BERNARDIS, L. L. & FROHMAN, L. A., 1970, Adipose tissue metabolism of weanling rats after destruction of ventromedial hypothalamic nuclei: effect of hypophyectomy and growth hormone, Metabolism. 19:995.

GOLDMAN, J. K., SCHNATZ, J. D., BERNARDIS, L. L. & FROMHAM, L. A., 1972, Effects of ventromedial hypothalamic destruction in rats with preexisting streptozotocin-induced diabetics, Metabolism 21:132.

GORDON, E. S., 1960, Non-esterified fatty acids in the blood of obese and lean subjects, Am. J. Clin. Nutr. 8:740.

GROSSIE, J. & TURNER, C. W., 1961, Effect of hyperthyroidism on body weight gain and feeding consumption in male and female rats, Proc. Soc. Exp. Bio. Med. 107:520.

GROSSIE, J. & TURNER, C. W., 1965, Effect of thyroxine, hydrocortisone and growth hormone on food intake in rats, Proc. Soc. Exp. Bio. Med. 118:28.

GROSSIE, J. & TURNER, C. W., 1965, Effect of thyro-parathyroidectomy and adrenalectomy on food intake in rats, Proc. Soc. Exp. Bio. Med. 118:25.

GROSSMAN, S. P., 1962, Direct adrenergic and cholinergic stimulation of hypothalamic mechanisms, Am. J. Physiol. 202:875.

GROSSMAN, S. P., 1972, Neurophysiologic aspects: extrahypothalamic factors in the regulation of food intake, Advances in Psychosomatic Medicine, 7:49.

GUSMAN, H. A., 1969, Chorionic Gonadotropin in obesity, Am. J. Clin. Nutr. 22:686.

HALES, C. N. & KENNEDY, G. C., 1964, Plasma glucose, non-esterified fatty acid and insulin concentrations in hypothalamic-hyperphagic rats, Biochem. J. 90:620.

HAN, P. W., MU, J., LEPKOVSKY, S., 1963, Food intake of parabiotic rats, Am. J. Physiol. 205:1139.

HAUSBERGER, F. X. & HAUSBERGER, B. C., 1960, The etiologic mechanism of some forms of hormonally induced obesity, Am. J. Clin. Nutr. 8:671.

HERBAI, G., 1970, Weight loss in obese-hyperglycaemic and normal mice following transauricular hypophysectomy by a modified technique, Acta Endococrinol. 65:712.

HERVEY, E. & HERVEY, G. R., 1965, The effects of progesterone on the body weight and fat content of castrated male rats bearing ovarian implants, J. Physiol. (Lond.) 179:20.

HERVEY, E. & HERVEY, G. R., 1967, The effects of progesterone on body weight and composition in the rat, J. Endocrinol. 37:361.

HERVEY, G. R., 1969, Regulation of energy balance, Nature 222:629.

HERVEY, G. R., 1959, The effects of lesions in the hypothalamus in parabiotic rats, J. Physiol. (Lond.), 145:336.

HIER, D. B., ARNASON, B. G. W. & YOUNG, M., 1973, Nerve growth factor: relationship to the cyclic amp system of sensory ganglia, Science, 182:79.

HINMAN, D. J. & GRIFFITH, D. R., 1973, Effects of ventromedial hypothalamic lesions on thyroid secretion rate in rats, Horm. Metab. Res. 5:48.

HOLLIFIELD, G., 1968, Glucocorticoid-induced obesity--a model and a challenge, Am. J. Clin. Nutr. 21:1471.

HUNTER, W. M., FRIEND, J. A. R. & STRONG, J. A., 1966, The diurnal pattern of plasma growth hormone concentration in adults, J. Endocrinol. 34:139.

HUSTVEDT, B. E. & LØVØ, A., 1972, Correlation between hyperinsulinemia and hyperphagia in rats with ventromedial hypothalamic lesions, Acta Physiol. Scand. 84:29.

ILLIANO, G., TELL, G. P. E., SIEGEL, M. I. & CUATRECASAS, P., 1973, Guanosine 3' : 5' - cyclic monophosphate and the action of insulin and acetylcholine, Proc. Nat. Acad. Sci. 8:2443.

JOHNSON, J. T. & LEVINE, S., 1973, Influence of water deprivation on adrenocortical rhythms, Neuroendocrinol. 11:268.

KAKOLEWSKI, J. W., COX, V. C. & VALENSTEIN, E. S., 1968, Sex differences in body weight change following gonadectomy of rats, Psychol. Rep. 22:547.

KANDUTSCH, A. A., COLEMAN, D. L. & ALPERT, S. E., 1972, Androgen effect on genetic and gold-thioglucose-induced obesity, Experientia 28:473.

KARAM, J. H., GRODSKY, G. M., PAVLATOS, F. C. & FORSHAM, P. H., 1965, Critical factors in excessive serum-insulin response to glucose, Lancet 1:286.

KENNEDY, G. C., 1966, Food intake, energy balance and growth, Br. Med. Bull. 22:216.

KENNEDY, G. C., 1957, The development with age of hypothalamic restraint upon the appetite of the rat, J. Endocrinol. 16:9.

KENNEDY, G. C., 1953, The role of depot fat in the hypothalamic control of food intake in the rat. Proc. Roy. Soc. Ser. B. 140:578.

KIM, K. S., MAGEE, D. F. & IVY, A. C., 1952, Mechanism of difference in growth rate between male and female rats, Am. J. Physiol. 169:525.

KING, J. M. & COX, V. C., 1973, The effects of estrogens on food intake and body weight following ventromedial hypothalamic lesions, Physiol. Psych. 1:261.

KRUG, U., KRUG, F. & CUATRECASAS, P., 1972, Emergence of insulin receptors in human lymphocytes during the vitro transformation, Proc. Nat. Acad. Sci. 67:2604.

KRUG, Z. L., 1973, Dopamine and 5-hydroxytryptamine inhibit feeding in rats, Nature (New Biology) 246:52.

KUMARESAN, P. & TURNER, C. W., 1965, Effect of alloxan on feed consumption in rats, Proc. Soc. Exp. Biol. Med. 119:400.

KURTZ, R. G., ROZIN, P. & TEITELBAUM, P., 1972, Ventromedial hypothalamic hyperphagia in the hyprophysectomized weanling rat. J. Comp. Physiol. Psych. 80:19.

LAMKI, L., EZRIN, C., KOVEN, I., & STEINER, G., 1973, L-thyroxine in the treatment of obesity without increase in loss of lean body mass, Metabolism, 22:617.

LIEBELT, R. A., ICHNIOE, S. & NICHOLSON, N., 1965, Regulatory influences of adipose tissue on food intake and body weight, Ann. N. Y. Acad. Sci. 131:559.

LIEBELT, R. A., & PERRY, J. N., 1967, Action of gold-thioglucose on the central nervous system, Handbook of Physiology. Sect. 6: Vol. 1. Food and Water Intake. pp. 271-285. Am. Physiol. Soc., Washington, D. C.

LEMAGNEN, J., 1969, Peripheral and systemic actions of food in the caloric regulation of intake, Ann. N. Y. Acad. Sci. 147:1126.

LIEBOWITZ, S. F., 1972, Central adrenergic receptors and the regulation of hunger and thirst, Neurotransmitters. 50:327.

LIKUSKI, H. J., 1967, Inhibition of gold thiglucose-induced hypothalamic obesity by glucose analogues, Am. J. Physiol. 212:669.

LIVINGSTON, J. N., CUATRECASAS, P. & LOCKWOOD, D. H., 1972, Insulin insensitivity of large fat cells, Science 177:626.

LOVETT, D. & BOOTH, D. A., 1970, Four effects of exogenous insulin on food intake, Quart. J. Exp. Psych. 22:406.

MACKAY, E. M., CALLAWAY, J. W. & BARNES, R. H., 1940, Hyperalimentation in normal animals produced by protamine insulin, J. Nutr. 20:59.

MARTIN, B., AGUILAR, E. & SCHIAFFINI, O., 1972, Oxidative metabolism of the limbic system in andregenized rats, Experientia 28:350.

MAYER, J., 1955, Regulation of energy intake and the body weight. The glucostatic theory and the lipostatic hypothesis, Ann. N. Y. Acad. Sci. 63:15.

MAYER, J., 1960, The hypothalamic control of gastric hunger contractions as a component of the mechanism of regulation of food intake, Am. J. Clin. Nutr. 8:547.

MAYER, J., MARSHALL, N. B., VITALE, J. J., CHRISTENSEN, J. H., MASHAYEKHI, M. B., & STARE, F. J., 1954, Exercise, food intake and body weight in normal rats and genetically obese adult mice, Am. J. Physiol. 177:544.

MAYER, J., ZOMZELY, C. & FURTH, J., 1956, Body composition and energetics in obesity induced in mice by adrenotropic tumors, Science 123:184.

MCLAUGHLIN, C. L., BAILE, C. A., TRUEHEART, P. A. & MAYER, J., 1973, Factors influencing the lesioning effect of gold-thioglucose on the ventromedial hypothalamus of bar harbor obese mice, Physiol. Behav. 10:339.

MILLER, E. A. & ALLEN, D. O., 1973, Hormone-stimulated lipolysis in isolated fat cells from "young" and "old" rats. J. Lipid Res. 14:331.

MOGENSON, G. K., RUSSEK, M. & STEVENSON, J. A. F., 1969, The effect of adrenaline on bar-pressing for food and self-stimulation, Physiol. Behav. 4:91.

MONTEMURRO, D. G., 1971, Inhibition of hypothalamic obesity in the mouse with diethylstilbestrol, Can. J. Physiol. Pharmacol. 49:554.

MOOK, D. G., KENNY, N. J., ROBERTS, S., NUSSBAUM, A. I., RODIER, W. I., III, 1972, Ovarian-adrenal interactions in regulation of body weight by female rats, J. Comp. Physiol. Psychol. 81:198.

MULLER, E. E., MIEDICO, D., GIUSTINA, G., PECILE, A., COCCHI, D. & MANDELLI, V., 1971, Impaired secretion of growth hormone in gold-thioglucose-obese mice, Endocrinol. 89:56.

MYERS, R. D., 1964, Emotional and autonomic responses following hypothalamic chemical stimulation, Canad. J. Psychol. 18:6.

NAESER, P., 1973, Effects of adrenalectomy on the obese-hypergly-cemic syndrome in mice, Diabetologia 9:376.

NANCE, D. M. & GORSKI, R. A., 1973, Effects of chronic diabetes on 2-deoxy-D-glucose induced feeding and drinking, Pharmacol. Biochem. Behav. 1:483.

NICOLAIDIS, S., 1969, Early systemic responses to orogastric stim-ulation in the regulation of food and water balance: functional and eleotrophysiological data, Ann. N. Y. Acad. Sci. 157:1176.

OOMURA, Y., 1973, Central mechanism of feeding, Advances in Biophys. 5:65.

PANKSEPP, J., 1971, A re-examination of the role of the ventromedial hypothalamus in feeding behavior, Physiol. Behav. 7:385.

PANKSEPP, J., 1971, Effects of fats, proteins and carbohydrates on food intake in rats, Psychon. Monog. Suppl. 4:85.

PANKSEPP., J., 1972, Hypothalamic radioactivity after intragastric glucose- 14_C in rats, Am. J. Physiol. 233:396.

PANKSEPP, J., 1973, A reanalysis of feeding patterns in the rat, J. Comp. Physiol. Psych. 82:78.

PANKSEPP, J., 1974, Hypothalamic Regulation of Energy Balance and feeding behavior, Fed. Proc. 33:1150.

PANKSEPP, J. & NANCE, D. M., 1972, Insulin, glucose and hypothalamic regulation of feeding, Physiol. Behav. 9:447.

PANKSEPP, J. & NANCE, D. M., 1974, The hypothalamic 14_C differential and feeding behavior, Bull. Psychon. Soc. In press.

PANKSEPP, J. & NANCE, D. M., 1974, Effects of para-chlorophenylalanine on food intake of rats, Physiol. Psych., In press.

PANKSEPP, J. & PILCHER, C. W. T., 1973, Evidence for an adipokinetic mechanism in the ventromedial hypothalamus, Experientia, 29:793.

PANKSEPP, J., TONGE, D. & OATLEY, K., 1972, Insulin and glucostatic control of feeding, J. Comp. Physiol. Psych. 78:226.

PARKER, D. C., ROSSMAN, L. G., VANDERLAAN, E. F., 1972, Persistence of rhythmic human growth hormone release during sleep in fasted and nonisocalorically fed normal subjects, Metabolism 21:241.

PFAFF, D., 1969, Sex differences in food intake changes following pituitary growth hormone or prolactin injections, Proc. 77th Ann. Conv. of Am. Psychol. Assoc. 77:211.

PICHICHERO, M., BEER, B. & CLODY, D. C., 1973, Effects of dibutyryl cyclic amp on resotration of function of damaged sciatic nerve in rats, Science, 182:724.

POWLEY, T. L. & KEESEY, R. E., 1970, Relationship of body weight to the lateral hypothalamic feeding syndrome, J. Comp. Physiol. Psych. 70:25.

POWLEY, T. L. & OPSAHL, C. A., 1974, Ventromedial hypothalamic obesity abolished by subdiaphragmatic vagotomy, Am. J. Physiol. 226:25.

RANDLE, P. J., GARLAND, P. B., HALES, C. N., NEWSHOLME, E. A., DENTON, R. M., & POGSON, C. I., Interation of metabolism and the physiological role of insulin, Rec. Prog. Horm. Res. 22:1.

REDDING, T. W., BOWERS, C. Y., & SCHALLY, A. V., 1966, Effects of hypophysectomy on hypothalamic obesity in CBA mice, Proc. Soc. Exp. Biol. Med. 121:727.

ROBERTS, S., KENNEY, N. J., & MOOK, D. G., 1972, Overeating induced by progesterone in the ovariectomized, adrenalectomized rat, Horm. Behav. 3:267.

ROSS, G. E., & ZUCKER, I., 1974, Progesterone and the ovarian-adrenal modulation of energy balance in rats, Horm. Behav. 5:43.

RUSSEK, M., MOGENSON, G. J. & STEVENSON, J. A. F., 1967, Calorigenic, hyperglycemic and anorexigenic effects of adrenaline and non-adrenaline, Physiol. Behav. 2:429.

SCHALLY, A. V., REDDING, T. W., LUCIEN, H. W. & MEYER, J., 1967, Enterogastrone inhibits eating by fasted mice, Science 157:210.

SCHEMMEL, R., MICKELSEN, O., PIERCE, S. A., JOHNSON, J. T., & SCHIER-
MER, R. G., 1971, Fat depot removal, food intake, body fat
and fat depot weights in obese rats, Proc. Soc. Exp. Biol.
Med. 136:1269.

SCHULMAN, J. L., CARLETON, J. L., WHITNEY, G. & WHITEHORN, J. C.,
1957, Effect of glucagon on food intake and body weight in
man, J. Applied Physiol. 11:419.

SCIORELLI, G., POLONI, M. & RINDI, G., 1972, Evidence of cholinergic
mediation of ingestive responses elicited by dibutyryladenosine-
3',5' - monophosphate in rat hypothalamus, Brain Res. 48:427.

SKIDMORE, I. F., SCHONHOFER, P. S., BOURNE, H. R. & KRISHNA, G.,
1972, Effect of adrenalectomy and cortisone replacement on
the lipolysis in fat tissue and fat cells, Naynyn-Schmiedeberg's
Arch. Pharmak. 274:113.

SIMS, E. A. H., DANFORTH, E., JR., HORTON, E. S., BRAY, G. A.,
GLENNON, J. A. & SALANS, L. B., 1973, Endocrine and metabolic
effects of experimental obesity in man. Rec. Prog. Horm. Res.
29:457.

SINGER, G. & KELLY, J., 1972, Cholinergic and adrenergic interaction
in the hypothalamic control of drinking and eating behavior,
Physiol. Behav. 8:885.

SMITH, C. J. V., 1972, Hypothalamic glucoreceptors--the influence of
gold-thioglucose implants in the ventromedial and lateral hypothalamic areas of normal and diabetic rats, Physiol. Behav.
9:391.

SMITH, G. P., GIBBS, J. & YOUNG, R. C., 1974, Cholecystokinin and
"Intestinal Satiety" in the rat, Fed. Proc. 33:1146.

SMITH, P. E., 1927, The disability caused by hypophysectomy and
their repair: the tuberal (hypothalamic) syndrome in the rat,
J. Am. Med. Association 88:158.

STEFFENS, A. B., 1970, Plasma insulin content in relation to blood
glucose level and meal pattern in the normal and hypothalamic
hyperphagic rat, Physiol. Behav. 5:147.

STEINBAUM, E. A. & MILLER, N. E., 1965, Obesity from eating elicited
by daily stimulation of hypothalamus, Am. J. Physiol. 208:1.

STERN, J. S. & HIRSCH, J., 1972, Obesity and pancreatic function,
Handbook of Physiology, Section 7: Vol. 1. Endocrine Pancreas.
pp. 641-651, Am. Physiol. Soc. Washington, D. C.

STEVENSON, J. A. F., BOX, B. M., FILEKI, V. & BOSTON, J. K., 1966, Bouts of exercise and food intake in the rat, J. Appl. Physiol. 21:118.

STEVENSON, J. A. F. & FRANKLIN, C., 1970, Effects of acth and corticosteroids in the regulation of food and water intake. Prog. Brain Res. Vol. 32 Pituitary, Adrenal and the Brain, pp. 515-152, Elsevier, Amsterdam.

STRAUTZ, R. L., 1970, Studies of hereditary-obese mice (ob/ob) after implantation of pancreatic islets in millipore filter capsules, Diabetologia 6:306.

STUMPF, W. E., 1970, Estrogen-neurons and estrogen-neuron systems in the periventricular brain, Am. J. Anat. 129:207.

STUNKARD, A. J. & BLUMENTHAL, S. A., 1972, Glucose tolerance and obesity, Metabolism 21:599.

SZABO, O. & SZABO, J., 1972, Evidence for an insulin-sensitive receptor in the central nervous system, Am. J. Physiol. 223:1349.

TARTTELIN, M. F. & GORSKI, R. A., 1973, The effects of ovarian steroids on food and water intake and body weight in the female rat, Acta Endocrinol. 72:551.

UNGERSTEDT, U., 1971, Adipsia and aphagia after 6-hydroxydopamine induced degeneration of the nigro-striatal dopamine system, Acta Physiol. Scand. Suppll. 367:95.

VALENSTEIN, E., COX, V. C. & KAKOLEWSKI, J. W., 1969, Sex differences in hyperphagia and body weight following hypothalamic damage, Ann. N. Y. Acad. Sci. 157:1030.

VALENSTEIN, E., WEBER, M. L., 1965, Potentiation of insulin coma by saccharin, J. Comp. Physiol. Psych. 60:443.

WADE, G. N., 1972, Gonadal hormones and behavioral regulation of body weight, Physiol. Behav. 8:315.

WADE, G. N. & ZUCKER, I., 1970, Modulation of food intake and locomotor activity in female rats by diencephalic hormone implants. J. Comp. Physiol. Psych. 72:328.

WADE, G. N. & ZUCKER, I., 1969, Taste Preferences of female rats: modification by neonatal hormones, food deprivation and prior experience, Physiol. Behav. 4:935.

WALKER, D. W. & REMLEY, N. R., 1970, The relationships among percentage body weight loss, circulating free fatty acids and consummatory behavior in rats, Physiol. Behav. 5:301.

WHEATLEY, M. C., 1944, The hypothalamus and affective behavior in cats, Archs. Neurol. Psychiat. 52:296.

WILLIAMS, R. H., 1968, Textbook of Endocrinology, W. B. Saunders, Co., Philadelphia.

WOODS, S. C. & SHOGREN, R. E., JR., 1972, Glycemic responses following conditioning with different doses of insulin in rats. J. Comp. Physiol. Psych. 81:220.

WOODS, S. C., DECKE, E. & WASSELLI, J. R., 1974, Metabolic hormones and regulation of body weight, Psychol. Rev. 81:26.

YAKSH, T. L. & MYERS, R. D., 1972, Neurohumoral substances released from hypothalamus of the monkey during hunger and satiety, Am. J. Physiol. 222:503.

YORK, D. A. & BRAY, G. A., 1972, Dependence of hypothalamic obesity on insulin, the pituitary and the adrenal gland. Endorinol. 90:885.

YORK, D. A., HERSHMAN, J. M., UTIGER, R. D. & BRAY, G. A., 1972, Thyrotropin secretion in genetically obese rats, Endocrinol. 90:67.

YOUNG, D. A. B., BENSON, B., ASSAL, J. P. & BALANT, L., 1969, A serum inhibitor of insulin action on muscle as a physiological control mechanism, Diabetes. Proceedings of the Sixth Congress of the International Diabetes Federation. Excerpta Med. Found. Intern. Congr. Ser. 172:248.

YOUNG, T. K. & LIU, A. C., 1965, Hyperphagia, insulin and obesity, Chinese J. Physiol. 19:247.

ZONDEK, H., 1944, The disease of the Endocrine Glands, Williams & Wilkins, Co., Baltimore.

CHAPTER 17

PINEAL GLAND AND BEHAVIOR

Roger A. Hoffman, Ph.D.

Department of Biology
Colgate University
Hamilton, New York   13346

CONTENTS

INTRODUCTION

Interest in and investigations of the pineal gland have waxed and waned over several centuries, but only in relatively recent times have convincing data been obtained hinting at its functions. Until the mid-1950's, the accumulated evidence was inconclusive, highly variable and often contradictory. From clinical evidence and various experimental studies, however, the consensus seemed to be that modification of reproductive activity was the most consistent finding following pineal manipulations. From anatomical considerations, expecially in lower vertebrates, and from associated experimental studies, it was also suspected, and sometimes demonstrated, that the pineal was responsive to changes in the photic environment.

Historically, the classical evidence required to label a particular organ as endocrine is the development of a specific set of abnormalties following its removal, the amelioration of these symptoms following its reimplantation into the organisms or following the administration of an extract prepared from it, and the subsequent isolation and identification of the specific compound(s) exerting the effects. On this basis, we still cannot state unequivocally that the pineal organ is endocrine in nature. Removal of the pineal in the higher vertebrates is not necessarily followed by a specific syndrome; effects noted have been inconsistent or species specific. The suspected biochemical products have not yet been isolated and definitively identified from blood, and administration of extracts or specific compounds found exclusively in the pineal have not yielded specific or consistent effects. Yet, in spite of these difficulties, the bulk of the evidence suggests that the pineal is indeed endocrine in nature, awaiting the necessary biochemical and physiological expertise, an appropriate animal model, and the specific set of environmental conditions for a conclusive demonstration. In the meantime, whether endocrine or not, whether sensory, secretory or both, rapidly expanding information focuses attention on this structure as probably posessing an important role in the adaptation of vertebrates to their environment.

At first blush, to include a chapter on the pineal gland in a book entitled Hormonal Correlates of Behavior seems a bit premature perhaps in view of a considerable paucity of published data on the subject or, at the very least, it shows a certain amount of courage or presumptuousness on the part of the editors. The rapidly expanding research efforts and literature on the pineal have focused on this gland as an endocrine organ having effects on other endocrine tissues, expecially the pituitary gland and more specifically on reproductive functions. Numerous recent reviews (Reiter & Frashini, 1969; Quay,

1969, 1970c, Reiter, 1972, 1973), two books (Wurtman, et al., 1968; Quay, 1974) and published symposia (Reiter, 1970; Wolstenholme & Knight, 1971) testify to the growing awareness of the pineal gland as a potentially critical modulator of endocrine activity. Yet, in spite of carefully collected and confirmed data showing specific and definite effects by the pineal gland in certain test animals under specific conditions, there remains a certain uneasiness on the part of many investigators that the responses measured may be once or twice removed from the main site of action, i.e., the effects which follow pineal removal, surpression, or stimulation may be but a consequence of a much more basic effect on higher centers, viz. central nervous system activity or sensitivity. Thus, it is not deemed premature to carefully consider the pineal gland as a potential modulator of neural activity. Enough data are already available to suggest that further investigations on the influence of the pineal gland on behavior offer considerable promise of significant and important information.

"From a phylogenetic point of view, few organs of vertebrates have shown such a plasticity of form and presumed function as has the epiphyseal complex. From paired, probably sensory, evaginations through the skulls of primitive vertebrates, the single remnant remaining in the higher vertebrates has evolved into a densely cellular, vascular organ with presumably secretory functions. Too few studies are available from throughout the vertebrates series to allow conclusions as to functions. Demonstrated effects on reproductive mechanisms, on phototaxis and pigment migration, on behavior, spontaneous activity, and a variety of other mechanisms are too inconsistent among and between the various groups to permit generalizations other than the likelihood that the epiphyseal complex directly or indirectly is responsive to some manifestations of light or its absence. Working backward from this assumption, it seems likely that the underlying activity of these complex structures will be a modulation of some basic, homeokinetic mechanism having much to do with the seasonal adjustment of the organism to its environment," (Hoffman, 1970).

At the moment, there seems little justification to alter, in any major way, the conclusions offered in the above quotation from a paper presented at the AIBS symposium in 1970. It will be the purpose of this chapter to look at the available information which supports the above generalization and specifically to review and correlate the evidence linking the pineal gland with neural activity and behavior. Effects of the pineal gland on other endocrine tissues and reproductive activities have been admirably reviewed in detail recently (see above references) and need not be repeated here. Behavioral changes as a consequence of variations in classical hormone balance are not considered germane to this chapter. Detailed information regarding the anatomy and biochemistry of this organ is likewise not considered pertinent to this particular review.

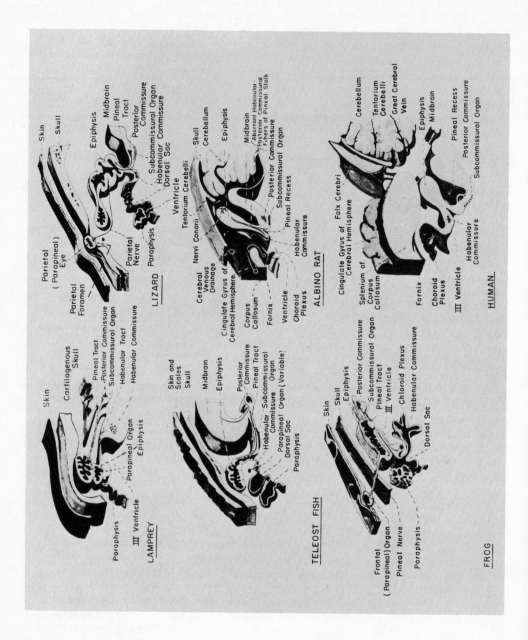

Fig. 1. (Opposite) A through F. Diagrammatic representations depicting longitudinal slices from the diencephalic roof region of the brains of several vertebrates. The facing surface of each slice has been taken at or near the median sagittal plane of the brain. Overlying cranial and/or integumental components are shown, particularly in relation to several pineal derivatives. These diagrams serve to illustrate the various pineal components as they appear in different species, their innervation, their vascularization, and their relationship to other diencephalic circumventricular organs. (Redrawn by Don Geyra from Fig. 1, The Pineal by Wurtman, Axelrod & Kelley, 1968, by permission of the authors and Academic Press.)

ANATOMY

In lower vertebrates, the pineal (epiphysis cerebri) is but one of several evaginations arising from the dorsal aspect of the diencephalon. The epiphyseal arch in the primitive condition gives rise to the anterior parapineal organ and the more posterior pineal organ. Generally speaking, the parapineal organ has persisted only in the cyslostomes, in certain reptiles as the parietal or "third" eye, and in amphibia as the frontal organ, while the pineal organ per se or portions of it has been retained in all species with a few notable exceptions.

A remarkable variability in form and structure is evident throughout the vertebrate species but the bulk of the evidence strongly suggests that in the lower forms, these two structures are sensory and directly responsive to photic input by virtue of classical photoreceptors, ganglion cells and neural fibers leading into the habenular commissure in the case of the parapineal organ and into the posterior commissure in the case of the pineal organ. Subsequent phylogenetic development has resulted in the apparent anatomical loss of the parapineal organ and the sensory function of the pineal, with a transformation of its proximal portion to a secretory body. Interested readers should refer to the published AIBS symposium held in Boston in 1969 (Reiter, 1970) or to the book by Wurtman et al. (1969) in which the anatomy and physiology of these structures are reviewed for all classes of vertebrates. The parapineal in various species has recently been reviewed and its physiological role as a monitor of solar radiation postulated in a fine new monograph by Eakin (1974). The anatomical differentiation and phylogenetic development of the epiphyseal complex of various classes of vertebrates is depicted in Fig. 1.

Fortunately, the pineal gland of most laboratory rodents is easily accessible, attached to the underside of the dura at the confluence of the superior sagital and transverse sinuses. The gland itself is connected via a stalk to the dorsal surface of the posterior commissure in these species. In carnivores, man and many other species, it has no stalk. Rather it lies deeply embedded, directly upon the posterior commissure and thus poses considerable surgical difficulties in studies where removal would be desirable without attendant damage to adjacent areas. In a series of South American bats from several families, the shape, size and spatial location of the pineal ranges from one extreme to another, even within the same family. In one species (Thyroptera sp.) no pineal was even evident (Hoffman, unpublished).

The technique of pinealectomy varies, of course, depending upon the species. In rodents, the technique we published in 1965 seems to be preferred by most investigators. (Hoffman & Reiter,

1965; Fig. 2). While rupture of the sinuses with concomitant bleeding is an unavoidable consequence of this technique, full apparent recovery is soon evident and the more laborious and time consuming procedures to avoid such vascular damage do not seem warranted at this time.

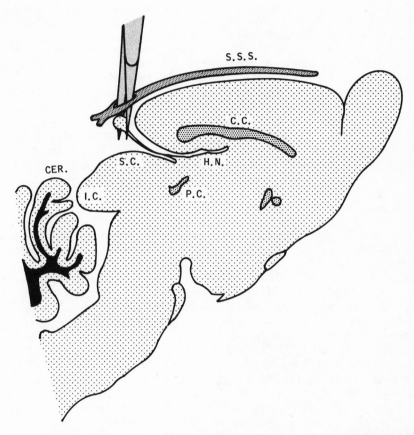

Fig. 2. Midsagital section through the brain of an adult hamster showing relationship of the pineal gland with surrounding structures and direction of approach for pinealectomy. CC, corpus callosum; CER, cerebellum; HN, habenular nuclei; IC, interior colliculus; PC, posterior commissure; SC, superior colliculus; SSS, superior sagital sinus. (Hoffman & Reiter, 1965. Reprinted by permission of the Wistar Press).

In careful studies made by Quay (1971a), section of the nervi conari, the sympathetic input to the pineal, or interruption of the tentorium cerebelli had no discernible affect on activity phase shifts

in rats. In a later report, however, he did find evidence that the
physical integrity of the cerebral meninges or the anterior dural
membrane was a factor to consider when activity entrainment to photic reversal was under investigation. Section of the pineal stalk
had only a transient effect (Quay, 1971b).

Over the years, a body of information has accumulated demonstrating that the pineal gland is responsive to photic information.
In rats, information on the daily photoperiod or the timing of light/
dark changes passes from the optic nerves into the inferior accessory
optic tracts, thence through the medial forebrain bundle and ultimately reaches the superior cervical ganglia (Moore et al., 1967).
From here, postsynaptic sympathetic fibers reach the pineal through
the paried nervi conari which enter the gland dorsally in association with the blood vessels. Thus, while the pineal of rats is derived from the brain embryologically, careful and methodical study
by Kappers (1960, 1965) indicates its neural input to be supplied
solely by the postsynaptic fibers from the superior cervical ganglia.

BIOCHEMISTRY

Historically, the function of the pineal has remained enigmatic,
due in large part to the fact that its removal does not necessarily
give rise to any consistent untoward effect and to the fact that any
presumed secretion is released in such minute amounts that it cannot
be easily detected in the blood. Indeed, a current controversy exists
as to whether the pineal secretes its products into the systemic circulation or into the cerebral spinal fluid of the third ventricle.
The early discovery of potent amphibian skin-lightening effects of
bovine pineal extracts, (McCord & Allen, 1917) and the subsequent
isolation and identification of the indoleamine, melatonin, (N-acetyl-
5-methoxytrytamine) by Lerner et al., (1958) which induced this effect soon opened the way for methodical biochemical studies on this
gland. Presumabley, melantonin has recently been demonstrated in
blood of chickens (Pelham et al., 1972) and possibly in humans (Pelham et al., 1973).

Biochemically, serotonin (5-hydroxytryptamine, 5HT), synthesized
in several steps from tryptophan, is acetylated by N-acetyl transferase to N-acetyl serotonin which is then O-methylated by hydroxyindole-O-methyl transferase (HIOMT) to melatonin. In mammals, HIOMT
seems to be localised almost exclusively within the pineal gland,
although it has also been reported in the Harderian glands and ret-
inae of rats (Vlahakes & Wurtman, 1972; Cardinelli & Wurtman, 1972).
In the lower vertebrates, HIOMT is more broadly distribued in many
tissues including brain. Pineal serotonin also serves as the precursor for several other indoleamimes, all of which utilize HIOMT
as the necessary enzyme for the final step on their synthesis. The
biosynthetic steps for these compounds are depicted in Fig. 3. Sev-

eral (N-acetylserotonin, melatonin, 5-hydroxytryptophol, 5-methoxy-
trytophol) show antigonadotropic properties in mammals. Indeed,
one (5-methoxytryptophol) appears to be at least as potent as melatonin in inhibiting gonadotropic activities (McIsaac et al., 1965;
Vaughan et al., 1972). Additionally, evidence is accumulating that
certain B-carbolines may be synthesized by pineal parenchymal cells
as metabolic products of 5-methoxytryptamine, 5-hydroxytryptamine
and melatonin. These compounds (6-hydroxytetrahydroharman, 6-meth-
oxytetrahydroharman and 6-methoxyharman) have definite neuropharma-
cologic effects at low doses and deserve careful study, expecially
by neurophysiologists and behaviorists.

Catecholamines, such as 3,4-dihydroxyphenylalanine (DOPA),
dopamine (DA) and norepinephrine (NE), are also found in pineal tissues and are obviously of considerable importance in its normal biochemical activities. Norepinephrine appears to be the neurotransmitter at the sympathetic nerve endings. Release of norepinephrine
increases and enhances melatonin formation apparently by stimulating adenyl cyclase which converts adenosine triphosphate to cyclic
AMP, the intracellular messenger of many hormones. Increased cyclic
AMP activity in turn stimulates the formation of N-acetyl transferase which then leads to increased melatonin production by a mass
action effect (Klein & Berg, 1970).

In addition to indoleamines, catecholamines and the B-carbolines,
evidence is accumulating that the pineal gland also synthesizes soluble proteins and peptides which may act as hormones or their precursors. A new monograph (Quay, 1974) has just been released on the
biochemistry of the pineal gland and should be referred to for detailed information in this field.

PINEAL-CENTRAL NERVOUS SYSTEM INTERACTIONS

Pineal extracts, melatonin

The early literature on pineal functions contains numerous reports purporting to show a relationship of this organ to brain function and mental health. This information, brought together in a comprehensive review by Kitay & Altschule (1954) pointed out rather
clearly the contraditions in the literature due to species differences and poorly designed or improperly controlled experiments. With
the isolation and characterization of melatonin and the subsequent
studies on pineal biochemistry from several laboratories, however,
much more valid data are now available lending substansive support
to the concept that the pineal may well have much to do with normal
neural activity.

Using bovine pineal extracts, Roldan et al., (1964) reported

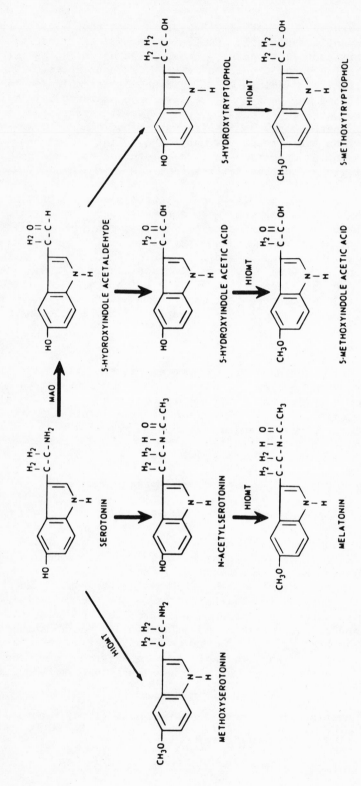

Fig. 3. Metabolism of pineal indoles from serotonin. Note that several pathways utilize hydroxyindole-0-methyl transferase (HIOMT).

a rapid (within 5 seconds after intravenous injection) increase in
frequency and voltage of the electrical activity of the paraventricular and periventricular nuclei which then spread to surrounding
areas and subsequently subsided toward normal by five minutes. Previously, Milcu & Demetrescu (1963) had reported that administration
of bovine extracts significantly modified the alpha rhythm in humans.
In a later study, again using relatively crude extracts, Roldan &
Anton-Tay (1968) reported that electrically-induced seizures in cats
were significantly surpressed within 20-45 minutes and this inhibition
persisted for as long as nine hours. Electroencephalographic (EEG)
tracings from several subcortical nuclear groups indicated the extract had increased the frequency but decreased the amplitude of the
electrical activity.

Crystalline melatonin itself has obvious effects on neural activity. Using unrestrained cats which had been chronically implanted
with stainless steel cannulae into several subcortical areas, Marczynski et al., (1964) recorded an obvious synchronization of the cortical leads, a remarkable increase in amplitude and a decrease in
frequency in the electrical activity when 15-30 μg of melatonin was
infused bilaterally into the preoptic area. [Note that these results
on electrical activity are contrary to those reported by Roldan &
Anton-Tay (1968)]. Associated with these electrical changes, the
animals lost interest in their surroundings, showed no reaction to
acoustic stimuli and promptly went to sleep. Similar but not so
dramatic effects were observed when the melatonin was infused into
the nucleus centralis medialis. No effects were elicited when the
brain stem reticular formation was the infusion site. The conclusions
drawn from this early report suggested that melatonin plays a neurohumeral role in the modulation of the states of wakefulness and sleep.
This conclusion was later shared by Barchas et al., (1967) who measured various physiological parameters following the administration of
huge doses of melatonin. While most measurements showed no changes,
consistently the hexobarbital sleeping-time in mice was markedly increased.

Later, Marini, (1961) also demonstrated that pentobarbitone-
induced sleep was significantly prolonged when male rats were simultaneously treated with melatonin or 5-methoxytryptophol. The effects
of either compound were dose-dependent. 5-hydroxytryptophol was
much less effective and serotonin completely so. Acquistition of
avoidance responses was unaffected by melatonin but extinction of the
learned avoidance response was significantly facilitated by melatonin.
It was pointed out, however, that this effect may have been mediated
indirectly by a melatonin surpression of pituitary adrenocorticotropin
secretion. De Wied (1966), for example, had reported ACTH to retard
extinction of avoidance responses. In young chicks, 2.5 mg of melatonin injected intravenously induced presumptive sleep (roosting) for
45 minutes, an effect later confirmed by Hishikawa et al., (1969).
In all these studies, however, it is important to be aware of the re-

latively huge, non-physiological, doses used. It has been estimated
for example that the pineal of rats contains only about 5×10^{-4} μg
of melatonin (Prop & Kappers, 1961), and a concentration of 0.2 -
11.5 μg/gm (Quay, 1974). Serum of chickens contains about 0.071 ±
0.007 ng/ml at night, and only about 0.002 ng/ml in mid-day (Pelham
et al., 1971, 1972).

In humans also, melatonin has been demonstrated to effect central nervous system activity and indeed even ameliorate some of the
symptoms of epilepsy and Parkinson's disease. In these studies,
Anton-Tay and colleagues (1971), administered 0.25 to 1.25 mg melatonin intravenously. In normal males and females, aged 18-25 years,
an increase in percentage and amplitude of alpha rhythm occurred as
well as abundant and vivid oniric episodes during the ensuing sleep.
On arousal, which was easily induced at 45 minutes, they reported a
sensation of well-being and moderate eleation. Five of the eleven
subjects experienced visual imagery. In epileptic patients, similar
behavioral and EEG results occurred with doses of 1.25 mg. In addition, rapid eye movement (REM) was quite evident during the sleep
as well as relaxation of the neck muscles. Paroxistic EEG activity
was markedly depressed for four hours following treatment. Two patients with advanced Parkinson's disease (stages 4,5), aged 69 and
71 years, received melatonin orally for four weeks, (1.2 gm/day)
followed by placebo. As the treatment progressed, the patients reported feelings of well-being associated with improvements in performance of daily tasks. By the third week, the chairbound patient
could walk and both patients showed marked improvement in the total
clinical picture. Rigidity and tremors decreased while sleep habits
were generally unaffected. The clinical improvement was paralleled
by improvement in the EEG tracings. Substitution of melatonin with
placebo was followed by a gradual return to the classical symptoms
of the disease. Briefly, the results from this study show melatonin
to slow EEG rhythm, increase REM and increase seizure-thresholds without gross deterioration of brain function.

There is now considerable evidence that brain catecholamines
and serotonin are involved with sleep-wakefullness cycles and also
that serotonin and γ-aminobutyric acid (GABA) have effects on seizure thresholds. It is known that serotonin is widely distributed
in the brain both in the serotonergic cell bodies in the midbrain
and within their peripheral nerve endings in the hypothalamus and
elsewhere. In a study of the effects of melatonin on brain serotonin,
Anton-Tay et al., (1968) showed that 150 μg intravenously decreased
serotonin concentrations in the cerebral cortex by 20 and 60 minutes
while that in the hypothalamus and midbrain increased. At 180 minutes, midbrain levels were still high while normal values were once
agin evident in the other two regions. Significantly, tritiated
melatonin has been shown to be selectively taken up by the midbrain
and hypothalamus (Anton-Tay & Wurtman, 1969) as well as in the pineal

gland itself. Significantly also, melatonin induces highly significant increases in brain pyridoxal phosphokinase, the enxyme which
catalyses the formation of pyridoxal phosphate in the brain (Anton-
Tay et al., 1970). Pyridoxal phosphate is a necessary cofactor for
the synthesis of 5-HT, DA and GABA. GABA is reported to double in
hypothalamic concentration in rabbits and to increase significantly
in the cortex as well following the intraperitoneal administration
of 50 μg/kg melatonin (Anton-Tay, 1971). In view of the known inhibitory effects of GABA on exitability of certain brain structures
and the apparent involvement of serotonin in sleep phenomena, it
seems logical to suggest that the pineal gland may have more than
a casual or coincidental relationship with these potent brain con-
stitiuents and their concentrations and activities.

Pinealectomy

     If the pineal gland is a modulator of nervous activity, then
its removal would be expected to modify behavior either directly or
indirectly. That this is the case is evident from the following reported data.

     Pinealectomy in rabbits is reported to be followed by convul-
sive electrical activity in the dorsal hippocampal neurons when the
contralateral side is stimulated. Intact animals showed no such hyperactivity (Bindoni & Rizzo, 1965). In 1969, Nir and colleagues
measured EEG activity of pinealectonized female rats in the arly
afternoon of the day of estrus two weeks after recovery from the
surgery. Control recordings were made on the same animals prior to
pinealectomy. The monopolar ball electrodes were placed on the dura
mater of the cortex in the left and right anterior and posterior areas.
Briefly, the recordings indicated that lack of the pineal gland was
associated with a shift to higher frequency, lower amplitude waves
and other manifestations indicative of alertness with intermittant
general paroxysmal outbursts of slow waves with high frequency of
centrocephalic origin. The authors suggested that because of the
state of constant estrus induced by pinealectomy, it was possible
that the effects were due to overactivity of the gonads and the subsequent increased estrogen levels. Later, Behroozi et al. (1970)
reported that time of death following lethal doses of sodium pentobarbital was significantly delayed in pinealectomized rats.

     Perhaps, the most interesting and potentially important clues
regarding pineal-brain relationships are found in a series of recent
reports by Reiter and his colleagues. In a study of the potential
influence of the thyroid gland on the antigonadal activity of the
pineal gland, rats were thyroidectomized and then pinealectomized
one week later. Surprisingly, many of these dually-operated animals
went into convulsive seizures within 4-8 hours after pinealectomy with
a mortality due to asphyxiation of about 50 percent within 48 hours

(Reiter et al., 1972). Subsequently, it was found that it was the
loss of the parathyroid gland alone which predisposed these animals
to seizures following pinealectomy (Reiter & Morgan, 1972), although
involvement of the thyroid was later suggested (Pomerantz & Reiter,
1973). Additional studies demonstrated that transection of the nervi
conari or removal of the superior cervical ganglia did not induce
seizures in previously parathyroidectomized animals. Convulsed animals
had unchanged brain concentrations of serotonin and dopamine but
norepinephrine levels were decreased. Convulsions were temporarily
inhibited by treatment with diazepam or chlordiazepoxide but not by
diphenylhydantion nor calcium lactate (Reiter & Morgan, 1972; Reiter
et al., 1973). Age of the animals did not affect the development of
seizures although the time of onset was delayed (Pomerantz & Reiter,
1973). The temporal sequence of the operations appears to important,
i.e., pinealectomy followed by parathyroidectomy one week later was
not followed by seizures.

    Since epileptiform seizures did not follow denervation of the
pineal gland, it must be concluded that the pineal gland modulates
the sensitivity or threshold of the neurons associated with the seizures by a mechanism exclusive of any peripheral neural input. Since
there are no known nerves from the pineal to the brain in these mamals (Kappers, 1965), we must conclude that its anticonvulsive activity is humeral in nature, the release of which is also regulated by
circulating chemical compounds. It is tempting to suggest that the
anticonvulsant substance in question is melatonin since it is known
to exhibit a circadian rhythm in total darkness (Ralph et al., 1971)
as well as in alternating light/dark cycles, thus displaying endogenous secretion in the absense of neural input. As noted above,
melatonin has inhibitory effects on certain areas of central nervous
system activity. Parenthetically, we have preliminary data from this
laboratory showing that melatonin also surpresses seizures in mice
susceptible to audiogenic seizures.

    The mechanism by which the dual operation induces convulsions
is far from clear, however. Generally, we know that the parathyroid
glands are primarily involved in the regulation of blood/bone calcium
and phosporus levels. Infusions of calcium had no ameliorating affects on the onset of convulsions. It seems unlikely that phosporus
levels are the predisposing condition necessary for seizure-induction.
Consequently, studies on the role of the parathyroid glands in brain
activity and the interaction of pineal/parathyroid glands seem war-
rarnted. It is known that parathyroidectomy is followed by heightened
neural activity. Significantly, loss of the pineal gland in sodium-
deficient rats consistently leads to small but significant decreases
in cerebral concentrations of potassium which could have profound effects on neural thresholds (Quay, 1969). Since this effect was duplicated by exposing the rats to constant light, it might be suspected
that peripheral input via the superior cervical ganglia was involved,

a condition not apparent in the parathyroidectomized/pinealectomized animal model as described by Reiter and colleagues.

It is interesting that parathyroidectomy must precede pineal-ectomy for convulsive activity to occur. This suggests that the af-fected neurons can adapt to the absence of pineal hormones, perhaps by shifting metabolic and biochemical activities through alternate enzymatic pathways. Similar adaptation to the loss of the parathy-roid secretion apparently does not occur.

It is not the purpose of this chapter to review the huge liter-ature linking the pineal gland to endocrine activities. It is suf-ficient to say that at least one locus for these affects appears to be on the hypothalamus and subsequently on the pituitary gland. More specifically, inhibitory influences on gonadotropins are well dem-onstrated (Reiter, 1972) with similar but perhaps not so dramatic nor consistent effects reported for the synthesis or release of other pituitary hormones. These data suggest that a site of action for the pineal secretion is likely to be on the neurons or terminals responsi-ble for the hypothalamic releasing or inhibiting factors. Signifi-cantly, Reiter & Sorrentino (1972) have reported that total or anteri-or hypothalamic deafferentation ("central sympathectomy") with the use of the Haláz brain knife prevents the gonadal atrophy that normally follows blinding in hamsters i.e., the effect of this operation is similar to the effects following pinealectomy in blinded animals. Presumabley, hypothalamic deafferentation results in a loss of sero-tonin- and catecholamine-rich terminals. The similarity of pineal-ectomy and deafferentation suggests that certain aminergic neurons may be a primary target site for pineal principles.

BEHAVIOR

Wheel Running Activity

It is well documented that given access to an activity wheel, most species spend a considerable portion of their daily active phase running in it. The timing of onset and termination of running are synchronized with onset and termination of light/dark input or in the absence of these daily cues (Zeitgebers), they may utilize tem-perature changes, social cues, or other periodic phenomena. In the absence of all cues, their cycles tend to free run with periods of about 24 hours (circadian).

The neural components responsible for the snychronization of these activity cycles to the environmental photoperiods or, in their absence, to maintain the endogenous rhythms are unknown. Undoubted-ly, however, they are the end result of a multitude of independent and interrelated component rhythms, the product or summation of which determines the neural output in terms of general spontaneous activity. Early reports on the influence of the pineal gland on activity cycles revealed a lack of consistent effects. Wong & Whiteside (1968), for example, reported a transient decrease in activity after administration of melatonin. Earlier, Reiss et al., (1963) had obtained similar effects with injections of pineal protein-free extracts. But other information was published showing a lack of effect by pinealectomy on locomotor activity of rats in cyclic or constant lighting conditions (Quay, 1965, 1968; Relkin, 1970). Menaker (1968) and Gaston & Menaker (1968) reported, however, that such operations modified circadian rhythms of locomotor activity of sparrows. In pinealectomized leghorn pullets, on the other hand, pinealectomy did not seem to affect circadian rhythms of oviposition (Harrison & Becker, 1969). However, in a series of later reports on phase shifting of activity rhythms in rats, Quay (1970a, 1970b) demonstrated that the pineal is indeed involved. Pinealectomized animals exposed to sudden reversal of light/dark schedules showed a precocious rate of phase-shifting as compared to sham-operated animals. Such differences were limited to the transient period between photoperiod reversal and entrainment to the new schedules, i.e., the efficiency of activity phase reversal in response to reversed photoperiod was greater in pinealectomized animals. Similar results were also reported by Kincl et al. (1970) who postulated that the pineal served as a "brake" on neural activity thereby preventing an easily attained asychrony with other light-dependent circadian rhythms such as are known to exist in brain, adrenal and thyroid glands. On the basis of his data, Quay (1970b) postulated a central interaction or counterbalancing of homeostatic or circadian mechanisms and peripheral input from cyclic zeitgebers. Removal of the pineal would tend to weaken the relative strength of the central homeostatic mechanism (or decrease the threshold to sensory input) thus favoring a more rapid or marked response to central/environmental asynchrony.

It is pertinent that many metabolic activities within the pineal gland show dramatic circadian rhythms of high amplitude. Norepinephrine, serotonin, melatonin and their requisite enzymes and precursors, total portein, RNA, lipids, nuclear and nucleolar size and a vareity of other components undergo dramatic daily fluctuations which may have much to do with certain behavioral differences so often reported in animals when tested at different times of day or night. The evidence suggests temporal differences in the peaks and troughs of these cycles between diurnal and nocturnal animals. Quay, in his recent book (1974), has brought these data together and charted the temporal sequencing of cellular and metabolic circadian rhythms within the pineal gland of the adult white rat. A review of this excellent monograph is highly recommended.

Sexual Activity

It has been well documented that neontal or prepubertal pineal-ectomy induces precocious sexual maturation while pineal extracts or melatonin can delay puberty by some days. Changes in sexual behavior are also a manifestation of pineal manipulations. Baum (1968), for example, reported that male hooded rats, pinealectomized at three days of age, maintained in total darkness and tested every four days after weaning, mounted receptive females more frequently and showed pelvic thrusting at an earlier age than their littermate, sham-oper-ated controls. After 42 days however, these differences disappeared.

In a later study, however, Tagliamonte et al., (1969) reported that the intense sexual excitement in adult male rats following treat-ment with p-chlorophenylalanine with or without pargyline was unaf-fected by prior pinealectomy. From these reports, it would appear that any influence of the pineal on sexual behavior is restricted to pre-pubertal animals and is an effect by virture of precocious sexual development and the subsequent modification of sex hormone levels which modify neural thresholds to those conditions eliciting copula-tory behavior.

Exploratory Behavior

Recently, Sampson & Bigelow (1971) tested open field explora-tory activity in 80-day-old female rats pinealectomized neonatally or treated with aqueous non-melatonin-containing pineal extracts or with physiological doses of melatonin. The results seem to demon-strate unequivocally that pineal ablation increases exploratory activ-ity under the experimental conditions posed while the pineal extract decreased it. Surprisingly, melatonin per se had no effect. Earlier, Stebbins (1960) removed the pineal body of the lizard (S. occidentalis) while attempting to leave the nerves from the parapineal organ intact. He reported marked fright reactions in these animals compared to con-trols or parietalectomized animals as well as increased locomotor activity and a three-fold increase in home-range.

Ethanol Preference

Exposure of rats to prolonged periods of darkness induces ethanol preference as compared to animals exposed to standard laboratory light-ing conditions (Geller, 1971; Blum et al., 1973). Since darkness en-hances pineal biosynthetic activities, it might be suspected that pineal indoleamines might have some influence on this particular ap-petite. Subsequently, data have been obtained confirming such a sup-position viz., melatonin (and a β-carboline, 1-methyl-6-methoxy-1,2,3,

4,-tetrahydro-2-carboline) enhanced ethanol preference in rats (Geller, 1971; Geller et al., 1973).

Recently, pineal involvement was found to be the case also in the golden hamster using the 3-bottle, 2-choice method of Myers & Holman, (1966). Reiter et al., (1974) found that by six weeks after pinealectomy, ethanol preference was significantly lower than that exhibited by sham-operated animals. Blinding of these animals did not change ethanol preference in the shamoperated group nor modify the lowered preference in the pinealectomized animals. Daily administration of large doses of melatonin to these animals had no effect. Water intake was unaffected by any treatment.

In further studies, these results were confimed, i.e., pineal ablation consistently reduced alcohol preference in blinded hamsters. The effect could also be duplicated by superior cervical ganglionectomy which effectively removes sensory input to the pineal gland. Thus dark-induced ethanol preference in the rat (Baum et al., 1973) and hamster seems to be modulated by pineal influence. Melatonin may be the active component in rats but not in hamsters. Indeed, a conclusive effect of melatonin administration on any parameter in hamsters has yet to be unequivocally demonstrated.

Feeding and Drinking

Feeding and drinking activities of rats are confined principally to the dark period under standard diurnal lighting conditions of the laboratory. Such feeding/drinking rhythms persist under conditions of constant light or dark (Richter, 1965). In an attempt to ascertain any potential influence of the pineal in modulating these activitites, Baum (1970) measured feeding activities of animals which had been superior cervical ganglionectomized or pinealectomized and exposed to various changes in the lighting regimen. Ganglionectomized animals ate significantly less food during darkness and required more days than controls to resynchronized their feeding patterns to shifts in lighting phases. Pinealectomized animals on the other hand, responded essentially the same as controls to such shifts. Since pineal ablation had no effect while removal of the ganglia significantly affected the feeding patterns, Baum concluded that other postsynaptic pathways from the superior cervical ganglia were responsible for the timing of feeding activity.

In studies on drinking behavior of rats, Bliss & Bates (1972) found that pinealectomy increased saline consumption compared to control animals under standard diurnal lighting conditions. In constant light, however, water intake of the pinealectomized animals remained constant while that of the control group decreased. Stephan & Zucker (1972), however, reported that pinealectomized animals also decreased their water intake inconstant light. In further studies, Donovick et al., (1973) tested intake of unpalatable solutions of KCl, NaCl or quinine in pinealectomized or septally-lesioned animals on sodium replete and sodium deplete diets. Ingestion of the two salts or of quinine was increased in all cases in the animals on sodium deplete diets. The increased intake of the aversive fluids was unaffected by the operations.

Thus, no strong indication of pineal influences on feeding and drinking behaviors of mamals can be marshalled as yet although suggestive data have recently been reported for hamsters by Zucker & Stephan (1973). The most apparent affect in all these studies and those on wheel running activities, however, seems to be on the rate of phase shifting when environmental lighting conditions are modified.

CONCLUDING REMARKS

This chapter has briefly reviewed only those relatively few published reports directly or indirectly relating the pineal gland to neural activities and thus to peripheral manifestations of behavior. It is emphasized again that a vast and rapidly expanding literature is available linking the pineal to various other functional activities as well. If we tentatively ascribe to the pineal a central role as a neurohumeral transducer by which environmental information of daily and seasonal time superimposed upon endogenous circadian rhythms is directly or indirectly received and transmitted to the appropriate central neural areas, then many of the observed and reported effects fall into place.

Antigonadal properties are perhaps the most often and best documented evidence of pineal activity. In retrospect, reproduction in almost all cases is cyclic and seasonal and, especially important in this context, is not characterized by gradations or degrees of activity (function), i.e., it is an all or none phenomenon. With inadequate hormonal support therefore, it is dramatically changed and thus easily observed and measured. Species survival depends upon reproductive integrity which is necessarily environmentally timed and thus a consequence of snychronized neural and humeral events. It is tempting to suggest a primary role of the pineal in this temporal synchrony of environmental and hormonal events. Other diurnally cyclic activities upon which survival depends, such as feeding, drinking, general activity, exploration, etc., also might be logically expected to respond to changes in pineal activity. The "solar dosimeter" function ascribed to the parietal eye of lizards by Glasser, (1958) and later elaborated upon by Eakin (1973) may not be too far removed from the function of the pineal body of higher vertebrates. By its interposition between the external photic environment and the functional activities within neural and endocrine structures, it may well serve to synchronize and time behavioral activities with daily and seasonal environmental changes.

ACKNOWLEDGEMENTS

Partial support for this review was furnished by the Colgate
Research Council.

REFERENCES

ANTON-AY, F., 1971, Pineal-brain relationships, in "The Pineal
    Gland" (G. E. W. Wolstenholme & J. Knight, eds.), p. 213,
    Churchill Livingstone, London.

ANTON-TAY, F., CHOU, C., ANTON, S., & WURTMAN, R. J., 1968, Brain
    serotonin concentration: Elevation following intraperitoneal
    administration of melatonin, Science 162:277.

ANTON-TAY, F., DIAZ, J. L., & FERNANDEZ-GUARDIOLA, A., 1971, On the
    effect of melatonin upon the human brain. Its possible thera-
    peutic implications, Life Sci. 10:841.

ANTON-TAY, F., SEPULVEDA, J., & GONZALEZ, S., 1970, Increase of brain
    pyridoxal phosphokinase activity following melatonin administra-
    tion, Life Sci. 9:1283.

ANTON-TAY, F., & WURTMAN, R. J., 1969, Regional uptake of H^3-melatonin
    from blood or cerebral spinal fluid by rat brain, Nature 221:474.

BARCHAS, J., DA COSTA, F., & SPECTOR, S., 1967, Acute pharmacology of
    melatonin, Nature 214:919.

BAUM, M. J., 1968, Pineal gland: Influence on development of copu-
    lation in male rats, Science 162:586.

BAUM, M. J., 1970, Light-synchronization of rat feeding rhythms fol-
    lowing sympathectomy or pinealectomy, Phisiol. Behav. 5:325.

BEHROOSI, K., ASSAEL, M., IVRIANI, I., & NIR, I., 1970, Electrocorti-
    cal reactions on pinealectomized and intact rats to lethal doses
    of pentobarbital, Neuropharmacology 9:219.

BINDONI, M., & RIZZO, R., 1965, Hippocampal-evoked potentials and
    convulsive activity after electrolytic lesions of the pineal
    body, in chronic experiments on rabbits. Arch. Sci. Biol. 49:223.

BLISS, R. K., & BATES, P. L., 1972, Choice intake of saline and water
    in pinealectomized rats under diurnal or constant lighting con-
    ditions, Physiol. Behav. 9:429.

BLUM, K., MERRITT, J. H., REITER, R. J., & WALLACE, J. E., 1973, A
    possible relationship between the pineal gland and ethanol pref-

erence in the rat, Cur. Ther. Res. 15:25.

CARDINELLI, R. P., & WURTMAN, R. J., 1972, Hydroxyindole-O-methyl transferases in rat pineal, Endocrinology 91:247.

DE WIED, D., 1966, Inhibitory effect of ACTH and related peptides on extinction of conditioned avoidance behavior in rats, Proc. Soc. Exp. Biol. Med., 122:28.

DONOVICK, P. J., BLISS, D. K., BURRIGHT, R. G., & WERTHEIM, D. M., 1973, Effect of pinealectomy or septal lesions on intake of un-palatable fluids in rats given sodium deplete or replete diets, Physiol. Behav. 10:1095.

EAKIN, R. M., 1974, "The Third Eye", University of Chicago Press, Illinois.

GASTON, S., & MENAKER, M., 1968, The biological clock in the sparrow, Science 160:1125.

GELLER, I., 1971, Ethanol preference in the rat as a function of photoperiod, Science 173:456.

GELLER, I., PURDY, R., & MERRITT, J. H., 1973, Alterations in ethanol preference in the rat; The role of brain biogenic amines. Pro-ceedings of the National Council on Alchoholism, Kansas City, Mo. (cited in Reiter et al., 1974).

GLASSER, R., 1958, Increase in locomotor activity following shielding of the parietal eye in night lizards, Science 128:1577.

HARRISON, P. C., & BECKER, W. C., 1969, Extraretinal photocontrol of oviposition in pinealectomized domestic fowl, Proc. Soc. Exp. Biol. Med. 132:161.

HISHIKAWA, Y., CRAMER, H., & KUHLO, W., 1969, Natural and melatonin-induced sleep in young chickens: A behavioral and electrographic study, Exp. Br. Res. 7:84.

HOFFMAN, R. A., 1970, The epiphyseal complex in fish and repitles, Amer. Zool. 10:191.

HOFFMAN, R. A., & REITER, R. J., 1965, Rapid pinealectomy in hamsters and other small rodents, Anat. Rec. 152:19.

KAPPERS, J. A., 1960, The development, topographical relations and innervation of the epiphysis cerebri in the albino rat, Zellforsch. Mikroskop Anat., 52:163.

KAPPERS, J. A., 1965, Survey of the epiphysis cerebi and accessory pineal organs of the vertebrates, Prog. Br. Res., 10:87.

KINCL, F. A., CHANG, C. C., & ZBUZKOVA, V., 1970, Observation on the influence of changing photoperiod on spontaneous wheel running activity of neonatally pinealectomized rats, Endocrinology 87:38.

KITAY, J. I., & ALTSCHULE, M. D., 1954, "The Pineal Gland, A Review of the Physiologic Literature", Harvard Univ. Press. Cambridge, Mass.

KLEIN, D. C. & BERG, G. R., 1970, Pineal Gland: Stimulation of melatonin production by norepinephrine involves AMP-mediated stimulation of N-acetyltransferase, Advanc. Biochem. Psychopharmalcol. 3:241.

LERNER, A. B., CASE, J. D., TAKAHASHI, Y., LEE, T. H., & MORI, W., 1958, Isolation of melatonin, the pineal gland factor that lightens melanocytes, J. Am. Chem. Soc., 80:2587.

MARCZYNSKI, T. J., YAMAJUCHI, N., LING, G. M., & GRODZINSKA, L., 1964, Sleep induced by the administration of melatonin (5-methoxy-N acetyltryptamine) to the hypothalamus in unrestrained rats, Experientia 20:435.

MARTINI, L., 1971, Behavioral effects of pineal principles, in "The Pineal Gland," (G. E. W. Wolstenholme & J. Knight, eds.) p. 368, Churchill Livingston, London.

MCCORD, C. R., & ALLEN, F. P., 1917, Evidences associating pineal gland function with alterations in pigmentation, J. Exptl. Zool. 23:207.

MCISAAC, N. M., FARRELL, G., TABORSKY, R. G., & TAYLOR, A. N., 1965, Indole compounds: Isolation from pineal tissue, Science 148:102.

MENAKER, M., 1968, Extraretinal light preception in the sparrow, I. Entrainment of the biological clock, Proc. Nat. Acad. Sci. 59:414.

MILCU, ST. M., & DEMETRESU, M., 1963, Decrease in alpha rhythm irradiation in the anterior leads following pineal extract administration, Electroencephalogr. Clin. Neurophysiol. 15:535.

MOORE, R. Y., HELLER, A., WURTMAN, R. J., & AZELROD, J., 1967, Visual pathway mediating pineal response to environmental light, Science 155:220.

MYERS, R. D., & HOLMAN, R. B., 1966, A procedure for eliminating position habit in preference-aversion tests for ethanol and other fluids, Psychon. Sci. 6:235.

NIR, I., BEHROOZI, K., ASSAEL, M., IVRIANI, I., & SULMAN, F. G., 1969, Changes in the electrical activity of the brain following pinealectomy, Neuroendocrinology 4:122.

PELHAM, R. W., RALPH, C. L., & CAMPBELL, I. M., 1972, Mass spectral identification of melatonin in blood, Biochem. Biophys. Res. Commun. 46:1236.

PELHAM, R. W., VAUGHAN, G. M., SANDOCK, K. L., & VAUGHAN, M. K., 1973, Twenty-four-hour cycle of a melatonin-like substance in the plasma of human males, J. Clin. Endocrinol. Metab. 37:341.

POMERANTZ, G., & REITER, R. J., 1973, Age-dependent changes in the susceptibility of parathyroidectomized, pinealectomized rats to seizures, Exp. Neurol 40:254.

PROP, N., & KAPPERS, J. A., 1961, Demonstration of some compounds present in the pineal organ of the albino rat by histochemical methods and paper chromatography, Acta. Anat., 45:90.

QUAY, W. B., 1965, Photic relations and experimental dissociation of circadian rhythms in pineal composition and running activity in rats, Photochem. Photobiol. 4:425.

QUAY, W. B., 1968, Individuation and lack of pineal effect in the rats circadian locomotor rhythm, Physiol. Behav. 3:109.

QUAY, W. B., 1969, The role of the pineal gland in environmental adaptation, in "Physiology and Pathology of Adaptation Mechanisms," (E. Bajusez, ed.) pp. 508-550, Pergamon Press, New York.

QUAY, W. B., 1970a, Physiological signifiacne of the pineal during adaptation to shifts in photoperiod, Physiol. Behav., 5:353.

QUAY, W. B., 1970b, Precocious entrainment and associated characteristics of activity patterns following pinealectomy and reversal of photoperiod, Physiol. Behav. 5:1281.

QUAY, W. B., 1970c, The signifiance of the pineal, in "Hormones and the Environment," Mem. Soc. Endocrinol. 18, (G. K. Benson & J. G. Phillips, eds.), pp. 423-444, Cambridge Univ. Press, London.

QUAY, W. B., 1971a, Dissimilar functional effects of pineal stalk and cerebral meningeal interruptions on phase shifts of circadian activity rhythms, Physiol. Behav. 7:557.

QUAY, W. B., 1971b, Effects of cutting nervi conarii and tentorium cerebelli on pineal composition and activity shifting following reversal of photoperiod, Physiol. Behav., 6:681.

QUAY, W. B., 1974, "Pineal Chemistry in Cellular and Physiological Mechanisms," Chas. C. Thomas, Springfield, Ill.

RALPH, C. L., MULL, D., LYNCH, H. J., & HEDLUND, H., 1971, A melatonin rhythm persists in rat pineals in darkness, Endocrinology 89:1361.

REISS, M., DAVIS, R. H., SIDEMAN, M. B., & PLICHTA, E. J., 1963, Pineal gland and spontaneous activity of rats, J. Endocrinol. 37:475.

REITER, R. J., (ed.) 1970, "The Pineal", A. I. B. S. Symposium, Boston, Mass., Publ. in Amer. Zool. 10, 1970.

REITER, R. J., 1972, The role of the pineal in reproduction, in "Reproductive Biology", (H. Balin & S. Glasser, eds.) pp. 71-114, Experpta Medica, Amsterdam.

REITER, R. J., 1973, Comparative Physiology: Pineal Gland, Ann Rev. Physiol. 35:305.

REITER, R. J., & FRASCINI, F., 1969, Endocrine aspects of the mammalian pineal gland: A review, Neuroendocrinology, 5:219.

REITER, R. J., & MORGAN, W. W., 1972, Attempts to characterize the convulsive response of parathyroidectomized rats to pineal gland removal, Physiol. Behav. 9:203.

REITER, R. J. & SORRENTINO, S. JR., 1972, Prevention of pineal-mediated reproductive responses in light-deprived hamsters by partial or total isolation of the medial basal hypothalamus, J. Neuro-Viscer, Rel., 32:355.

REITER, R. J., BLASK, D. E., TALBOT, J. A. & BARNETT, M. P., 1973, Nature and time course of seizures associated with surgical removal of the pineal gland from parathyroidectomized rats, Exp. Neurol, 38:386.

REITER, R. J., BLUM, K., WALLACE, J. E. & MERRITT, J. H., 1974, Pineal gland: Evidence for an influence on ethanol preference in male Syrian hamsters, Comp. Biochem. Physiol. 47:11.

REITER, R. J., SORRENTINO, S. JR., & HOFFMAN, R. A., 1972, Muscular spasms and death in thyroparathryroidectomized rats subjected to pinealectomy, Life Sci. 11:123.

RELKIN, R., 1970, Influence of prepubertal and postpubertal pinealectomy on treadwheel activity. Physiol. Behav. 5:341.

RICHTER, C. P., 1965, "Biological Clocks in Medicine and Psychiatry." Chas. C. Thomas, Springfield, Ill.

ROLDAN, E. & ANTON-TAY, F., 1968, EEG and convulsive threshold changes produced by pineal extract administration, Br. Res., 11:238.

ROLDAN, E., ANTON-TAY, F., & ESCOBAR, A., 1964, Studies on the pineal gland. IV. The effect of pineal extract on the electroencephalo- gram, Biol. Inst. Estud. Med. Biol., 22:145.

SAMPSON, P. H., & BIGELOW, L., 1971, Pineal influence on exploratory behavior of the female rat, Physiol. Behav. 7:713.

STEBBINS, R. C., 1960, Effects of pinealectomy in the Western Fence Lizard, Sceloporus occidentalis, Copeia 4:276.

STEPHAN, F. K. & ZUCKER, I., 1972, Rat drinking rhythms: Central visual pathway and endocrine factors mediating responsiveness to environmental illumination, Physiol. Behav. 8:315.

TAGLIAMONTE, A., TAGLIAMONTE, P., GESSA, G. L. & BRODIE, B. B., 1969, Compulsive sexual activity induced by p-chlorophenylalanine in normal and pinealectomized male rats, Science 166:1433.

VAUGHAN, M. K., REITER, R. J., VAUGHAN, G. M., BIGELOW, L., & ALT- SCHULE, M. D., 1972, Inhibition of compensatory ovarian hyper- trophy in the mouse and vole: A comparison of Altschule's pineal extract, pineal indoles, vasopressin, and oxytocin, Gen. Comp. Endocrinol, 18:372.

VLAHAKES, G. J. & WURTMAN, R. J., 1972, A Mg^{+2} dependent hydroxyindole- O-methyl transferase in rat Harderian gland, Biochem. Biophys. Acta. 261:194.

WOLSTENHOLME, G. E. W. & KNIGHT, J. (eds.), 1971, "The Pineal Gland", Ciba Foundation Symposium, Churchill Livingstone, London.

WONG, R. & WHITESIDE, C. B. C., 1968, The effect of melatonin on the wheel-running activity of rats deprived of food, J. Endocrinol, 40:383.

WURTMAN, R. J., AXELROD, J. & KELLY, D. E., 1968, "The Pineal", Academic Press, New York.

ZUCKER, I. & STEPHAN, K. K., 1973, Light-dark rhythms in hamster eat- ing, drinking and locomotor behaviors, Physiol. Behav., 11:239.

CHAPTER 18

BIOGENIC AMINES AND BEHAVIOR: ACTIVITY AND AVOIDANCE LEARNING

Karen L. Stavnes, Ph.D.

Department of Psychiatry and Behavioral Sciences
University of Oklahoma Health Sciences Center
800 N. E. 13th Street
Oklahoma City, Oklahoma   73190

CONTENTS

INTRODUCTION

Interest in the biochemical basis of behavior has led to extensive research attempts to relate biogenic amines to a wide variety of behaviors ranging from mental illness in humans, through social behavior, to investigation of activity levels in animal models. Discovery of the presence of these amines in specific regions of the brain and general acceptance of their involvement in neurotransmission or neuromodulation in the central nervous system (CNS) has created much interest in what role they may play in learning and memory. Thus, a large portion of the current literature, which has attempted to link biogenic amines and behavior, has been concerned with learning and memory functions.

The first part of this chapter will be devoted to a cursory review of the biogenic amines, dopamine (DA), norepinephrine (NE), 5-hydroxytryptamine (5-HT), and their characteristics. The remaining portion of the chapter will be limited in scope to investigations that have attempted to relate DA, NE and 5-HT to behavior. The specific behaviors that will be covered are locomotor activity and aversively motivated learning.

Two approaches have commonly been used in investigation of the neurochemical correlates of behavior. In the first approach the effects of experimental manipulation of the metabolism of biogenic amines on behavior are observed. Methods such as drug administration, lesions or dietary means are used to modify amine metabolism. The second approach investigates the effect of environmental variables or the effect of the behavior itself on changes in biogenic amine metabolism. Little research using this second method has been conducted in the study of locomotor activity and avoidance learning. Causal relationships between biogenic amines and behavior have been difficult to establish. Correlations can be observed between specific amines and behaviors; as a function of depleting or enhancing amine levels or turnover rates in whole brain or parts of brain, as a function of dose of the treatment (usually pharmacological), as a function of time after the treatment, and as a function of individual differences between animals or strains. However, experimental manipulations that alter a biogenic amine system in an organism result in effects on many aspects of an organism's behavior aside from the specific aspects of interest. For instance, in research related to the neurochemical basis of learning and memory, it is difficult to distinguish the effect the amine system has on learning from the effect it has on other behaviors involved in the performance of the learning task such as sensory processes, motivation, or motor activity. It may be most parsimonious to view these amine systems as exerting excitatory or inhibitory effects on behavior. These opposed effects may interact to produce a central arousal state in the organism that leads to appropriate behavioral responsiveness to the environment under normal conditions. In addition, many of the pharmacological agents used to modify biogenic amine systems have multiple effects on the organism which can result in behavioral changes that are not mediated by the amine of interest. Finally, an often ignored problem concerns the separation of the influence of peripherally located biogenic amines on behavior from the influence of centrally located amines on behavior.

CHARACTERISTICS OF BIOGENIC AMINES

Catecholamines

The catecholamines (CA), dopamine and norepinephrine are thought to be involved in neurotransmission in the brain and have been located in specific neuronal tracts in the brain. CAs are organic compounds that consist of a benzene ring with two adjacent hydroxyl groups (catechol) and an amine group (Fig. 1). Compounds must fulfill a variety of established criteria to meet the requirements of a chemical transmitter in the brain. To date, none of these amines have conclusively been shown to be neurotransmitter in the CNS. For a more detailed discussion of both CAs and indoleamines and of evidence leading to their acceptance as putative neurotransmitters, refer to McLennan 1970; Cooper et al., 1974; and Barchas et al., 1972.

Dopamine. Recently, the histochemical fluorescence technique has led to the identification of pathways in the brains of several species, including cell bodies, axons and nerve terminals, that contain either DA or NE. Investigators are continuing to use this method in search of more detailed information (See Ungerstedt, 1971). DA cell bodies are found in four main areas in the brain: 1) the zona compacta of the substantia nigra, 2) caudal to the substantia nigra, 3) near the interpeduncular nucleus, and 4) in the arcuate nucleus and anterior periventricular nucleus in the hypothalamus (Fig. 2). Axons arising from cell bodies found caudal to and in the substantia nigra terminate in the nucleus caudatus and putamen of the corpus striatum. This pathway is known as the nigro-striatal DA system and appears to be important in Parkinson's disease in which symptoms of motor rigidity and tremor are present. The disease is thought to be related to DA deficiency resulting from degeneration of this tract and is therapeutically treated by administration of dihydroxyphenylalanine (DOPA), the immediate precursor of DA. The meso-limbic DA system originates from cell bodies found near the interpeduncular nucleus. Axons from these cell bodies ascend together with axons of the nigro-striatal DA system and later diverge to terminate in the nucleus accumbens and tuberculum olfactorium. A third system, the tuberoinfundibular DA system, be-

gins from the cell bodies located in the arcuate and periventricular
nuclei of the hypothalamus and descends to the median eminence (anterior portion of the beginning of the pituitary stalk).

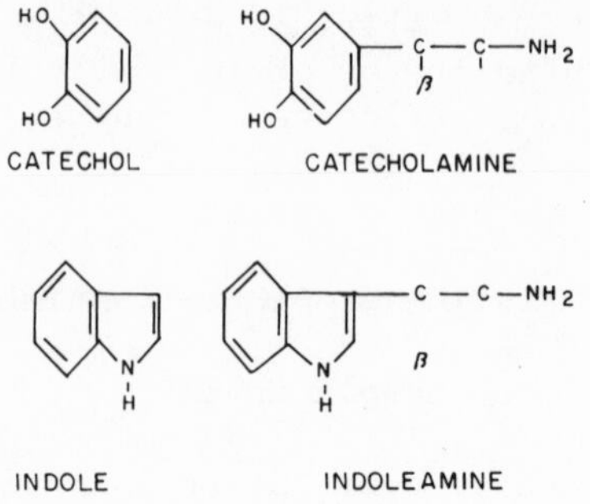

Fig. 1.   Catecholamine and indoleamine structure.

Norephinephrine.   NE pathways are more widely distributed
than those of DA.   The ventral NE pathway, one of the two major
ascending pathways, originates from several groups of NE cell
bodies which are located in the medulla oblongata and pons.
Their axons ascend through the reticular formation and medial forebrain bundle and terminate along this pathway in many areas of the
brain including the lower brain stem, mesencephalon and diencephalon.
There is major innervation of the hypothalamus by this ventral NE
pathway.   In the locus coeruleus in the pons, NE cell bodies are
very densely packed.   The locus coeruleus is the origin of the dorsal ascending pathway.   This dorsal pathway also ascends through
the medial forebrain bundle and appears to innervate nearly all
parts of the brain, especially the cerebellum, hippocampus and
cerebral cortex.   There is some speculation that single cells in
the locus coeruleus may send collateral innervation to all three
of these areas (Ungerstedt, 1971).   Researchers interested in the
biochemical basis of learning and memory have recently begun to investigate the role neurons arising from the locus coeruleus may have
in learning and memory.   A descending NE pathway arises from the
medulla oblongata and terminates in the spinal cord.   It should be
noted that the distribution of DA pathways is quite different from
that of NE pathways suggesting that DA has functions other than its
role as a precursor for NE.

Biosynthesis.   Fig. 3 depicts the biosynthesis of DA and NE.
The dietary amino acid tyrosine, the precursor of both DA and NE,
is taken up into neurons by an active transport mechanism.   The relatively slow hydroxylation of tyrosine by the enzyme, tyrosine hydroxylase, to form DOPA appears to be the rate limiting step in the
synthesis of both DA and NE.   Administration of a commonly used com-

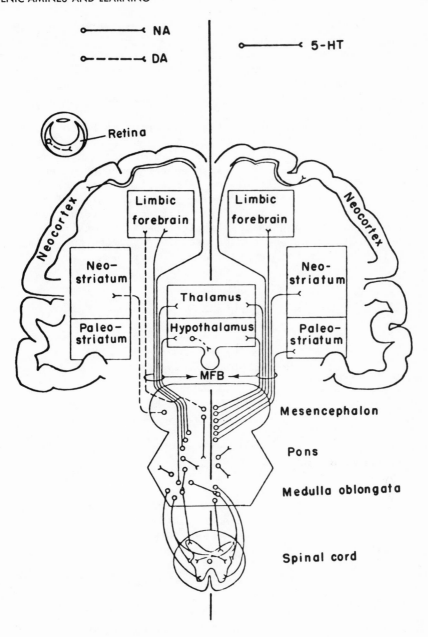

Fig. 2. Schematic drawing of the location of the biogenic amine systems, DA, NE and 5-HT, in the CNS. The median forebrain bundle of the hypothalamus is symbolized by MFB. This figure is taken from Anden et al. (1966).

pound, α-methyltyrosine (α-MT), inhibits this enzymatic step causing inhibition of the synthesis of DA and NE with a resultant drop
in levels of these CAs. The next step in CA synthesis is the decarboxylation of DOPA by the enzyme, aromatic amino acid decarboxylase (DOPA decarboxylase), to form DA. These preceding steps in
CA synthesis occur in the cytoplasm of NE neurons and some fraction
of DA is then probably taken up into the storage granules by an
active transport mechanism and the transformation of DA to form NE,
mediated by the enzyme, DA-β-hydroxylase (DA-β-oxidase), appears to
occur in these storage granules (Axelrod, 1965). DA-β-hydroxylase
is lacking in those parts of brain such as the caudate nucleus,
in which DA is the predominant CA and little NE is present. Inhibition of the synthesis of DA and NE is most successful if the rate
limiting step is affected by inhibition of tyrosine hydroxylase.
Disulfiram and other compounds that inhibit DA-β-hydroxylase selectively lower levels of NE and can be used to determine the relative
roles DA and NE have in the expression of behavior.

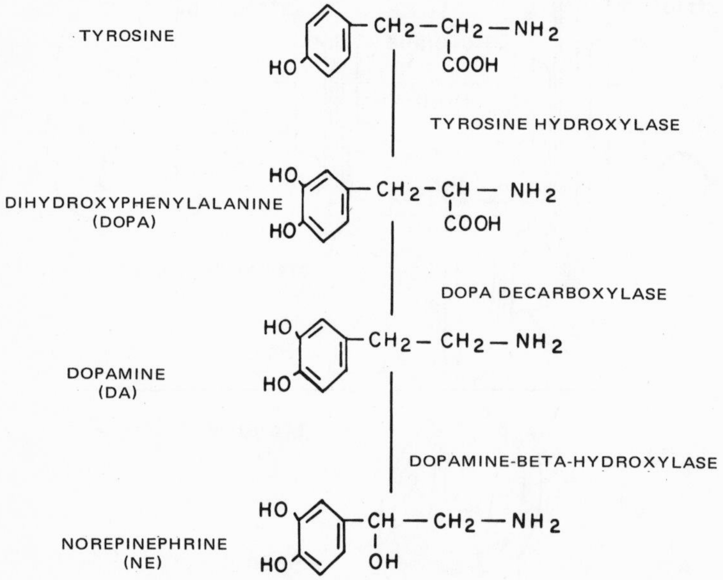

Fig. 3. Biosynthesis of dopamine and norepinephrine.

Degradation. The degradation of the CAs is summarized in Fig.
4. Monoamine oxidase (MAO) and catechol-o-methyl transferase (COMT)
are the two primary enzymes involved in the degradation of the CAs
and are both relatively non-specific to their substrates. DA and
NE are deaminated by MAO to their corresponding aldehydes; DA is
converted to 3, 4-dihydroxyphenylacetaldehyde and NE is converted
to 3, 4-dihydroxyphenylglycolaldehyde. The aldehydes are then
rapidly converted to the corresponding acids, 3, 4-dihydroxyphenyl-

acetic acid (DOPAC) and 3, 4-dihydroxymandelic acid (DOMA) by the
enzyme, aldehyde dehydrogenase. COMT catalyzes the acid products
of DA and NE to homovanillic acid (HVA) and 3-methoxy-4-hydroxymandel-
ic acid (VMA), respectively, which are then excreted in the urine.
The aldehydes formed in the first MAO catalyzed degradative step
for CAs may also be reduced by the enzyme, aldehyde reductase, to
form alcohols. There is evidence that this may be the major route
for NE metabolism in the brain (Maas & Landis, 1968; Schanberg et al.,
1968a and 1968b). The main alcohol derivative of NE, 3-methoxy-4-
hydroxy-phenylglycol (MOPEG), which in some species is conjugated
to a sulfate, is able to diffuse from the brain into general circulation. Measurement of MOPEG in humans with affective disorders
has been used as an index of NE utilization in the CNS (Shopsin et
al., 1974).

In an alternative metabolic pathway DA and NE are first methyl-
ated to 3-methoxytyramine (MTA) and normetanephrine (NM) respectively. These products are then catalzyed by MAO to form the DA derivative, 3-methoxy-4-hydroxyphenylacetaldehyde and the NE derivative
3-methoxy-4 - hydroxyphenylglycolaldehyde. Aldehyde dehydrogenase
then converts these aldehydes to the major metabolites of the CAs,
HVA and VMA. Thus, the metabolic product of whichever enzyme (COMT
or MAO) acts first on the CAs is converted by the other enzyme
(COMT or MAO) into HVA or VMA. Traditionally, MAO is thought to
degrade CAs intraneurally and COMT appears to act first on CAs in
the synapse. Slow release of CAs by drugs or low frequency nerve
impulses results in degradation first by MAO, while rapid release
of CAs by neurons or exogenous administration results in degradation by COMT first (Koelle, 1970).

5-Hydroxytryptamine

5 - Hydroxytryptamine (serotonin) is an indoleamine consisting
of an indole group and an amine group (Fig. 1). Like the CAs, it
is synthesized in the brain, but does not easily pass into the brain
via the blood supply (blood-brain barrier). There is ample evidence
to suggest that 5-HT has a role in neural functioning in the brain.

The cell bodies of neurons that contain 5-HT are located in the
brain stem as are the cell bodies of DA and NE. Specificially,
5-HT cell bodies are found in the raphe nuclei in the pons and midbrain. From the raphe nuclei the axons ascend via the medial forebrain bundle through the lateral hypothalamus to the limbic system
and cortical areas (Fig. 2). The most caudal 5-HT cell groups in
the medulla oblongata descend to innervate the spinal cord. The
distribution of pathways for 5-HT is somewhat similar to that observed for NE. For more extensive coverage of the location of DA,
NE and 5-HT pathways, refer to Ungerstedt, 1971; Dahlstrom & Fuxe,
1965; Fuxe et al., 1968 and 1970.

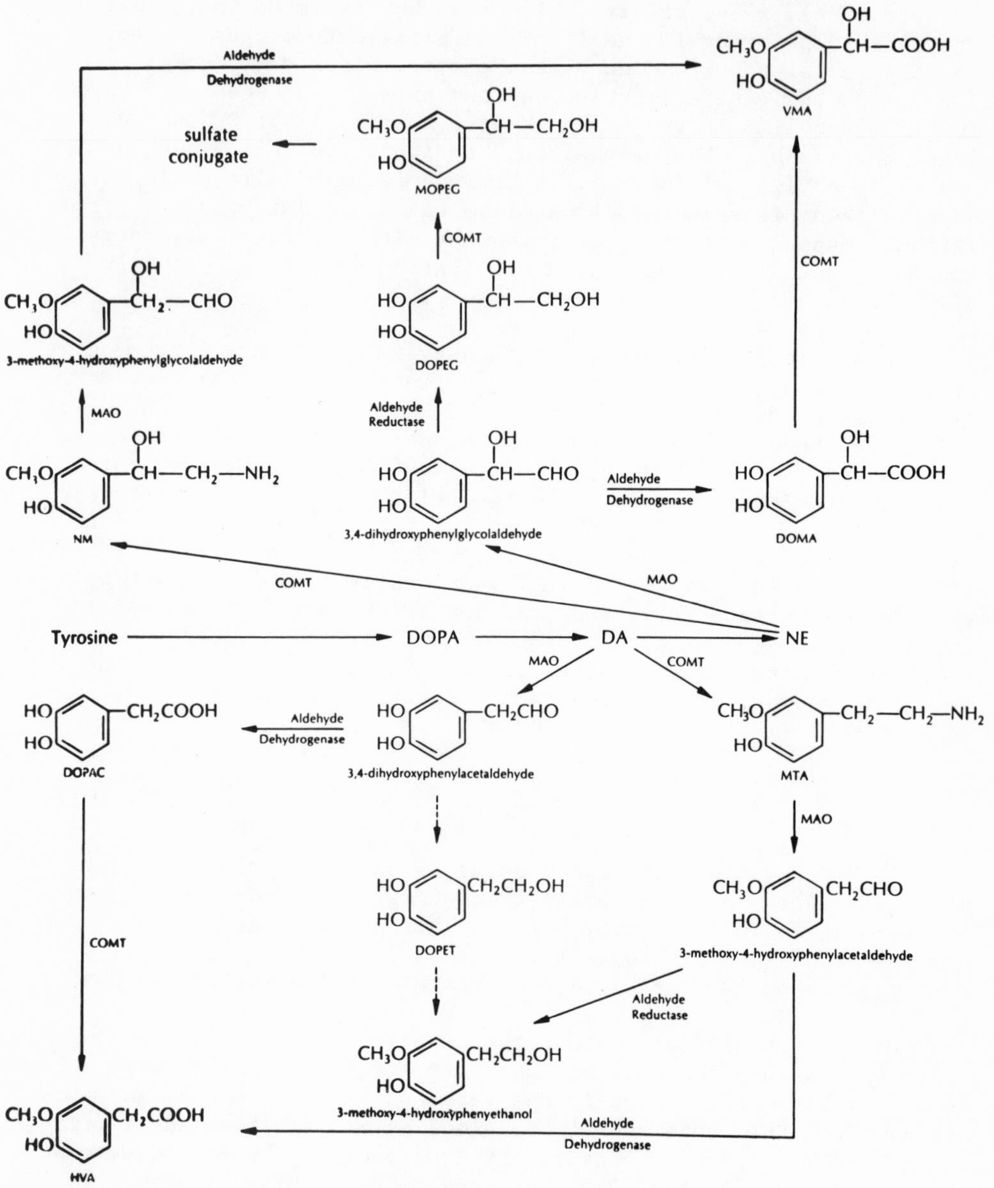

Fig. 4. Degradation of dopamine and norepinephrine. Abbreviations are described in the text. This figure is taken from Cooper et al., (1974).

Biosynthesis. The synthetic pathway of 5-HT is summarized in Fig. 5. In mammals 5-HT is synthesized from dietary tryptophan. As with tyrosine in the synthesis of DA and NE, there is active uptake of the precursors into the neuron. However, certain other amino acids can compete with precursors for uptake and thus inhibit uptake of tryptophan and tyrosine. Hydroxylation of tryptophan by the enzyme, tryptophan hydroxylase, leads to the formation of 5-hydroxytryptophan (5-HTP), the immediate precursor of 5-HT. This step is so slow in comparison to the others that it is widely considered to be rate-limiting in the formation of 5-HT. 5-HTP is then rapidly converted to 5-HT by the enzyme aromatic amino acid decarboxylase. This is a non - specific enzyme, also known as 5-HTP decarboxylase and DOPA decarboxylase and is the same enzyme that decarboxylates DOPA to DA. Some of the newly synthesized 5-HT is then actively taken up into storage granules in the neuron. Inhibition of 5-HT synthesis can be accomplished by interfering with the rate limiting step which is most susceptible to pharmacological manipulations. The compound, p-chloro-phenylalanine (PCPA) is often used to deplete 5-HT in the brain and elsewhere since it inhibits tryptophan hydroxylase.

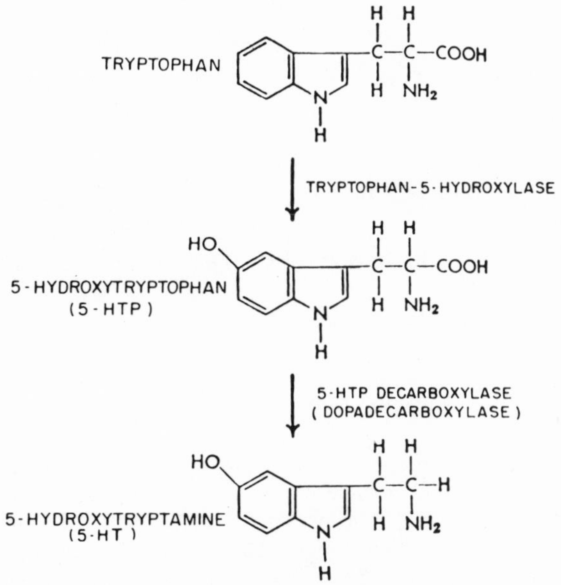

Fig. 5. Biosynthesis of 5-hydroxytryptamine. This figure is taken from Douglas (1970).

Degradation. The main route for degradation of 5-HT is via the enzyme, MAO, which deaminates 5-HT. This enzyme appears to be identical to that which degrades the CAs. 5-HT is transformed by

MAO to 5-hydroxyindoleacetaldehyde which usually is rapidly oxi-
dized to 5-hydroxyindoleacetic acid (5-HIAA) by aldehyde dehydrogenase or in an alternative route which is less likely under normal
conditions, the aldehyde is reduced to 5-hydroxytryptophol (5-HTOL)
by alcohol dehydrogenase (Fig. 6). These metabolites are excreted
in the urine. Compounds that inhibit MAO such as nialamide and
tranylcypromine are often used to raise levels of both CAs and 5-
HT.

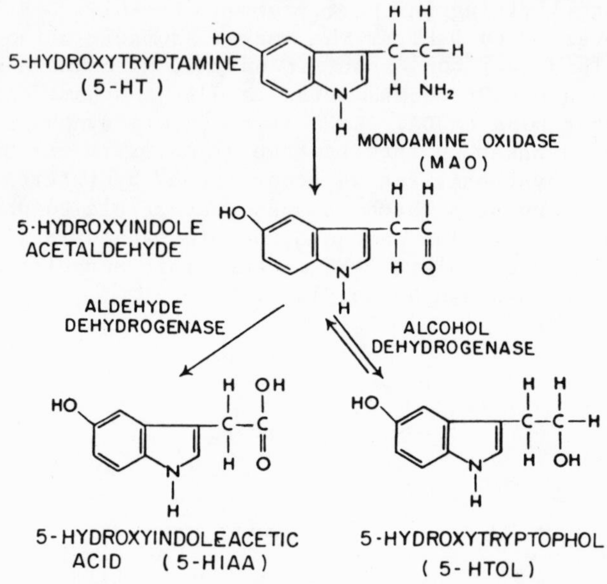

Fig. 6. Degradation of 5-hydroxytryptamine. This figure is taken
from Douglas (1970).

PHARMACOLOGICAL MANIPULATION OF BIOGENIC AMINES

Familiarity with the metabolism of DA, NE and 5-HT is necessary
to understand many of the experimental manipulations used in research on biogenic amines and behavior. Drugs may act at a variety
of sites in the metabolic pathways of the biogenic amines. Besides
inhibiting the enzymatic steps in either the synthesis or degradation of the biogenic amines, drugs can interfere with precursor
transport, storage mechanisms that bind the monoamines within the
neuron, release from these storage pools in the presynaptic nerve
terminal and normal receptor function on which these monoamines have
their effects. Compounds that decrease synthesis, compete for
storage sites, or block release of biogenic amines, decreasing the
availability of the amines at the synapse. Administration of precursors, drugs which activate release or prevent inactivation of

synthetic enzymes increase the availability of monamines at the synapse. Because the CA and indoleamine systems have enzymes in common, pharmacological manipulation of these enzymes has effects on both systems. Often more than one drug is used to achieve the desired result with each drug having its main effect on different aspects of the metabolism. One of the principle techniques for distinguishing the role of indoleamine and CA function is to pharmacologically inhibit tyrosine hydroxylase and tryptophan hydroxylase which will stop synthesis and thus eventually deplete the nerve endings of DA, NE and 5-HT. This can be accomplished with α-MT and PCPA. Then the nerve endings can be replenished by administering the precursors, either DOPA or 5-HTP (both pass the blood-brain barrier), and thus, bypass the rate-limiting step. Reserpine blocks uptake of amines into the storage particles making them susceptible to degradation by MAO and is also often used to deplete major stores of CAs and 5-HT in this type of design. To separate the function of CNS monoamines from peripherally acting monoamines, some investigators have attempted to inhibit their synthesis in the periphery with drugs that do not easily pass the blood-brain barrier while pharmacologically manipulating amines in the CNS.

Once a biogenic amine is released into the synaptic cleft, it has to be inactivated. Although enzymes can degrade these amines, the principle route of inactivation for DA, NE and 5-HT appears to be reuptake by an active transport system into the nerve terminals that released them. Certain drugs selectively block this uptake process and thus increase the quantity of amine that is available to stimulate the receptors. Table 1 summarizes the effects of some drugs that are commonly used to manipulate biogenic amine systems. More information of the metabolism of biogenic amines and drug effects on these systems can be found in Glowinski, 1966; Weiss & Laties, 1969; Koelle, 1970 and Douglas, 1970.

Recently, 6-hydroxydopamine (6-OHDA), which does not pass the blood-brain barrier, has been used frequently in behavioral research. Injection of 6-OHDA into the cerebral ventricals of experimental animals results in chemically produced lesions by destroying DA and NE nerve terminals and sometimes also destroying the cell bodies of these neurons. 5-HT and cholinergic neurons are apparently not affected. Selective destruction of either NE or DA neurons can be accomplished by manipulation of dose (NE neurons are more susceptible to 6-OHDA than DA neurons) or pretreatment with drugs that protect either DA or NE neurons. A review by Thoenen & Tranzer (1973) further characterizes the pharmacology of 6-OHDA.

Search for an analogous tool for use in the 5-HT system has led to experimentation with the agent, 5,6-dihydroxytryptamine (5,6-DHT) (Baumgarten & Schlossberger, 1973). Intraventricular injections of

5,6-DHT in rats appear to selectively affect 5-HT neurons and have been shown to destroy 5-HT nerve terminals with a resultant, relatively long-lasting depletion of 5-HT throughout the CNS.

A great deal of recent research on biogenic amines and behavior attempts to separate the effects each of the monamines, DA, NE and 5-HT have on behavior. Accumulating evidence indicates that the CA and indoleamine systems interact with each other and with other systems involved in neurotransmission such as the cholinergic system (Carlton, 1963; Mabry & Campbell et al., 1969; Swonger & Rech, 1972). Pharmacological manipulation of one of these systems is likely to affect the functioning of another system thus making it more difficult to interpret the relation of the monoamine of interest to the observed behavioral effects.

Two main methods of measuring endogenous monoamines or the effects of experimental manipulations on monoamines in the brain are available. The first approach measures levels of DA, NE or 5-HT in the brain to see if they deviate from normal levels. However, an increase in the amount of biogenic amine present in brain tissue does not necessarily mean that more is released by nervous activity or that more is stimulating receptors. MAO inhibitors given alone in single doses to laboratory animals may have little obvious effect on behavior while producing significant increases in brain amine levels. On the other hand, levels of a monoamine can remain the same while the entire metabolism of the amine can increase or decrease associated with higher or lower rates of utilization of the amine in neurotransmission. Thus, the second method of measuring monoamines in the brain estimates the dynamic states of brain amine systems based on utilization rate over time. For example, alpha-MT can be injected into an experimental animal and levels of CAs measured as a function of time after injection. Since new DA and NE are not being synthesized, the brain will eventually become depleted of DA and NE. The speed with which this depletion occurs is indicative of the turnover rate of DA and NE under the specific experimental conditions. Injection of radioactive labeled monoamines or precursors of monoamines allows investigators to measure the amount of radioactivity present at points along the metabolic pathways in newly formed metabolites or in the monoamine itself. This also results in information on rate of turnover of these amines. However, measures of turnover rate assume that the amount of biogenic amine being used is functionally active. Recently, Grahame-Smith (1971, 1973) has developed a hypothesis in which 5-HT may be noramlly synthesized in excess of functional needs and both functionally active and functionally inactive 5-HT may be degraded to 5-HIAA. Thus, depending on the proportion of functionally active 5-HT to functionally inactive 5-HT, measurement of turnover rates may or may not be a good estimate of functional activity.

Table 1. Action and results of action of some drugs that are
commonly used in biogenic amine research.

DRUG	ACTION	RESULT
α-MT	inhibition of tyrosine hydroxylase	CA depletion
PCPA	inhibition of tryptophan hydroxylase	5-HT depletion
diethyldithiocarbamate disulfiram (disulfide)	inhibition of DA-β-hydroxylase	NE depletion, DA accumulation?
pargyline nialamide tranylcypromine	inhibition of MAO	CA and 5-HT accumulation
reserpine	blocks uptake into storage particles and depletes major stores leaving amines susceptible to MAO	CA and 5-HT depletion
amphetamine	releases CAs from neuron and prevents reuptake?	CA accumulation
6-OHDA	neurochemical lesions in CA system	CA depletion
5,6-DHT	neurochemical lesions in 5-HT system	5-HT depletion

BIOGENIC AMINES AND BEHAVIOR

Activity

Catecholamines. The majority of investigations attempting to
relate CAs and behavior have observed increased locomotor activity
or excitation in animals when drugs are administered that accelerate
the activity of synthesis or decrease the rate of degradation leading to increased levels or turnover rates of DA and NE. In contrast,

drugs that lower levels of DA and NE have usually resulted in behavioral depression. The open field apparatus in which the animal
is able to explore a large environment and stabilimeter cages are
most commonly used to measure activity. Activity measures have
often been used as a behavioral index of the state of general
arousal or excitation of the CNS in organisms. This central arousal
state is thought to have important effects on many behaviors including learning and memory (Kety, 1970; Routtenberg, 1968).

Attempts have been made to enhance the central effects and decrease the peripheral effects of injecting the precursor DOPA, on
CAs and behavioral excitation. Low doses of trihydroxyphenylhydra-
zine (Ro 4-4602) selectively inhibit decarboxylation of DOPA in
extra-cerebral tissues while high doses also inhibit cerebral DOPA
decarboxylase (Bartholini et al., 1969). Locomotor activity has
not been affected by low doses but has been completely inhibited
by high doses of Ro 4-4602 (Reichenberg & Vetulani, 1973). Injections of DOPA in combination with small doses of Ro 4-4602 increased spontaneous locomotor activity and this increase in activity appeared to correlate most closely with increased activity of
DA and not NE (Benkert et al., 1973a and 1973b; Bartholini et al.,
1969). In contrast, injections of DOPA with high doses of Ro 4-
4602 has yielded no increase in activity. Butcher & Engel (1969)
have found that the suppression of spontaneous motor activity that
is sometimes seen after low doses of DOPA disappears when a small
dose of Ro 4-4602 is given in conjunction with DOPA suggesting
a pheripheral effect of DOPA and probably DA on activity. This
peripheral effect may account for some of the discrepant results
that have been observed in efforts to relate CAs to activity.

Recently, investigators have attempted to determine if both
DA and NE are important in locomotor activity or if one or the
other of these CAs has the major effect. There currently is not
a consensus of opinion as to the relative importance of DA and NE
in activity. One of the main problems is the ability of DA to
both act as a precursor for NE and to itself influence neurotransmission. Some researchers have presented evidence that DA and NE
may control different types of motor activity. DA has been implicated in stereotyped hyperactivity characterized by compulsive
gnawing and sniffing in rodents (Randrup & Munkvad, 1967). This
has been observed after administration of amphetamine or DOPA
(Randrup & Munkvad, 1970). Lesions in the corpus striatum have
eliminated sterotyped behavior (Fog et al., 1970). Stereotyped
postural deficits have also been observed with changes in DA.
Unilateral intrastriatal injections of DA into rat brain have resulted in asymmetrical posture leading to turning movements contralateral to the side of injection (Ungerstedt et al., 1969).
Bilateral DA denervation in rats due to administration of 6-OHDA
has led to catalepsy, rigidity and tremor reminiscent of symptoms

of Parkinson's disease in humans (Ungerstedt, 1974). Since these denervated rats also exhibited a variety of other behaviors indicating inability to respond appropriately to sensory stimuli. Ungerstedt has proposed that the nigro-striatal DA system is involved in sensory-motor integration.

On the other hand, NE neurons have been thought to influence nonstereotyped locomotor activity to a greater extent than DA neurons. D-amphetamine has been found to have its main effect on NE systems and d- and l-amphetamine appear to have relatively equal effects on the nirgro-striatal DA system (Taylor & Snyder, 1971; Phillips & Fibiger, 1973). Taylor & Snyder (1971) found that d-amphetamine increased spontaneous locomotor activity to a much greater extent than l-amphetamine but was only twice as active in evoking stereotyped gnawing behavior. These data indicated NE had a major role in locomotor activity and DA systems were related to stereotyped behavior. However, more recent evidence suggests that brain DA is important in both locomotor activity and stereotyped behavior produced by d-amphetamine (Hollister et al., 1974). In these experiments, differential 6-OHDA treatments induced chronic depletions of brain NE, DA or both. Locomotor activity and stereotyped behavior produced by d-amphetamine was antagonized by depletion of DA, both DA and NE, but not NE alone. Other evidence also suggests that DA and not NE has a relatively major influence on locomotor activity (Svensson & Waldeck, 1970).

Intraventricular infusion of CAs into the brain is also being used to investigate the relative roles of DA and NE in activity. Segal and his colleagues have used this infusion technique and have found increases in spontaneous locomotor activity of rats given either DA or NE (Segal & Mandell, 1970; Geyer et al., 1972). When pretreated with imipramine which prevents the uptake of CAs into adrenergic neurons, rats infused with DA did not show the activity increase while rats given NE still exhibited an increase in activity. In addition, haloperidol, which blocks DA receptors, did not affect the activity increase observed after infusion of either DA or NE. This indicated that infused DA had to get into the neuron to increase locomotor activity and did not need to interact with its own DA receptors to have this effect. Based on these results, the authors suggested that DA indirectly influenced activity by either 1) increasing the release of NE by displacing it in the neuron or by 2) acting as a precursor and thus increasing the quantity of NE. Subsequently, reserpine which blocks uptake of amines into the storage granules, significantly reduced the hyperactivity response to infused DA and not to infused NE (Geyer & Segal, 1973). Although these results did not completely rule out the displacement hypothesis, since DA is converted to NE in the storage vesicles, these results indicated DA produced its effect on activity by its conversion to NE. Chronic administration of α-MT enhanced the hyperactivity

effect of NE but did not change the hyperactivity effect of DA.
Under these conditions the conversion of DA to NE was not altered
but less NE was available for displacement indicating that DA has
its major effect on activity by acting as a precursor to NE, not by
displacing NE or by acting directly.

Recent behavioral evidence suggests the existance of a feedback mechanism between activity at the adrenergic receptor level
and the rate-limiting step involving tyrosine hydroxylase (Segal
et al., 1972). Five inbred strains of rats, ACI, BN, BUF, 5344,
LEW and random bred Sprague Dawley rats were measured for spontaneous locomotor activity and tyrosine hydroxylase activity. A
high negative correlation was found between tyrosine hydroxylase
activity in the striatal and midbrain regions of the CNS and locomotor activity. According to these authors, the results suggested
a direct relationship between behavioral activity and central adrenergic receptor activity which could influence the rate-limiting
step in CA biosynthesis; high receptor activity being associated
with low tyrosine hydroxylase activity and vice versa. Evidence
for feedback from receptors or metabolic end products to synthetic
mechanisms has been observed on a biochemical level also (Costa
& Meek, 1974). A subsequent study has indicated that this adrenergic receptor activity which is correlated with behavioral activity
in these strains of rats may be elicited by NE acting on adenosine
3',5'-monophosphate (cyclic AMP) systems that are sensitive to
NE in the midbrainstriatal region (Skolnick & Daly, 1974). Cyclic
AMP appears to be involved in neurotransmission and associated with
adrenergic receptors.

5-Hydroxytryptamine. A great deal of evidence indicates that
5-HT is involved in the production of sleep and that depletion of
5-HT leads to wakefulness (Jouvet, 1968 and 1969). The proposition
that the 5-HT system is inhibitory in nature, and thus, depletion
of 5-HT leads to behavioral excitation and arousal has led to a
great deal of research in which the relationship 5-HT has to activity in experimental animals has been explored. Lesions in the midbrain raphe nuclei have been associated with lowered levels of 5-
HT and its metabolites in brain, increased spontaneous locomotor
activity and behavioral excitation, and an electroencephalographic
arousal pattern characterized by high frequency, low amplitude
waves (Kostowski et al., 1968; Steranka & Barrett, 1974). Likewise,
in pharmacological investigations an increase in spontaneous locomotor activity when 5-HT levels are lowered by PCPA has often been
observed and these effects have been reversed with injections of
the precursor, 5-HTP (Fibiger & Campbell, 1971; Mabry & Campbell,
1973; Chrusciel & Herman, 1969). Rats treated only with 5-HTP have
shown a decrease in activity (Fibiger & Campbell, 1971; Jacobs &
Eubanks, 1974). However, attempts to reduce brain 5-HT have not
consistently led to increases in activity in laboratory animals.

Rats have been treated with the precursor, tryptophan, resulting in
no observable changes in motor activity but when tryptophan was
administered with an MAO inhibitor, an increase in activity was observed (Grahame-Smith, 1971; Jacobs et al., 1974). These results
could be interpreted to mean that the serotonergic system might be
involved in hyperactivity and behavioral excitation, not inhibition.

   Several investigators have made attempts to reconcile these
inconsistencies in the association of 5-HT and activity. Studies
have shown that depletions of 5-HT lead to hyperreactivity to stimuli which under certain conditions, may result in increased locomotor activity. Depletion of 5-HT levels by injections of PCPA has
resulted in decreased locomotor activity in rats, but when external
stimuli such as tones and flashing lights were presented these rats
showed a larger increase in activity than undrugged control rats
(Brody, 1970; Ellison & Bresler, 1974). Opposed behavioral syndromes have been observed in rats with partial and more complete
lesions in 5-HT axons and terminals produced by small multiple doses
of 5,6-DHT (Diaz et al., 1974). Partially lesioned rats which were
given three intracerebral injections were initially more active
than control rats in the open field, reared less, and exhibited
exaggerated responsivity. On the other hand, rats that were given
6 injections of 5,6-DHT to produce more complete lesions, were initially less active in the open field and reared more. When lights
and tones were presented, both partially and more completely
lesioned rats increased their rearing behavior. Diaz et al., suggested that partial lesions resulted in supersensitivity of the 5-HT system, a phenomenon which has also been observed in the CA system with
partial and more complete lesions produced by 6-OHDA (Sorenson & Ellison, 1973).

   In addition, since 5-HT is also metabolized outside of the CNS,
peripheral effects of pharmacologically administered substances may
account for some of the inconsistencies in this area of research.
Modigh (1972) has attempted to separate the peripheral and central
effects of 5-HTP administration on spontaneous locomotor activity in
mice. Treatment with large doses of 5-HTP was associated with a decrease in activity, but when 5-HTP was given in combination with a 5-
HTP decarboxylase inhibitor that did not pass the blood-brain barrier, a large increase in activity was associated with the increase
in brain 5-HT levels. These data implied that central effects of
5-HTP were excitatory and probably due to excessive stimulation of
5-HT receptors while the peripheral effects were inhibitory.
Rats have also been peripherally injected with a wide range of
doses of 5-HT or 5-HTP and their locomotor activity observed (Jacobs
& Eubanks, 1974). Since 5-HT which does not easily pass the blood-
brain barrier had a greater inhibitory effect on locomotor activity
than 5-HTP, which can get into brain, these authors suggested that
inhibition of motor activity observed after 5-HTP administration

was due to the peripheral action of 5-HT.

Besides the difficulty of distinguishing peripheral from central effects, there are several other problems involved in pharmacological studies that attempt to relate the central serotonergic system to behavior. The precursors, the amine itself, or its metabolites could possibly be active in influencing behavior. Recent evidence indicates that the inhibitory effect of large doses of tryptophan on locomotor activity is not mediated by any of its metabolites including 5-HT (Modigh, 1973). In addition, after large doses of 5-HTP, 5-HT is also formed in the brain outside of the serotonergic neurons and is present in other cells including CA-containing neurons from which it can displace CAs which may then act on receptors (Modigh, 1972; Chase & Murphy, 1973). Finally, PCPA which as been thought to exclusively inhibit tryptophan hydroxylase has recently been associated with depletions of CAs (Chase & Murphy, 1973) which may have effects on activity (Welch & Welch, 1967; Fibiger & Campbell, 1971). All of these effects should be taken into account in the interpretation of results.

Several researchers have presented evidence indicating that putative neurotransmitter systems interact with each other. This interaction has been detected in observations of locomotor activity. Hutchins & Rogers (1973) measured the circadian rhythm of locomotor activity after depletion of monoamines by α-MT and PCPA. α-MT abolished most nocturnal activity but did not affect the short spurt of activity that occurred just after light onset. PCPA increased activity overall and inhibited the activity decrease that normally occurred just before the short spurt of activity mentioned above. The authors concluded that intact CA systems were necessary for nocturnal activity and its termination depended on 5-HT. Chrusciel & Herman (1969) have suggested that 5-HT and CA systems are in dynamic equilibrium such that depletion of 5-HT increases CAs and depletion of CAs increases 5-HT. They observed that DOPA increased locomotor activity in mice and increased NE levels and PCPA potentiated this increase in activity and in NE levels. These data suggested that CAs stimulated locomotor activity centers and 5-HT inhibited them. Spiroperidol, a DA receptor blocking agent, has been found to inhibit the increase in locomotor activity and hyperreactivity observed by Jacobs et al. (1974) after concurrent administration of tryptophan and the MAO inhibitor, pargyline. NE receptor blockers had no effect, and thus, the DA receptor was somehow involved in the effect the serotonergic system had on locomotor activity. Based on pharmacological manipulations of three putative neurotransmitter systems, serotonergic, adrenergic and cholinergic, and their subsequent effects on locomotor activity, Campbell and his associates (Mabry & Campbell, 1973; Fibiger et al., 1970) have suggested the existance of an inhibitory system that is mediated by 5-HT which influences an adrenergic excitatory system in the reticular formation.

This adrenergic excitatory system can interact with a cholinergic
inhibitory system which may exert its influence from the cerebral
cortex and thus influence behavioral arousal of the organisms.

Avoidance Learning

Since the initial finding by Wooley & Van Der Hoeven (1963)
that increased cerebral 5-HT was associated with decreases in maze
learning ability and decreases of 5-HT and that CAs slightly increased maze learning ability in mice, a substantial literature
has arisen implicating these biogenic amines in the acquisition,
maintenance and retention of a wide range of learning tasks. Since
much of this research has used avoidance training procedures, the
following discussion will be limited to this area. For detailed
discussion of methodological issues involved in learning paradigms
refer to Chapter 19.

Catecholamines. Hanson and his coworkers have pharmacologically investigated active avoidance behavior in cats and rats (Fuxe &
Hanson, 1967; Hanson, 1965, 1967a and 1967b; Seiden & Hanson, 1964).
These findings indicated that depletion of CAs by such drugs as
α-MT and reserpine, produced a deficit in maintenance of active
avoidance responding in either a shuttlebox or lever press task.
Sufficient doses of DOPA reversed this deficit and restored levels
of CAs. Amphetamine reversed the behavioral effect of reserpine.
Seiden & Carlsson (1965) have also observed DOPA reversal of reserpine induced behavioral depression of shuttlebox avoidance performance in mice and rats, although this reversal was partial. The
majority of studies, in agreement with this work, indicate that depletions of CAs impair acquisition, maintenance and retention of
avoidance responding. Increasing the levels of CAs by MAO inhibitors
has improved poor shuttlebox avoidance behavior in hamsters (Sansone
et al., 1972). Likewise, rats that were poor performers in shuttlebox avoidance improved after injection of amphetamine (Rech & Moore,
1968). Evidence has indicated that the deficit observed in shuttlebox avoidance performance after α-MT injections was due to the action
of this drug on the adrenergic system and occurred when toxic effects
of the drug itself were absent (Rech et al., 1966 & 1968). In these
studies behavioral effects correlated well with CA levels over time,
poor avoidance performance being associated with low DA and NE levels. However, peripheral effects of the drugs themselves or drug
induced changes in peripheral CAs could account for some of the observed results in the studies discussed in this section so far. Evidence exists, in fact, that peripheral depletion of NE is associated
with a depressed rate of acquisition in a passive avoidance task
(Guisto, 1972).

Up to this point in the discussion, the relative roles of DA

and NE have not been made clear. Recently much research has been
conducted untilizing 6-OHDA to produce central sympathectomy and
this has opened up new vistas concerning the relative importance
of DA and NE in avoidance learning.

    Breese, Cooper & associates have extensively investigated
the effects of intracisternal injections of 6-OHDA on the behavior of rats. 6-OHDA depletes central CAs without appearing
to influence peripheral CAs (Breese & Traylor, 1970, 1971). In general
after 6-OHDA injection initial behavioral depression is observed
with subsequent recovery within a few days even though central
CAs remain depleted (Breese et al., 1973; Cooper & Breese, 1974;
Taylor & Laverty, 1972; Herman et al., 1972). Several explanations for this observed dissociation between brain CAs and behavior have been presented. Taylor & Laverty (1972) have suggested an initial transitory action of 6-OHDA not based on neuronal
destruction, e.g. inhibition of tyrosine hydroxylase or action
of a false transmitter, may be responsible for the transitory behavioral depression. On the other hand, initial behavioral changes
may reflect a new state of balance between the CA system and other
putative transmitter systems (Herman et al., 1972) or compensatory
mechanisms such as enhanced receptor sensitivity or increased amine
synthesis may be involved in the recovery of normal behavior (Breese
et al., 1973; Cooper & Breese, 1974). However, 6-OHDA treated rats
that had recovered from behavioral depression and were given low
doses of reserpine or α-MT which had no effect on controls have
shown severe decrements in shuttlebox avoidance responding (Breese
et al., 1973). In addition, double doses of 6-OHDA produced chronic
loss of acquisition and avoidance performance associated with drastic
depletions of CAs. These investigators have developed 6-OHDA treatments by combined use of additional drugs and scheduling of injections that moderately or drastically reduce both NE and DA or preferentially reduce NE or DA. The more drastic the reduction of CAs, the
larger and more permanent the behavioral effects which have been
observed to extend to 72 days after injection (Cooper et al., 1973).
Reduction of both NE and DA has led to impaired acquisition of a
two-way shuttlebox avoidance task and a one-way avoidance task but
did not impair acquisition of a one-trial passive avoidance task
(Cooper et al., 1972 and 1973). Similar deficits were observed for
the effects of 6-OHDA treatments on established shuttlebox active
avoidance responding. In contrast, preferential depletion of NE
significantly improved active avoidance acquisition whereas preferential depletion of DA resulted in performance that was not significantly different from control rats that received vehicle injections.
The effect of reserpine or α-MT injections on the maintenance of
shuttlebox performance in these rats preferentially depleted of NE
or DA by 6-OHDA treatments, resulted in relatively large decrements
in avoidance responding in those rats depleted by DA compared to
those preferentially depleted of NE. These findings suggested that

DA was playing and important role in the maintenance of avoidance responding and that a critical amount of DA must be depleted before this avoidance performance deficit was observable. Preferential depletion of DA in infant rats has resulted in impairment of shuttlebox avoidance behavior whereas rats depleted of NE during development did not show a deficit and, in fact, performed better than controls (Smith et al., 1973) again implicating DA in active avoidance behavior.

To more specifically examine the role DA has in active avoidance performance, chemical lesions have been selectively produced by injections of 6-OHDA specifically into DA pathways. Bilateral injections into the substantia nigra significantly reduced striatal DA levels, tyrosine hydroxylase activity and hypothalamic NE levels, and prevented acquisition of a shuttlebox avoidance response (Fibiger et al., 1974). These rats learned the escape response but not the avoidance response. To determine whether damage to the ventral noradrenergic projection was involved in this effect, 6-OHDA was injected bilaterally into the ventral bundle which depleted hypothalamic NE. These rats were not significantly different from controls that were treated with an empty injection needle in the substantia nigra and acquired the avoidance response. Rats were also extensively trained in the shuttlebox prior to 6-OHDA injections and subsequently tested for retention. Rats with lesions in the substantia nigra exhibited a relatively slight deficit in the retention of this overtrained task, although they performed significantly less well than the control rats on retention tests. Other researchers have administered 6-OHDA to rats through cannuli implanted bilaterally into the ventral anterior striatum (Neill et al., 1974b). Administration of 6-OHDA resulted in a decrement in pre-established active avoidance responding in the shuttlebox. The severity of the avoidance deficit was positively correlated with the degree of forebrain DA but not NE depletion.

Electrolytic lesions similarly have implicated DA in avoidance learning. Kirkby & Kimble (1968) reported that bilateral lesions in the corpus striatum impaired both active avoidance and escape behavior. In addition, water deprived rats with lesions that had been well trained to run to water reinforcement were unable to acquire inhibition of this response when shocked as they approached the water reward. However, water deprived rats with lesions that were relatively untrained to approach water reward were able to acquire this passive avoidance response. Mitcham & Thomas (1972) found that lesions of the substantia nigra or caudate nucleus resulted in poor avoidance performance in the shuttlebox when the task was a two-way active avoidance, one-way active avoidance or required inhibition of the previously acquired one-way active avoidance (passive avoidance). Local administration of scopolamine, an anticholinergic agent, to the ventral caudate, but not the dorsal

caudate, has been observed to facilate active avoidance in the
shuttlebox whereas lesions in the ventral or dorsal caudate impaired avoidance acquisition (Neill & Grossman, 1970). These
findings indicated to the authors that the ventral caudate contained pathways that were not subject to cholinergic interference
and that were involved in avoidance learning. Subsequently, ventral striatal lesions were found to deplete forebrain DA to a significantly greater extent than dorsal striatal lesions (Neill et
al., 1974a). Neither lesion produced a significant change in levels of NE when compared to operated controls. Rats with dorsal
lesions were able to reaquire preoperative shuttlebox avoidance
performance to a significantly greater extent than ventrally
lesioned rats.

Electrical stimulation of brain areas that involve the DA
system have been reported to disrupt memory of passive avoidance
tasks. Pouttenberg & Holzman (1973) observed that electrical
stimulation of the substantia nigra and pars compacta but not
several other brain areas resulted in memory disruption of a
pretrained step-down passive avoidance task. Stimulation was
administered before and during the retest. Likewise, stimulation of the caudate nucleus through electrode implants has been
found to impair passive avoidance learning (Wyers et al., 1968).
In this experiment, thirsty rats were pretrained to press a lever
for water and were subsequently shocked as they approached the
lever. Brain stimulation administered immediately after the
shock interfered with passive avoidance of the lever 24 hours
later when given in the caudate nucleus or hippocampus but not
other regions of the brain that were tested.

5-Hydroxytryptamine. The relation of 5-HT to avoidance learning has been less extensively investigated than that of the CAs
and its functional role in avoidance learning still remains obscure.
The agent, 5,6-DHT, which is thought to selectively produce neurochemical lesions in the 5-HT system as 6-OHDA does in the adrenergic
system is a needed tool. The recent discovery of its action may
stimulate research in this area and help to distinguish the central
effects of 5 - HT from the peripheral effects on behavior.

Numerous investigators have observed an increase in avoidance
performance and depletion of brain 5-HT after administration of
PCPA. Tanaka et al. (1972) have reported a dose dependent PCPA induced increase in a pretrained lever press sidman avoidance task
and a decrease in number of shocks received by rats. Administration
of 5-HTP was observed to reverse this effect. PCPA has also facilitated the acquisition of a pole climb avoidance task in rats, however, chronic administration of PCPA from birth decreased jump-up
avoidance acquisition in mice (Schlesinger et al., 1968). These
authors suggested that chronic PCPA during development mimics the

inherited disease in humans, phenylketonuria, which is characterized
by chronically high levels of phenylalanine, low levels of 5-HT and
behavioral symptoms including mental retardation. This experimental
result is in general agreement with other work that has attempted to
investigate learning in experimentally produced animal models of
phenylketonuria (Chamove & Harlow, 1973; Kilbey & Harris, 1971;
Butcher et al., 1970). PCPA has facilitated avoidance acquisition
of a jump-up avoidance task in rats (Tenen, 1967) and this behavioral effect has been demonstrated to be independent of phenalalanine
changes or of PCPA itself (Brody, 1970). 5-HTP reversed this facilitation (Tenen, 1967). PCPA has resulted in good passive avoidance
in a step-down task (Brody, 1970), however, Stevens & Fechter (1969)
found that PCPA retarded passive avoidance learning. Water deprived
rats were pretrained to run to a drinking spout which was subsequently electrified. PCPA injected rats showed poor inhibition of the pretrained response. These authors suggested that depletion of 5-HT reduced emotionality in the rats and thus affected performance.

Depletion of brain 5-HT by selective lesions has also
been associated with increased acquisition in avoidance learning
tasks. Lorens et al., (1970) produced electrolytic lesions in the
nuclei accumbens septi of rats which is part of the striatum and an
important contributer of fibers to the descending component of the
medial forebrain bundle. Telencephalic 5-HT was lowered with no
significant effect on NE levels and active avoidance acquisition in
the shuttlebox was enhanced. Lesions in the raphe nuclei have also
resulted in reduced brain 5-HT levels and superior performance in a
shuttlebox active avoidance task (Lorens et al., 1971) and a discrimination avoidance task in a Y-maze (Steranka & Barrett, 1974). In
the Y-maze raphe lesioned, sham lesioned and non-handled rats did
not differ in number of correct discriminations made, but raphe
lesioned rats avoided more and escaped less than the control groups.

Tenen (1967) found that depletion of brain 5-HT by PCPA only
increased avoidance performance over controls at low but not high
shock intensities and decreased the jump threshold in response to
shock. 5-HTP reversed these effects. These findings implied that
depletion of 5-HT was producing an effect on shock sensitivity and
not on learning per se which increased performance in the learning
situtation. Several researchers have extensively investigated this
phenomenon. Harvey & Lints (1971) have found that lesions in the
medial forebrain bundle decreased both the jump threshold to foot-
shock and levels of 5-HT in the telencephalon of rats. Injections
of 5-HTP produced a dose dependent increase in 5-HT in both lesioned
and sham operated rats. Within limits this was associated with a
dose dependent increase in jump threshold only in lesioned rats.
PCPA decreased both jump threshold and 5-HT levels in both sham and
lesioned rats. Furthermore, Yunger & Harvey (1973) have found that
bilateral lesions in the medial forebrain bundle decreased the shock
detection threshold and 5-HT levels while the magnitude of response

to shock was increased.   Injections of 5-HTP given to these lesioned
rats brought the magnitude of response back to normal but the shock
detection threshold was still below normal.   This implied that 5-HT
was related to increased reactivity to painful stimuli but not to
changes in detection threshold.   Experiments with PCPA have also indicated that reactivity to footshock and not changes in aversion
thresholds to footshock is affected by depletion of 5-HT (Fibiger
et al., 1972).

     Several studies have attempted to influence the labile phase
of memory that is thought to occur immediately after an animal is
trained but before it becomes more permanent long term memory.   Essman (1971 and 1972) has found that increased 5-HT in brain produced
by intracranial injections of 5-HT when injected following a single
training trial in as passive avoidance task produced amnesia in mice
that decreased as the amount of time between the training trial and
injection increased.   Recently similar experiments have been conducted by Rake and his associates (Dismukes & Rake, 1972; Rake, 1973;
Allen et al., 1974).   Mice were trained in an active avoidance task,
the shuttlebox, or in a one trial passive avoidance task in which
they were placed in a small lighted compartment and shocked when
they entered an adjoining larger, dark compartment through a hole.
Immeidately after active or passive avoidance training the mice
were injected with one or more drugs that affected serotonergic or
adrenergic systems and were retested later.   Neither training nor
testing occurred under the influence of drugs.   Reserpine injected
after training in the shuttlebox or passive avoidance task produced
amnesia when the mice were tested later but amnesia did not occur if
the injection was delayed to 24 hours after training.   Injections
of DOPA along with the reserpine injection reversed the amnesia to
a relatively much greater extent in the active avoidance than in the
passive avoidance task.   On the other hand, 5-HTP reversed the effect on the passive avoidance task.   In a subsequent experiment the
active task was made more similar to the passive task.   The passive
avoidance apparatus was used to train mice to a criterion of one
avoidance in which they were trained to leave the larger dark compartment and enter the safe compartment before shock onset.   The results again suggested CAs had a relatively larger role in memory of
active avoidance whereas 5 - HT was more important in the memory of
passive avoidance.   In addition, immediately after training in the
shuttlebox injections of diethyldithiocarbamate which prevents the
hydroxylation of DA to NE, produced amnesia as did dichloroisoproter-
enal which blocks β-NE receptors.   This indicated that NE might influence memory of active avoidance performance.   However, another
study in which mice were injected with diethydithiocarbamate immediately after training on a one trial passive avoidance task resulted
in amnesia 24 hours later which was associated with a decrease in
brain NE (Randt et al., 1971). According to the authors, this implicated NE also in passive avoidance memory.

The work of Rake and his colleagues also suggests biogenic amine systems may have opposing roles and thus interact to produce excitatory or inhibitory behavior. Other researchers have presented evidence supporting the hypothesis that these systems interact. The Kamin effect, in which memory for a previously learned active avoidance task is poorest at intermediate times after training and best immediately after or 24 hours after training has recently been explained in terms of an interaction between central cholinergic and adrenergic mechanisms (Anisman & Kokkinidis, 1974). Shock is thought to release CAs which increases general activity of the organism immediately after training and stimulates the cholinergic system which subsequently leads to inhibition of general activity resulting in poor performance at intermediate times after training. Swonger & Rech (1972) have presented a model which attempts to integrate the serotonergic, adrenergic and cholinergic systems in terms of facilitory or inhibitory processes. In their model, stimulation of the adrenergic system increases arousal and when the organism is in a low or moderate arousal state the cholinergic inhibitory system adequately functions to maintain appropriate behavioral responsiveness to the environment. The serotonergic system, however, responds to high arousal states of the organism and can increase the inhibition of the cholinergic system under these conditions. As these authors point out, the evidence presented earlier in this chapter that indicates locomotor activity is not changed by 5-HT depletion until arousal stimuli are presented implicates 5-HT in high but not low arousal states. This hyperreactivity to arousal stimuli also occurs in response to shock as indicated by response magnitude when 5-HT levels are depleted (see above discussion).

State-dependent Learning

In the last 10 years, much research has been directed toward understadning the state-dependent learning or dissociation phenomenon. Simply stated, dissociation is present if responses acquired when an organism is drugged are performed during subsequent test trials only when the drug state is reinstated, while responses acquired under undrugged conditions are subsequently performed only without administration of a drug (Overton, 1964). A commonly used technique in state-dependent learning studies is to train the animal to perform one response in the drug state and another response in the undrugged state. After good discriminative response control has been established based on drug state, other drugs may either be substituted for the original drugs or injected along with the original drugs to determine if they produce a decrement in responding and thus are unlike the original drug state or disrupt it. An additional procedure used in state-dependent learning investigations to directly test whether amnesia for the learned response is produced by a change in drug conditions is the 2 x 2 design. In this

procedure 2 groups of animals are trained under either drugged or
undrugged conditions. Each group is then subsequently divided
and tested under either the same drug conditions (no state change)
or under the alternative drug conditions (state change). Dissociation has occurred if the state change groups perform poorly or do
not respond when compared to the 2 groups for which drug conditions
have not changed during testing.

Recent evidence implicates biogenic amines in state-dependent
performance. Based solely on drug state, rats were trained to
perform a spatial discrimination in a T-maze (Schechter & Rosecrans,
1972). One side of the maze was reinforced as the correct side
after a saline injection and the other side was reinforced after a
nicotine injection. After this discrimination based on drugged
and undrugged states was clearly established by means of both foot-
shock and milk reinforcement, PCPA or α-MT were administered to the
rats in each of the 2 established drug states. PCPA did not interrupt the discrimination, however, α-MT disrupted the cueing effect
of nicotine but not saline. Because of the well known effect nicotine has on the cholinergic system, these authors concluded that
the CNS cueing effect produced by nicotine was mediated by NE via
the cholinergic system in which nicotine acted on a cholinergic
receptor which resulted in the release of NE. This produced the
interoceptive cue that allowed the response associated with the
nicotine state to occur. Similarly, 5-HT was demonstrated to be
involved in a situation in which rats were trained to escape shock
by choosing the correct compartment in a three compartment box based
on a morphine or saline state (Rosecrans et al., 1973). After the
two choice discrimination was established, PCPA or α-MT were administered to the rats whle in the morphine or saline state. PCPA
disrupted responding in the morphine but not the saline state,
while α-MT had no effect. Schechter (1973) has also reported involvement of the 5-HT system in a task where ethanol was used as
a discriminative cue. After establishment of a discrimination response in the three compartment box based on the ability to discriminate between ethanol and saline, PCPA was administered. The
rats were then injected with either saline or ethanol and tested.
PCPA did not alter the saline cue but eliminated the ethanol cue
resulting in chance choices of the correct compartment after ethanol
injections. To determine the relationship of brain amines to an
amphetamine state, Roffman & Lal (1972) trained rats in a jump-up
avoidance task under the influence of amphetamine and subsequently
retested them with appropriate novel drugs administered alone or
superimposed upon the amphetamine state. When the rats were retested with the peripherally acting drug, hydroxyamphetamine, a
decrement in performance was observed that was not seen when retested with amphetamine which has effects both centrally and peripherally. Depletion of peripheral amines with syrosingopine did
not prevent responses from occurring in the amphetamine state, while

depletion of both central and peripheral amines with reserpine disrupted performance. On the basis of these findings the authors concluded that the amines involved in the amphetamine state were located in the CNS. If either DOPA or 5-HTP were given in conjunction with reserpine, the amphetamine state remained disrupted while if both DOPA and 5-HTP were given, the amphetamine state was left intact. No response decrement was noted in either a state produced by concurrent administration of three compounds, 5-HTP, PCPA and amphetamine, or DOPA, α-MT and amphetamine, whereas both PCPA and α-MT disrupted responding in the amphetamine state. DOPA but not 5-HTP was found to substitute for amphetamine. Both the adrenergic blocking agent, chlorpromazine and the serotonergic blocking agent, cyproheptadine, resulted in reduced responding of amphetamine treated rats. These pharmacological manipulations indicated that both CAs and indoleamines were involved in the CNS state produced by amphetamine.

An attempt to more directly investigate the role biogenic amines have in state-dependent performance was carried out by Zornetzer et al. (1974). Mice were trained in a one trial passive avoidance task after injection of either α-MT or saline and retested either 30 minutes later in the same state or 24 hours later in the same state or in the alternative state. No significant differences in performance were observed during initial training. Since state change groups performed significantly worse than groups that were trained and tested in the same state, a state-dependent effect was present. Groups tested at 30 minutes did not differ from each other or from their respective nonstate change groups tested at 24 hours. The authors concluded that α-MT did not prevent establishment of either short- or long-term retention. However, investigation of the state-dependent effects of α-MT which significantly lowered brain DA and NE levels and bis-(4-methyl-1-homopeperazinylthiocarbonyl) disulfide (FLA-63) which reduced brain NE and resulted in an increase in brain DA levels yielded different results (Ahlenius, 1973). Mice were trained to avoid shock in a shuttlebox in one of the two drug states or a saline state. Retest occurred in either the same or alternative state. α-MT did not exhibit a state-dependent learning effect but FLA-63 did. α-MT appeared to produce a decrement in responding during retest. The reason for the discrepancy in the effects of α-MT between these two studies is not immediately apparent, although the different learning tasks, one active and one passive, and the different modes of injection and dose of α-MT may be responsible.

It should be noted that many of the studies mentioned in previous sections in this chapter that have attempted to determine relationships between conditioned behavior and biogenic amines using pharmacological techniques have failed to control for state-dependent learning effects. Recent evidence indicates that the state-

dependent learning phenomenon can also be demonstrated when drugs
are administered immediately after, instead of prior to, training
and reinstated later prior to testing (Chute & Wright, 1973). Since
the articles discussed above implicate brain amines in state-dependent performance, future research exploring neurochemical correlates
of behavior should attempt to control for dissociation effects
whether injections are given prior to or immediately after training.

Effects of Behavior on Biogenic Amines

Although few studies have been concerned with the effects behavior, specificially activity and aversively conditioned behavior,
may have on neurochemistry, there currently appears to be some interest in this area. Seiden and his coworkers (Seiden et al., 1973;
Seiden & Campbell, 1974) have emphasized the mutual interaction between behavior and the adrenergic system. They have presented a
model in which biogenic amine metabolism may be influenced by internal and external factors of the organism including drugs, environment and behavior. They have postulated an interaction between behavior and the environment in which behavior can modify the environment and the environment can reinforce behavior. Biogenic amines
can influence behavior and either behavior or the environment can
alter endogenous amine metabolism resulting in feedback relationships. This model predicts a biochemical basis for drug effects
which depend on the nature of the ongoing behavior. For example,
a constant dose of a drug such as amphetamine can facilitate low
behavior rates associated with low turnover of CAs while in the
presence of high CA turnover, amphetamine may flood the synapse
with CAs, and thus, produce a block resulting in inhibition of high
rates of behavior. As these authors point out, this model could
account for observations such as those made by Evans (1971) in
which a constant dose of methamphetamine decreased high lever pressing rates and high activity levels but increased low lever pressing rates and low activity levels.

A few studies have observed changes in endogenous amine concentrations as a function of behavior. Elo & Tirri (1972) have
reported changes in endogenous biogenic amine levels in rats due
to forced motility in a treadwheel. Both 5-HT and NE increased
in parts of brain and 50 minutes of rest after the forced exercise nearly restored 5-HT to control levels. He suggested this increase might be associated with a high arousal state. Endogenous
levels of NE and 5-HT have also been measured in rats trained in an
active avoidance jump-up task, yoked shock controls and non-shock
controls (Weiss et al., 1970). Brain NE levels were determined 20
or 40 minutes after training. Rats in the experimental group which
could either avoid or escape the shock exhibited a significant rise

in NE levels when compared to control groups. No changes in 5-HT
level were observed. Under more stressful conditions in a task
where rats could avoid or escape shock by turning a wheel, the
yoked shock control group had significantly lower brain NE levels
than the non-shock control group which is in agreement with the
effects of stress on brain NE. In support of their previous results using the jump-up task, rats that could avoid or escape
exhibited a significant rise in brain NE. Weiss et al. also attempted to control for activity differences between the trained
group and yoked shock control group. Different groups of animals
were shocked under either free-moving or immobile conditions for
three hours and no difference between these two groups in brain
NE levels were found.

In an attempt to relate the performance decrement observed
in the Kamin effect to brain NE and 5-HT levels, Bauer (1973)
partially trained rats in a one-way active avoidance task or
subjected them to approximately the same amount of inescapable
shock which the experimental group received and either trained
them or assayed for brain NE and 5-HT 10 minutes, 3.5 or 24 hours
after original training. Both the partially trained and shock
control group showed the Kamin effect by performing the avoidance
task better at 10 minutes and 24 hours when compared to 3.5 hours.
However, a similar U-shaped function was not observed for either
5-HT or NE. Brain 5-HT levels showed no changes while NE levels
were significantly lower at 10 minutes and 3.5 hours. Bauer concluded endogenous levels of these amines present after partial
avoidance training or exposure to inescapable shock were not related to poorer avoidance at intermediate retest intervals. The
apparent discrepancy between this study and the study by Weiss
et al. in the effects of training produced on NE levels may be
due to differences in amount of training. Bauer trained his rats
to only one avoidance response before assaying for NE levels whereas Weiss et al. trained his rats for 70 trials in the jump-up task
and 48 hours in the wheel-turning task resulting in performance
of many more avoidance and escape responses. Thus, Bauer may
have been only observing an effect of shock on NE levels, while
Weiss et al. was observing what he called "copying behavior".

Whole brain analysis of biogenic amines can mask important
changes occurring in specific areas of the brain as a result of behavior. Wimer et al. (1973) investigated the effects of behavioral manipulations of NE and 5-HT levels in parts of brain. Inbred
strains of mice, C57BL/6J and DBA/2J, were subjected to one of a
variety of treatments including training in a shock-motivated jump-
up task. Unhandled control C57BL/6J mice had significantly less
5-HT in hippocampus than DBA/2J mice. Changes in levels of NE and
5-HT observed in parts of brain after treatments were in the same
direction for both strains except for the hippocampus in which the
treatments resulted in a decrease of 5-HT in DBA/2J mice and an in-

crease in C57BL/6J mice, 42% and 266% respectively of control values. This approach to the study of the relationship between biogenic amines and behavior may help to implicate specific areas of the brain and specific amines that play important roles in conditioned behavior. In addition, it expresses the importance of individual differences in behavioral effects on neurochemistry.

DISCUSSION

There is sufficiently extensive evidence that the CNS biogenic amines, DA, NE and 5-HT have a role in activity and aversively conditioned behavior, although their specific function in these behaviors and their relative importance remain obscure. Much of the research to date has been plagued with several problems represented by unwanted side effects of drugs, peripheral effects of monoamines and the possibility that active metabolities of amines may conceal the interaction between CNS monoamines and behavior. NE has been observed to stimulate DA receptors (Ungerstedt et al., 1969), and thus, the likelihood that monoamines can stimulate receptors other than their own further complicates interpretations of experimental results. On the other hand, in a complex behavior pattern like avoidance learning it is difficult to determine whether monoamine changes are altering learning itself or variables that contribute to avoidance performance such as motivation, sensory capacity, shock sensitivity or activity. In spite of these drawbacks, much research progress has been made in the last few years partially due to the discovery of tools such as 6-OHDA. More investigators are beginning to examine parts of brain instead of whole brain for changes in maonoamine concentration or turnover rate. This is advantageous since whole brain assays can mask important changes in parts of brain which may lead to implication of specific brain areas or monoamines in certain types of behavior. Much more information is needed on the mutual interaction of biogenic amines and behavior. Behavioral states can probably trigger neurochemical changes and the nature of this association needs to be investigated. Seiden & Campbell (1974) have pointed out that drug effects can be a function of the ongoing behavioral and neurochemical state of the organism. Some of the discrepant experimental results that have been found could be accounted for by this phenomenon.

A much neglected approach to the study of amines and behavior is the use of genetic studies. Several recent studies have reported that inbred strains of mice differ in neurochemistry (Eleftheriou, 1971 and 1974; Kempf et al., 1974; Kessler et al., 1972; Barchas, et al., 1974) and the evidence that strains differ in behavior is extensive (Sprott & Staats, 1975). Correlations between monoamines and behavior can be determined with the use of inbred strains and subsequent behavioral analysis carried out by environmental manipulation. For example, differences between strains of mice in the time course for DOPA reversal of reserpine induced depression have been noted and levels of brain DA and NE were found to correlate with the behavioral recovery period in each strain (Seiden et al., 1973). Similarly, DA concentrations in nervous tissue have been found to be negatively correlated with spontaneous locomotor activity in strains of Drosophila melanogaster (fruit flies) (Rick & Fulker, 1972). Following administration of γ-hydroxybutyric acid, nervous tissue DA increased in one strain and was not altered in another. The effects of the drug on locomotor activity were consistent with the neurochemical changes. Subsequent genetic analysis can also be applied to the study of monoamines and behavior. This approach has been utilized by Mandel et al. (1974) in an attempt to investigate cholinergic parameters and learning ability in inbred strains of mice and their F_1 offspring produced by crossing the parental strains. Appropriate crossing of parental strains can produce offspring generations in which genes segregate. Correlations between biogenic amines and behavioral characters that are not due to chance will remain correlated in these segregating populations. This approach has been used to investigate behavioral correlates of the γ-aminobutyric acid system (Rick & Fulker, 1972).

Finally, evidence is accumulating that suggests biogenic amine systems interact with each other. Manipulation of one system most likely will produce a disturbance in other systems. Tunnicliff et al. (1973) have observed correlations between the activity of pairs of enzymes in the adrenergic, cholinergic and γ-aminobutyric acid systems in inbred strains of mice. Enzyme activity is often used as a measure of the dynamic state of monoamine systems. Significant differences in enzyme activity were observed between strains and certain behaviors correlated with the activity of particular enzymes. Understanding of the putative neurotransmitters and their association to behavior may best be realized by manipulation of two or more of these amine systems simultaneously and the study of the interaction between them and the behavior.

ACKNOWLEDGEMENTS

The preparation of this manuscript was supported by training grants C-1216500 and MH-12126 from the National Institute of Mental Health.

REFERENCES

ANDEN, N.-E., DAHLSTROM, A., FUXE, K., LARSSON, K., OLSON, L. & UNGERSTED, U., 1966, Ascending monoamine neurons to the telencephalon and diencephalon, Acta Physiol. Scand. 67:313.

AHLENIUS, S., 1973, Inhibition of catecholamine synthesis and conditioned avoidance acquisition, Pharmacol. Biochem. Behav. 1:347.

ALLEN, C., ALLEN, B. S. & RAKE, A. V., 1974, Pharmacological distinctions between "active" and "passive" avoidance memory formation as shown by manipulation of biogenic amine active compounds, Psychopharmacologia, 34:1.

ANISMAN, H. & KOKKINIDIS, L., 1974, Effects of central and peripheral adrenergic and cholinergic modification on time-dependent processes in avoidance performance, Behav. Biol. 10:161.

AXELROD, J., 1965, The metabolism, storage, and release of catecholamines, Rec. Prog. Horm. Res. 21:597.

BARCHAS, J. D., CIARANELLO, R. D., STOLK, J. M., BRODIE, K. H. & HAMBERG, D. A., 1972, Biogenic amines and behavior, in "Hormones and Behavior," (S. Levine, ed.), pp. 235-329, Academic Press, New York.

BARCHAS, J. D., CIARANELLO, R. D., DOMINIC, J. A., DEGUCHI, T., ORENBERG, E., RENSON, J. & KESSLER, S., 1974, Genetic aspects of monoamine mechanisms, in "Neuropsychopharmacology of Monoamines and Their Regulatory Enzymes," (E. Usdin, ed.), pp. 195-204, Raven Press, New York.

BARTHOLINI, G., BLUM, J. E. & PLETSCHER, A., 1969, Dopa-induced locomotor stimulation after inhibition of extracerebral decarboxylase, J. Pharm. Pharmacol. 21:297.

BAUER, R. H., 1973, Brain norepinephrine and 5-hydroxytryptamine as a function of time after avoidance training and footshock, Pharmacol. Biochem. Behav. 1:615.

BAUMGARTEN, H. G. & SCHLOSSBERGER, H. G., 1973, Effects of 5,6-dihydroxytryptamine on brain monoamine neurons in the rat, in "Serotonin and Behavior," (J. Barchas & E. Usdin, eds.), pp. 209-224, Academic Press, New York.

BENKERT, O., GLUBA, H. & MATUSSEK, N., 1973a, Dopamine, noradrenaline and 5-hydroxytryptamine in relation to motor activity, fighting and mounting behavior. I. L-DOPA and DL-threo-dihydroxyphenyl-serine in combination with Ro 4-4602, pargyline and reserpine, Neuropharmacol. 12:177.

BENKERT, O., RENZ, A. & MATUSSEK, N., 1973b, Dopamine, noradrenaline and 5-hydroxytryptamine in relation to motor activity, fighting and mounting behavior. II. L-DOPA and DL-threo-dihydroxyphenyl-serine in combination with Ro 4-4602 and parachlorophenylalanine, Neuropharmacol. 12:187.

BREESE, G. R. & TRAYLOR, T. D., 1970, Effect of 6-hydroxydopamine on brain norepinephrine and dopamine: evidence for selective de-generation of catecholamine neurons, J. Pharmacol. Exp. Therap. 174:413.

BREESE, G. R. & TRAYLOR, T. D., 1971, Depletion of brain noradrena-line and dopamine by 6-hydroxydopamine, Brit. J. Pharmacol. 42:88.

BREESE, G. R., COOPER, B. R. & SMITH, R. D., 1973, Biochemical and behavioral alterations following 6-hydroxydopamine administra-tion into brain, Abstracts of papers presented at Frontiers in Catecholamine Research. III. International Catecholamine Symposium. University of Strasbourg, Strasbourg, France.

BRODY, J. F., JR., 1970, Behavioral effects of serotonin depletion and of p-chlorophenylalanine (a serotonin depletor) in rats, Psychopharmacologia 17:14.

BUTCHER, L. L. & ENGEL, J., 1969, Peripheral factors in the media-tion of the effects of L-DOPA on locomotor activity, J. Pharm. Pharmacol. 21:614.

BUTCHER, R., VORHEES, C. & BERRY, H., 1970, Alearning impairment associated with induced phenylketonuria, Life Sci. 9:1261.

CAMPBELL, B. A., LYTLE, L. D. & FIBIGER, H. C., 1969, Ontogeny of adrenergic arousal and cholinergic inhibitory mechanisms in the rat, Science 166:635.

CARLTON, P. L., 1963, Cholinergic mechanisms in the control of be-havior by the brain, Psychol. Rev. 70:19.

CHAMOVE, A. S. & HARLOW, H. F., 1973, Avoidance learning in phenyl-ketonuric monkeys, J. Comp. Physiol. Psychol. 84:605.

CHASE, T. N. & MURPHY, D. L., 1973, Serotonin and central nervous system function, Ann. Rev. Pharmacol. 13:181.

CHRUSCIEL, T. L. & HERMAN, Z. S., 1969, Effect of dopalanine on be-
    havior in mice depleted of norepinephrine or serotonin, Psycho-
    pharmacologia 14:124.

CHUTE, D. L., & WRIGHT, D. C., 1973, Retrograde state dependent
    learning, Science 180:878.

COOPER, B. R. & BREESE, G. R., 1974, Relationship of dopamine neural
    systems to the behavioral alterations produced by 6-hydroxydo-
    pamine administration into the brain, in "Neuropsychopharma-
    cology of Monoamine and Their Regulatory Enzymes. Advances
    in Biochemical Psychopharmacology," pp. 353-368, Raven Press,
    New York.

COOPER, B. R., BREESE, G. R., HOWARD, J. L. & GRANT, L. D., 1972,
    Effect of central catecholamine alterations by 6-hydroxydopa-
    mine on shuttle box avoidance acquisition, Physiol. Behav. 9:
    727.

COOPER, B. R., BREESE, G. R., GRANT, L. D. & HOWARD, J. L., 1973,
    Effects of 6-hydroxydopamine treatments on active avoidance
    responding: evidence for involvement of brain dopamine, J.
    Pharmacol. Exp. Therap. 185:358.

COOPER, J. R., BLOOM, F. E. & ROTH, R. H., 1974, "The Biochemical
    Basis of Neuropharmacology," Oxford University Press, New York.

COSTA, E. & MEEK, J. L., 1974, Regulation of biosynthesis of cate-
    cholamine and serotonin in the CNS. Ann. Rev. Pharmacol. 14:491.

DAHLSTROM, A. & FUXE, K., 1965, Evidence for the existance of mono-
    amine neurons in the central nervous system. II. Experimental-
    ly induced changes in the intraneuronal amine levels of bulbo-
    spinal neuron systems, Acta Physiol. Scand. Suppl. 247:1.

DIAZ, J., ELLISON, G. & MASUOKA, D., 1974, Opposed behavioral syn-
    dromes in rats with partial and more complete central serotoner-
    gic lesions made with 5,6-dihydroxytryptamine, Psychopharmacolo-
    gia 37:67.

DISMUKES, R. K. & RAKE, A. V., 1972, Involvement of biogenic amines
    in memory formation, Psychopharmacologia 23:17.

DOUGLAS, W. W., 1970, Histamine and antihistamines; 5-hydroxytrypta-
    mine and antagonists, in "The Pharmacological Basis of Thera-
    qeutics," (L. S. Goodman & A. Gilman, eds.), pp. 621-662, Mac-
    millan, New York.

ELEFTHERIOU, B. E., 1971, Regional brain norepinephrine turnover rates in four strains of mice, Neuroendocrinology 7:329.

ELEFTHERIOU, B. E., 1974, A gene influencing hypothalamic norepinephrine levels in mice, Brain Res. 70:538.

ELLISON, G. & BRESLER, D. E., 1974, Tests of emotional behavior in
rats following depletion of norepinephrine, of serotonin, or
of both, Psychopharmacologia 34:275.

ELO, H. & TIRRI, R., 1972, Effect of forced motility on the noradrenaline and 5-hydroxytryptamine metabolism in different parts
of the rat brain, Psychopharmacologia 26:195.

ESSMAN, W. B., 1971, Drug effects and learning and memory processes,
Adv. Pharmacol. Chemotherap. 9:241.

ESSMAN, W. B., 1972, Retrograde amnesia and cerebral protein synthesis: initiation by 5-hydroxytryptamine, Totus Homo 4:61.

EVANS, H. L., 1971, Behavioral effects of methamphetamine and α-
methyltyrosine in the rat, J. Pharmacol. Exp. Therap. 176:244.

FIBIGER, H. C. & CAMPBELL, B. A., 1971, The effect of para-chlorophenylalanine on spontaneous locomotor activity in the rat,
Neuropharmacol. 10:25.

FIBIGER, H. C., LYTLE, L. D. & CAMPBELL, B. A., 1970, Cholinergic
modulation of adrenergic arousal in the developing rat, J.
Comp. Physiol. Psychol. 72:384.

FIBIGER, H. C., MERTZ, P. H. & CAMPBELL, B. A., 1972, The effect of
para-chlorophenylalanine on aversion thresholds and reactivity
to footshock, Physiol. Behav. 8:259.

FIBIGER, H. C., PHILLIPS, A. G. & ZIS, A. P., 1974, Deficits in
instrumental responding after 6-hydroxydopamine lesions of the
nigro-neostriatal dopaminergic projection, Pharmacol. Biochem.
Behav. 2:87.

FOG, R., RANDRUP, A. & PAKKENBERG, H., 1970, Lesions in the corpus
striatum and cortex of rat brains and the effect on pharmacologically induced stereotyped, aggressive and cataleptic behavior,
Psychopharmacologia 18:346.

FUXE, K. & HANSON, L. C. F., 1967, Central catecholamine neurons
and conditioned avoidance behavior, Psychopharmacologia 11:439.

FUXE, K., HOKFELT, T. & UNGERSTEDT, U., 1968, Localization of indole-
alkylamines in CNS, Adv. Pharmacol. 6:235.

FUXE, K., HOKFELT, T. & UNGERSTEDT, U., 1970, Central monoaminergic tracts, Princ. Psychopharmacol. 6:87.

GEYER, M. A. & SEGAL, D. S., 1973, Differential effects of reserpine and α-methyl-p-tyrosine on norepinephrine and dopamine induced behavioral activity, Psychopharmacologia 29:131.

GEYER, M. A., SEGAL, D. S. & MANDELL, A. J., 1972, Effect of intraventricular infusion of dopamine and norepinephrine on motor activity, Physiol. Behav. 8:653.

GIUSTO, E. L., 1972, Adrenaline or peripheral noradrenaline depletion and passive avoidance in the rat, Physiol. Behav. 8:1059.

GLOWINSKI, J., & BALDESSARINI, R. J., 1966, Metabolism of norepinephrine in the central nervous system, Pharmacol. Rev. 18:1201.

GRAHAME-SMITH, D. G., 1971, Studies in vivo on the relationship between brain tryptophan, brain 5-HT synthesis and hyperactivity in rats treated with a monoamine oxidase inhibitor and 1-tryptophan, J. Neurochem. 18:1053.

GRAHAME-SMITH, D. G., 1973, Does the total turnover of brain 5-HT reflect the functional activity of 5-HT in brain?, in "Serotonin and Behavior," (J. Barchas & E. Usdin, eds.), pp. 5-7, Academic Press, New York.

HANSON, L. C. F., 1965, The disruption of conditioned avoidance response following selective depletion of brain catechol amines, Psychopharmacologia 8:100.

HANSON, L. C. F., 1967a, Evidence that the central action of (+)-amphetamine is mediated via catecholamines, Psychopharmacologia 10:289.

HANSON, L. C. F., 1967b, Biochemical and behavioral effects of tyrosine hydroxylase inhibition, Psychopharmacologia 11:8.

HARVEY, J. A. & LINTS, C. E., 1971, Lesions in the medial forebrain bundle: relationship between pain sensitivity and telencephalic content of serotonin, J. Comp. Physiol. Psychol. 74:28.

HERMAN, Z. S., KMIECIAK-KOLADA, K. & BRUS, R., 1972, Behavior of rats and biogenic amine level in brain after 6-hydroxy-dopamine, Psychopharmacologia 24:407.

HOLLISTER, A. S., BREESE, G. R. & COOPER, B. R., 1974, Comparison of tyrosine hydroxylase and dopamine-beta-hydroxylase inhibition with the effects of various 6-hydroxydopamine treatments on d-amphetamine induced motor activity, Psychopharmacologia 36:1.

HUTCHINS, D. A. & ROGERS, K. J., 1973, Some observations on the circadian rhythm of locomotor activity of mice after depletion of cerebral monoamines, Psychopharmacologia 31:343.

JACOBS, B. L. & EUBANKS, E. E., 1974, A comparison of the locomotor effects of 5-hydroxytryptamine and 5-hydroxytryptophan administered via two systemic routes, Pharmacol. Biochem. & Behav. 2:137.

JACOBS, B. L., EUBANKS, E. E. & WISE, W. D., 1974, Effect of indolealkylamine manipulations on locomotor activity in rats, Neuropharmacol. 13:575.

JOUVET, M., 1968, Insomnia and decrease of cerebral 5-hydroxytryptamine after destruction of the raphe system in the cat, Adv. Pharmacol. 6:265.

JOUVET, M., 1969, Biogenic amines and the states of sleep, Science 163:32.

KEMPF, E., GREILSAMER, J., MACK, G. & MANDEL, P., 1974, Correlation of behavioral differences in three strains of mice with differences in brain amines, Nature 247:483.

KESSLER, S., CIARANELLO, R. D., SHIRE, J. G. M. & BARCHAS, J. D., 1972, Genetic variation in activity of enzymes involved in synthesis of catecholamines, Proc. Nat. Acad. Sci. 69:2448.

KETY, S. S., 1970, The biogenic amines in the central nervous system: their possible roles in arousal, emotion, and learning, in "The Neurosciences Second Study Program," (F. O. Schmitt, ed.) pp. 324-336, Rockefeller University: New York.

KILBEY, M. M. & HARRIS, R. T., 1971, Behavioral, biochemical and maturational effects of early dl-para-chlorophenylalanine treatment, Psychopharmacologia 19:334.

KIRKBY, R. J. & KIMBLE, D. P., 1968, Avoidance and escape behavior following striatal lesions in the rat, Exp. Neurol. 20:215.

KOELLE, G. B., 1970, Neurohumoral transmission and the autonomic nervous system, in "The Pharmacological Basis of Therapeutics," (L. S. Goodman & A. Gilman, eds.), pp. 402-441, Macmillan, New York.

KOSTOWSKI, W., GIACALONE, E., GARATTINI, S. & VALZELLI, L., 1968, Studies on behavioral and biochemical changes in rats after lesion of midbrain raphe, Eur. J. Pharmacol. 4:371.

LORENS, S. A., SORENSEN, J. P. & HARVEY, J. A., 1970, Lesions in
    the nuclei accumbens septi of the rat: behavioral and neuro-
    chemical effects, J. Comp. Physiol. Psychol. 73:284.

LORENS, S. A., SORENSEN, J. P. & YUNGER, L. M., 1971, Behavioral
    and neurochemical effects of lesions in the raphe system of
    the rat, J. Comp. Physiol. Psychol. 77:48.

MAAS, J. W. & LANDIS, D. H., 1968, In vivo studies of the metabolism
    of norepinephrine in the central nervous system. J. Pharmacol.
    Exp. Therap. 163:147.

MABRY, P. D. & CAMPBELL, B. A., 1973, Serotonergic inhibition of
    catecholamine-induced behavioral arousal, Brain Res. 49:381.

MANDEL, P., AYAD, G., HERMETET, J. C. & EBEL, A., 1974, Correlation
    between choline acetyltransferase activity and learning ability
    in different mice strains and their offspring, Brain Res. 72:
    65.

MCLENNAN, H., 1970, "Synaptic Transmission," W. B. Saunders, Phila-
    delphia.

MITCHAM, J. C. & THOMAS, R. K., 1972, Effects of substantia nigra
    and caudate nucleus lesions on avoidance learning in rats, J.
    Comp. Physiol. Psychol. 81:101.

MODIGH, K., 1972, Central and peripheral effects of 5-hydroxytrypto-
    phan on motor activity in mice, Psychopharmacologia 23:48.

MODIGH, K., 1973, Effects of L-tryptophan on motor activiity in
    mice, Psychopharmacologia 30:123.

NEILL, D. B. & GROSSMAN, S. P., 1970, Behavioral effects of lesions
    or cholinergic blockade of the dorsal and ventral caudate of
    rats, J. Comp. Physiol. Psychol. 71:311.

NEILL, D. B., BOGGAN, W. O. & GROSSMAN, S. P., 1974a, Behavioral
    effects of amphetamine in rats with lesions in the corpus
    striatum, J. Comp. Physiol. Psychol. 86:1019.

NEILL, D. B., BOGGAN, W. O. & GROSSMAN, S. P., 1974b, Impairment
    of avoidance performance by intrastriatal administration of
    6-hydroxydopamine, Pharmacol. Biochem. Behav. 2:97.

OVERTON, D. A., 1964, State-dependent or "dissociated" learning
    produced with pentobarbital, J. Comp. Physiol. Psychol. 57:3.

PHILLIPS, A. G. & FIBIGER, H. C., 1973, Dopaminergic and noradrener-
    gic substrates of positive reinforcement: differential effects

of d- and l-amphetamine, Science 179:575.

RAKE, A. V., 1973, Involvement of biogenic amines in memory formation: the central nervous system indole amine involvement, Psychopharmacologia 29:91.

RANDRUP, A. & MUNKVAD, I., 1967, Stereotyped activities produced by amphetamine in several animal species and man, Psychopharmacologia 11:300.

RANDRUP, A. & MUNKVAD, I., 1970, Biochemical, anatomical and psychological investigations of stereotyped behavior induced by amphetamines, in "Amphetamines and Related Compounds," (E. Costa & S. Garattini, eds.), pp. 695-713, Raven Press, New York.

RANDT, C. T., QUARTERMAIN, D., GOLDSTEIN, M. & ANAGNOSTE, B., 1971, Norepinephrine biosynthesis inhibition: effects on memory in mice, Science 172:498.

RECH, R. H. & MOORE, K. E., 1968, Interactions between d-amphetamine and α-methyltyrosine in rat shuttle-box behavior, Brain Res. 8:398.

RECH, R. H., BORYS, H. K. & MOORE, K. E., 1966, Alterations in behavior and brain catecholamine levels in rats treated with α-methyltyrosine, J. Pharmacol. Exp. Therap. 153:412.

RECH, R. H., CARR, L. A. & MOORE, K. E., 1968, Behavioral effects of α-methyltyrosine after prior depletion of brain catecholamines, J. Pharmacol. Exp. Therap. 160:326.

REICHENBERG, K. & VETULANI, J., 1973, Intraventricular injections of L-DOPA: the effect on rat locomotor activity and body temperature, Eur. J. Pharmacol. 22:376.

RICK, J. T. & FULKER, D. W., 1972, Some biocehmical correlates of inherited behavioral differences, Prog. Brain Res. 36:105.

ROFFMAN, M. & LAL, H., 1972, Role of brain amines in learning associated with "amphetamine-state," Psychopharmacologia 25:195.

ROSECRANS, J. A., GOODLOE, M. H. & BENNETT, G. J., 1973, Morphine as a discriminative cue: effects of amine depletors and naloxone, Eur. J. Pharmacol. 21:252.

ROUTTENBERG, A., 1968, The two-arousal hypothesis: reticular formation and limbic system, Psychol. Rev. 75:51.

ROUTTENBERG, A. & HOLZMAN, N., 1973, Memory disruption by electrical
    stimulation of substantia nigra, pars compacta, Science 181:83.

SANSONE, M., RENZI, P. & MESSERI, P., 1972, Effects of monoamine
    oxidase inhibitors on shuttle-box avoidance behavior of ham-
    sters, Pharmacol. Res. Comm. 4:357.

SCHANBERG, S. M., SCHILDKRAUT, J. J., BREESE, G. R. & KOPIN, I. J.,
    1968a, Metabolism of normetanephrine-H^3 in rat brain-identifica-
    tion of conjugated 3-methoxy-4-hydroxyphenylglycol as the major
    metabolite, Biochem. Pharmacol. 17:247.

SCHANBERG, S. M., BREESE, G. R., SCHILDKRAUT, J. J., GORDON, E. K.
    & KOPIN, I. J., 1968b, 3-methoxy-4-hydroxyphenlglycol sulfate
    in brain and cerebrospinal fluid, Biochem. Pharmacol. 17:2006.

SCHECHTER, M. D., 1973, Ethanol as a discriminative cue: reduction
    following depletion of brain serotonin, Eur. J. Pharmacol.
    24:278.

SCHECHTER, M. D. & ROSECRANS, J. A., 1972, Nicotine as a discrimina-
    tive stimulus in rats depleted of norepinephrine or 5-hydroxy-
    tryptamine, Psychopharmacologia 24:417.

SCHLESINGER, K., SCHREIBER, R. A. & PRYOR, G. T., 1968, Effects of
    p-chlorophenylalanine on conditioned avoidance learning,
    Psychon. Sci. 11:225.

SEGAL, D. S. & MANDELL, A. J., 1970, Behavioral activation of rats
    during intraventricular infusion of norepinephrine, Proc. Nat.
    Acad. Sci. 66:289.

SEGAL, D. S., KUCZENSKI, R. T. & MANDELL, A. J., 1972, Strain differ-
    ences in behavior and brain tyrosine hydroxylase activity,
    Behav. Biol. 7:75.

SEIDEN, L. S. & CAMPBELL, A. B., 1974, Catecholamines, drugs, and
    behavior: mutal interactions, in "Neuropsychopharmacology of
    Monoamines and Their Regulatory Enzymes. Advances in Biochem-
    ical Psychopharmacology," (E. Usdin, ed.), pp. 325-338, Raven
    Press, New York.

SEIDEN, L. S. & CARLSSON, A., 1963, Temporal and partial antagonism
    of L-DOPA of reserpine-induced suppression of a conditioned
    avoidance response, Psychopharmacologia 4:418.

SEIDEN, L. S. & HANSON, L. C. F., 1964, Reversal of the reserpine-
    induced suppression of the conditioned avoidance response in
    the cat by L-DOPA, Psychopharmacologia 6:239.

SEIDEN, L. S., BROWN, R. M. & LEWY, A. J., 1973, Brain catecholamines and conditioned behavior: mutual interactions, in "Chemical Modulation of Brain Function," (H. C. Sabelli, ed.), pp. 261-275, Raven Press, New York

SHOPSIN, B., WILK, S., SATHANANTHAN, G., GERSHON, S. & DAVIS, K., 1974, Catecholamines and affective disorders revised: a critical assessment, J. Nerv. Ment. Dis. 158:369.

SKOLNICK, P. & DALY, J. W., 1974, Norepinephrine-sensitive adenylate cyclases in rat brain: relation to behavior and tyrosine hydroxylase, Science 185:175.

SMITH, R. D., COOPER, B. R. & BREESE, G. R., 1973, Growth and behavioral changes in developing rats treated intracisternally with 6-hydroxydopamine: evidence for involvement of brain dopamine, J. Pharmacol. Exp. Therap. 185:609.

SORENSON, C. A. & ELLISON, G. D., 1973, Nonlinear changes in activity and emotional reactivity scores following central noradrenergic lesions in rats, Psychopharmacologia 32:313.

SPROTT, R. L. & STAATS, J., 1975, Behavioral studies using genetically defined mice- a bibliography, Behav. Genetics 5:27.

STERANKA, L. R. & BARRETT, R. J., 1974, Facilitation of avoidance acquisition by lesion of the median raphe nucleus: evidence for serotonin as a mediator of shock-induced suppression, Behav. Biol. 11:205.

STEVENS, D. A. & FECHTER, L. D., 1969, The effects of p-chlorophenylalanine, a depletor of brain serotonin, on behavior: II. Retardation of passive avoidance learning, Life Sci. 8:379.

SVENSSON, T. H. & WALDECK, B., 1970, On the role of brain catecholamines in motor activity: experiments with inhibitors of synthesis and of monoamine oxidase, Psychopharmacologia 18:357.

SWONGER, A. K. & RECH, R. H., 1972, Serotonergic and cholinergic involvement in habituation of activity and spontaneous alternation of rats in a Y-maze, J. Comp. Physiol. Psychol. 81:509.

TANAKA, C., YOH, Y.-J. & TAKAORI, S., 1972, Relationship between brain monoamine levels and sidman avoidance behavior in rats treated with tyrosine and tryptophan hydroxylase inhibitors, Brain Res. 45:153.

TAYLOR, K. M. & LAVERTY, R., 1972, The effects of drugs on the behavioral and biochemical actions of intraventricular 6-hydroxydopamine, Eur. J. Pharmacol. 17:16.

TAYLOR, K. M. & SNYDER, S. H., 1971, Differential effects of D-
and L-amphetamine on behavior and on catecholamine disposition
in dopamine and norepinephrine containing neurons of rat brain,
Brain Res. 28:295.

TENEN, S. S., 1967, The effects of p-chlorophenylalanine, a serotonin depletor on avoidance acquisition, pain sensitivity and
related behavior in the rat, Psychopharmacologia 10:204.

THOENEN, H. & TRANZER, J. P., 1973, The pharmacology of 6-hydroxy-
dopamine, Ann. Rev. Pharmacol. 13:169.

TUNNICLIFF, G., WIMMER, C. C. & WIMER, R. E., 1973, Relationships
between neurotransmitter metabolism and behavior in seven inbred strains of mice, Brain Res. 61:428.

UNGERSTEDT, U., 1971, Stereotaxic mapping of the monoamine pathways in the rat brain, Acta Physiol. Scand. Suppl. 367:1.

UNGERSTEDT, U., 1974, Brain dopamine neurons and behavior, in "The
Neurosciences Third Study Program," (F. O. Schmitt & F. G.
Worden, eds.), pp. 695-703, MIT Press, Cambridge.

UNGERSTEDT, U., BUTCHER, L. L., BUTCHER, S. G., ANDEN, N.-E. &
FUXE, K., 1969, Direct chemical stimulation of dopaminergic
mechanisms in the neostriatum of the rat, Brain Res. 14:461.

WEISS, B. & LATIES, V. G., 1969, Behavioral pharmacology and toxi-
cology, Ann. Rev. Pharmacol. 9:297.

WEISS, J. M., STONE, E. A. & HARRELL, N., 1970, Coping behavior
and brain norepinephrine level in rats, J. Comp. Physiol.
Psychol. 72:153.

WELCH, A. S. & WELCH, B. L., 1967, Effect of p-chlorophenylalanine
on brain noradrenaline in mice, J. Pharm. Pharmacol. 19:632.

WIMER, R. E., NORMAN, R. & ELEFTHERIOU, B. E., 1973, Serotonin level
in hippocampus: striking variations associated with mouse
strain and treatment, Brain Res. 63:397.

WOOLLEY, D. W. & VAN DER HOEVEN, T. H., 1963, Alternation in learning ability caused by changes in cerebral serotonin and catecholamines, Science 139:610.

WYERS, E. J., PEEKE, H. V. S., WILLISTON, J. S. & HERZ, M. J.,
1968, Retroactive impairment of passive avoidance learning by
stimulation of the caudate nucleus, Exp. Neurol. 22:350.

YUNGER, L. M. & HARVEY, J. A., 1973, Effect of lesions in the medial forebrain bundle on three measures of pain sensitivity and noise-elicited startle, J. Comp. Physiol. Psychol. 83:173.

ZORNETZER, S. F., GOLD, M. S. & HENDRICKSON, J., 1974, α-methyl-p-tyrosine and memory: state-dependency and memory failure, Behav. Biol. 12:135.

CHAPTER 19

HORMONES AND AVOIDANCE LEARNING

Richard L. Sprott, Ph.D.

The Jackson Laboratory
Bar Harbor, Maine   04609

CONTENTS

INTRODUCTION

Hormonal involvement in learning processes is most likley to
take one of two forms. First, as the previous chapter has shown,
hormones in the form of neurotransmitters could underlie the formation and maintenance of memory traces themselves and play a major
role in the neural organization of information as well. Second,
hormones can affect the learning process by altering the "internal
state" of an organism in learning situations. Effects of this
type are most obvious in avoidance learning situations.

METHODOLOGICAL ISSUES

Previous reviews (e.g., Levine, 1968; Endroczi, 1972; DeWied et al., 1972) have thoroughly discussed the potentially exciting literature in the hormones and avoidance learning area, but have almost completely ignored some of the thorny methodological problems involved in learning research of this kind. As a consequence, this chapter will be devoted largely to a discussion of possible approaches rather than an exhaustive review of the literature.

The major problem with learning paradigms is that they are apparently easy to arrange and often appear to provide simple, straightforward results. In fact, it is difficult to arrange learning situations which are free from unwanted contamination, and the results are almost never straightforward. Definitions of learning range from "...a change in performance which occurs under the conditions of practice" (McGeoch & Irion, 1952), to "...the process by which an activity originates or is changed through reacting to an encountered situation, provided that the characteristics of the change in activity cannot be explained on the basis of native response tendencies, maturation, or temporary states of the organism (e.g., fatigue, drugs, etc.)" (Hilgard, 1956). Most of the sticky problems in learning research are contained in the second half of the second definition; "native response tendencies, maturation, or temporary states of the organism." If our interest were simply hormonal correlates of behavior change, then these variables would not be problems, but our interest in this chapter is hormonal correlates of learning. While we hope to achieve some understanding of the biological basis of learning processes, we often engage in research which deals only with performance, not learning.

Shock-motivated avoidance procedures are commonly used in research on the hormonal correlates of learning for at least two reasons. First, avoidance situations presumably induce fear, anxiety, or stress responses in human or rodent subjects. Since fear, anxieity, and stress almost invariably invoke hormonal responses (Selye's "general adaptation syndrome" for example) these situations are the logical place to start a search for hormonal effects on learning processes. Secondly, the use of electric shock in a learning situation should provide sufficient motivation for all subjects so that performance differences will reflect differences in learning ability even if small differences in response to shock are observed. Certainly it should be easier to adjust motivation levels with shock by adjusting intensity, than to adjust motivation levels in food reinforced situations by adjusting deprivation levels or subjective "quality" of the food reward. If a task is used which requires little movement, such as a passive-avoidance task or the conditioned emotional response (Estes & Skinner, 1941), then performance measures may be even more representative of learning differences, since differences in motor capacities should play a relatively small role.

However, the assumptions just stated are not as reasonable as they seem to be. Paré (1969) has shown that there are systematic age-related differences in the average foot-shock threshold of <u>adult</u> rats. In this study, young and old female rats had lower shock thresholds than did older male rats. Body weight, which is of course age-related, was the major determinant of threshold, but activity level may also have played a role. In addition, performance, even in a passive situation, may depend to some degree on reaction time, which has been shown to systematically differ with age. Performance in active-avoidance and passive-avoidance situations has been shown to vary as a function of genotype (Collins, 1964; Wimer <u>et al</u>., 1968; Oliverio <u>et al</u>., 1973; Sprott, 1972). While these effects are interesting problems in their own right (hormonal correlates of aging are discussed in chapters 10 and 11 and the effects of genotype in chapter 12), they are major contributors to error variance in learning research.

Avoidance learning situations are relatively easy to implement and quickly produce stable behavioral changes. In these situations, the subject is trained to avoid a noxious stimulus, quite often electric foot-shock, by emitting a behavioral response. Initially the response that is to be emitted is not a likely one, and thus, there is a period of investigation and trial and error behavior. Exposure to the noxious stimulus is delayed or terminated by the subject's response.

Avoidance learning is usually divided into two classes, active- and passive- (or inhibitory) avoidance. In active avoidance, the subject must learn to emit an active response, such as a bar press or a leap to safety to avoid the noxious stimulus. In passive-avoidance situations the subject learns to inhibit a natural or "species-specific" response, such as jumping when confronted by dangers, or retreat to darkened "safe" areas, usually by remaining relatively motionless in a small area designated as safe by the investigator. Entry into unsafe areas results in exposure to the noxious stimulus. The processes underlying passive-avoidance, however, are not necessarily passive. They quite likely involve active inhibition of preferred responses, and in fact the subjects often engage in approach-avoidance or displacement behavior while remaining in the safe area.

The choice of an avoidance task is often critical. Tasks which appear to be similar often place very different demands upon the subject and thus have a significant impact upon the behavior which is observed. By far the most commonly used active-avoidance task uses the shuttle-box, first described by Warner (1932). To avoid or escape foot-shock, administered through a grid floor, the subject must run from one compartment of a two compartment box to the other. In two-way active-avoidance designs, first one compartment and then the other is designated as the safe area and the subject is therefore required to respond in two directions. While this is a useful task, it does present problems in that it is difficult to determine whether performance differences are the result of differences in learning, response speed, or motivation.

Another commonly used device is the jump-box. When used for active-avoidance, the subject is placed in a box with a grid floor and can escape or avoid the foot-shock by leaping to a platform or shelf mounted above the grid floor (e.g., Maatsch, 1959). Here again motivation and speed of response variables may be difficult to control. The same device can be used for passive-avoidance training by simply placing the subject on the platform and requiring that it not step down to the grid floor (Wimer et al., 1968). Other active-avoidance apparati such as the shuttle-box (Fuller, 1966) can also be adapted to passive-avoidance. In addition, various types of "hole-in-the-wall" or "step-through" tasks are commonly used (e.g., Kurtz & Pearl, 1960). These tasks often result in single-trial learning and thus are often used in memory research.

Both active and passive tasks can be modified to include a discrimination response. With a discrimination requirement the correct avoidance response is based on the presence or absence of a stimulus. Tasks of this variety offer several advantages. Once the basic avoidance response is learned, different stimuli may be used to test different sensory modalities. After the initial avoidance learning has taken place, subsequent tests with new stimuli will be relatively free of the problems encountered in initial learning such as species-specific responses which impede learning. These problems will have been either been overcome, or their contribution to performance will be known and can be accounted for in data analysis. On the other hand, this type of testing precludes the possibility of using naive subjects, and this may be unacceptable for many experiments.

As the possibilities for increased behavioral control offered by the operant conditioning techniques developed by Skinner (Ferster & Skinner, 1957) have become apparent to investigators outside the "operant tradition," these techniques have been incorporated as research tools in other disciplines. Many of the tests described above can also be arranged in a "Skinner-box" with simpler response requirements and less contamination by speed of response, motor skill, and other extraneous variables. The most commonly used operant situation for hormonal studies has been called the CAR (conditioned avoidance response) technique. The subject is placed in a conditioning chamber and taught to press a bar for a food pellet reward. After this response has been acquired, the bar itself and the grid floor of the chamber are electrified, so that a subsequent bar-press results in the administration of a foot-shock. Several performance measures are possible including acquisition, the number of shock trials needed for the subject to learn to avoid the bar (acquire the CAR), and extinction. Once the CAR has been acquired the shock contingency can be removed and the amount of time or number of trials needed for the subject to return to bar-pressing can be used as a measure of extinction. The Conditioned Emotional Response (CER) technique (or more properly, the Estes-Skinner Procedure, Estes & Skinner, 1941) is an analytically more powerful modification of this technique. The subject is first trained to bar-press for a food reward until a stable baseline of bar press behavior is developed. Then a warning stimulus (Conditioned Stimulus - CS) is introduced on an aperiodic basis. Termination of the CS is paired with the occurrence of a foot-shock. The suppression of bar press behavior which quickly develops in the presence of the CS is the CER. The amount of suppression is easily quantified and the procedure can be used with a variety of stimuli (Sidman et al., 1968). Administration of pharmacologic agents which affect "anxiety" will have predictable effects upon suppression and the efficacy of a variety of agents can easily be compared. The procedure can also be further developed so that one-trial tests can be accomplished (Sprott & Waller, 1966). Foot-shock intensities can easily be adjusted to account for individual difference, thus removing one of the major contaminants of avoidance research.

The use of a Sidman avoidance procedure removes the necessity to develop a food reward baseline of bar-press behavior. In this procedure (Sidman, 1960) the subject is trained to bar-press to postpone the onset of foot-shock. Programmed foot-shocks occur on a regular temporal schedule (e.g., once very 10 sec.) unless a bar-press occurs. Each bar-press postpones foot-shock for a fixed period (e.g., 20 sec.). Generally this procedure produces relatively stable behavior which can then be manipulated to assess the effects of stimulus changes or pharmacologic agents. This procedure is the operant equivalent of the active avoidance tasks.

Once an investigator has selected any one of the above procedures, he must also decide which performance measures are most likely to provide the data that is most relevant to his problem. The two most commonly used classes of performance measures are rate measures and probability of response measures. Rate measures, such as latency to jump in active avoidance and bar-presses per minute in the CER, generally are more indicative of the motivational or arousal state of the organism than of its learning ability. Obviously, then these are the measures of choice when motivational states are the focus of interest. However, some care must be exercised since rate measures are also influenced by motor speed and skill, and to a small degree by neural speed. Probability of response measures, such as error scores in avoidance tasks or number

of bar-presses in extinction, are usually used as an index of
learning ability or retention. However, in many test situations,
such as the active and passive tasks, response rate and response
probability are positively correlated, and it is difficult or impossible to pin down the source of changes in performance.

AVOIDANCE CONDITIONING

By far the most important studies of hormones and learned
behaviors are those dealing with the effects of hormones of the
pituitary-adrenal system on avoidance behavior.

The evidence for pituitary-adrenal involvement in the acquisition of avoidance responses is suggestive, but not convincing.
ACTH administration has been shown to facilitate avoidance acquisition in some situations, e.g., a CAR procedure (Bohus & Endroczi,
1965); in a shuttle-box situation (Beatty et al., 1970), and a
Sidman avoidance procedure (Wertheim et al., 1967). On the other
hand ACTH has been shown to be without effect on avoidance acquisition in a CAR situation (Bohus & Lissak, 1968) and in the shuttlebox (Murphy & Miller, 1955). The effects of adrenalectomy are
equally contradictory. Applezweig & Baudry (1955) found that adrenalectomy interfered with avoidance acquisition, while Beatty et al.,
(1970) report improved acquisition in some conditions, and other
investigators report no effect (Moyer, 1958a, 1958b; Bohus & Endroczi, 1965). Levine (1968) has suggested that "...the increase in
adrenocortical activity which is associated with improved acquisition of an avoidance response may merely reflect a generalized difference in arousal" while DeWied (DeWied et al., 1972) concluded
that normal pituitary-adrenal function is not a necessary condition
for avoidance learning,but that the activity of the pituitary-adrenal system has some association with avoidance behavior. Since
rather minor variations in experimental parameters can have a major
effect on performance in avoidance situations (Sprott, 1972), the
lack of agreement among these studies is not very surprising. It
does suggest however that the influence of ACTH in avoidance acquisition may be no greater than that of many other variables.
Certainly more precise experiments are needed before ACTH's role in
acquisition can be understood.

While the role of the pituitary-adrenal system in the extinction of avoidance behavior is not necessarily better understood, it
is clear that its influence is important. It has been clearly shown
(Murphy & Miller, 1955; Miller & Ogawa, 1962; DeWied, 1966) that
ACTH administered before or during extinction trials interfers with
the extinction process. In additional studies (summarized in De-
Wied et al., 1972) DeWied was able to show that administration of
corticosterone during extinction, which should reduce circulating
ACTH, facilitated extinction performance. On the basis of these

and other studies (see Levine, 1968) it seems clear that high
levels of circulating ACTH interfere with extinction of active-
avoidance responses and that the administration of ACTH inhibitors
(e.g., dexamethasone) facilitates active-avoidance extinction.

Several interpretations of the extinction effects are possible. Levine (1968) argues that the pituitary-adrenal system
is involved in the development and maintenance of internal inhibition. Glucocorticoids are assumed to be necessary for development of internal inhibition, while "ACTH disinhibits the inhibitory process." While this is an attractive hypothesis since it
provides some real basis for an hypothetical construct, and it may
in fact be the best available explanation of the data, it is certainly not the only possibility. It is also possible to account
for these results on the basis of motivational concepts (see
Chapter 20) such as fear (e.g., Brady, 1967). The possibility of
effects upon the emission of species-specific defense reactions
which might occur if pituitary-adrenal hormones affect the subject's perception have been given little attention. Similarly,
extinction of avoidance responses presupposes that the subject
emits (or inhibits) a non-avoidance response and thereby "dis-
covers" that the noxious stimulus has been removed. Any manipulation which changes the probability of this discovery would have
a corresponding effect on performance during extinction. Thus if
ACTH reduces the probability that the subject will change its behavior, while glucocorticoids increase this probability, this
would account for the results which have been observed. Opera-
tionally this hypothesis is not different from Levine's, but it
does not rest upon the assumption of an internal inhibitory process, but could merely reflect changes in activity level.

Some support for this last possibility can be derived from
the reported effects of ACTH upon passive-avoidance performance
(Lissak & Endroczi, 1961; Levine & Jones, 1965; Anderson et al.,
1968), which suggest that high levels of ACTH facilitate passive-
avoidance acquisition and low levels of ACTH facilitate the extinction of passive-avoidance performance. This is exactly what
would be expected if ACTH affects the subjects activity level,
since the activity requirements in passive-avoidance are the reverse of those in active.

DISCUSSION

It is obvious that hormones play an imporant role in the determination of behavior which occurs in learning situations. However, it is not at all clear whether hormones such as those of
the pituitary-adrenal system have an effect on the "learning process" itself or act only indirectly by affecting the motivation,

perception, and motor coordination of the subjects in these experiments. The distinction between these possibilities is probably of only secondary importance to the endocrinologist whose major interest is to elucidate the role of hormones in behavior. On the other hand, the distinction is of primary importance to the experimental psychologist in search of the physiological basis of learning. The weight of the evidence presently available seems to suggest that the major role of hormones in learning situations is motivational (see Brush, this Volume) and that the direct effects of hormones upon learning occur through their interaction with biogenic amines as the evidence in the previous chapter clearly demonstrates. As more powerful behavioral techniques (such as the CER or Estes-Skinner procedure) come into common use, so that behavioral technique more closely matches the precision of endocrine analysis, it should become possible to assess the roles of hormones in the determination of the many aspects of performance.

ACKNOWLEDGEMENTS

Preparation of this chapter was supported by NIH Research Grants NIH HD-05523 from the National Institute of Child Health and Human Development and GM-21266 from the Division of General Medical Sciences.

REFERENCES

ANDERSON, D. C., WINN, W., & TAM, T., 1968, Adrenocorticotrophic hormone and acquisition of a passive avoidance response: a replication and extension, J. Comp. Physiol. Psychol. 66:497.

APPLESWEIG, M. H., & BAUDRY, F. D., 1955, The pituitary-adrenocortical system in avoidance learning, Psych. Rep. 1:417.

BEATTY, P. A., BEATTY, W. W., BOWMAN, R. E., & BILCHRIST, J. C., 1970, The effects of ACTH, adrenalectomy and dexamethasone on the acquisition of an avoidance response in rats, Physiol. Behav. 5:939.

BOHUS, B., & ENDROCZI, E., 1965, The influence of pituitary-adrenocortical function on the avoidance reflex activity in rats, Acta Physiol. 26:183.

BOHUS, B., & LISSAK, K., 1968, Adrenocortical hormones and avoidance behavior of rats, Int. J. Neuropharmacol. 7:301.

BRADY, J. V., 1967, Emotion and the sensitivity of psychoendocrine systems, in "Neurophysiology and Emotion," (D. C. Glass, ed.) pp. 70-95, Rockefeller University and Russell Sage Foundation, New York.

COLLINS, R. L., 1964, Inheritance of avoidance conditioning in mice:

A diallel study, Science 143:1188.

DEWIED, D., 1966, Inhibitory effect of ACTH and related peptides on extinction of conditioned avoidance behavior in rats, Proc. Soc. Exp. Biol. Med. 122:28.

DEWIED, D., VAN DELFT, A. M. L., GISPEN, W. H., WEIJNEN, J. A. W. M., & VAN WIMERSMA GREIDANUS, TJ. B., 1972, The role of pituitary-adrenal system hormones in active avoidance conditioning, in "Hormones and Behavior," (S. Levine, ed.), pp. 135-171, Academic Press, New York.

ENDROCZI, E., 1972, Pavlovian conditioning and adaptive hormones, in "Hormones and Behavior," (S. Levine, ed.), pp. 173-207, Academic Press, New York.

ESTES, W. K., & SKINNER, B. F., 1941, Some quantitative properties of anxiety, J. Exp. Psychol. 29:390.

FERSTER, C. B., & SKINNER, B. F., 1957, "Schedules of Reinforcement," Appleton-Century-Crofts, New York.

HILGARD, E. R., 1956, "Theories of Learning," (2nd ed.), p. 3, Appleton-Century-Crofts, New York.

KURTZ, K. H., & PEARL, J., 1960, The effects of prior fear experiences on acquired-drive learning, J. Comp. Physiol. Psychol. 53:201.

LEVINE, S., 1968, Hormones and conditioning, in "Nebraska Symposium on Motivation, 1968," Vol. XVI (W. J. Arnold, ed.), pp. 85-101, University of Nebraska Press, Lincoln.

LEVINE, S., & JONES, L. E., 1965, Adrenocorticotrophic hormone ACTH) and passive avoidance learning, J. Comp. Physiol. Psychol. 59:357.

LISSAK, K., & ENDROCZI, E., 1961, Neurohumoral factors in the control of animal behavior, in "UNESCO Symposium, Brain Mechanisms and Learning," pp. 293-308, Oxford University Press, Blackwell.

MAATSCH, J. L., 1959, Learning and fixation after a single shock trial, J. Comp. Physiol. Psychol. 52:408.

MCGEOCH, J. A., & IRION, A. L., 1952, "The Psychology of Human Learning," p. 5, Longmans, Green & Co., New York.

MILLER, R. E., & OGAWA, N., 1962, The effect of adrenocorticotrophic hormone (ACTH) on avoidance conditioning in the adrenalectomized rat, J. Comp. Physiol. Psychol. 55:211.

MOYER, K. E., 1958(a), The effect of adrenalectomy on anxiety motivated behavior, J. Genet. Psychol. 92:11.

MOYER, K. E., 1958(b), The effect of adrenalectomy on emotional elimination, J. Genet. Psychol. 92:17.

MURPHY, J. V., & MILLER, R. E., 1955, The effect of adrenocortico-trophic hormone (ACTH) on avoidance conditioning in the rat, J. Comp. Physiol. Psychol. 48:47.

OLIVERIOU, A., ELEFTHERIOU, B. E., & BAILEY, D. W., 1973, A gene influencing active avoidance performance in mice, Physiol. and Behav. 11:497.

PARÉ, W. P., 1969, Age, sex and strain differences in the aversive threshold to grid shock in the rat, J. Comp. Physiol. Psychol. 69:214.

SIDMAN, M., 1960, Normal sources of pathological behavior, Science 132:61.

SIDMAN, M., RAY, B. A., SIDMAN, R. L., & KLINGER, J. M., 1966, Neurological mutant mice: a method for the preliminary evaluation of hearing and vision, Exp. Neurol. 16:377.

SPROTT, R. L., 1972, Passive-avoidance conditioning in inbred mice: effects of shock intensity, age, and genotype, J. Comp. Physiol. Psychol. 80:327.

SPROTT, R. L., & WALLER, M. B., 1966, The effects of electroconvulsive shock on the action of a reinforcing stimulus, J. Exp. Anal. Behav. 9:663.

WARNER, L. H., 1932, The association span of the white rat, J. Genet. Psychol. 52:408.

WERTHEIM, G. A., CONNOR, R. L., & LEVINE, S., 1967, Adrenocortical influences on free-operant avoidance behavior, J. Exp. Anal. Behav. 10:555.

WIMER, R. E., SYMINGTON, L., FARMER, H., & SCHWARTZKROIN, P., 1968, Differences in memory processes between inbred mouse strains C57BL/6J and DBA/2J, J. Comp. Physiol. Psychol. 65:126.

CHAPTER 20

MOTIVATIONAL EFFECTS OF THE PITUITARY AND ADRENAL HORMONES

F. R. Brush, Ph.D.

and

J. C. Froehlich, Ph.D.
Experimental Psychology Laboratory
Syracuse University
Syracuse, New York   13210

CONTENTS

INTRODUCTION

Although it has been accepted as fact for many years that the hormones of reproduction affect a variety of reproductive as well as non-reproductive behaviors, only recently have the hormones of the pituitary and adrenal glands been viewed as behaviorally significant, thanks largely to the pioneering work of De Wied and his co-workers. As an index of the burgeoning interest in this area, review articles, conference summaries or major portions thereof, and entire volumes devoted to this topic have been appearing at an accelerating rate (James & Landon, 1968 Ganong & Martini, 1969; De Wied & Weijnen, 1970; Di Giusto et al., 1971; Sawyer & Gorski, 1971; Levine, 1972; Brodish & Redgate, 1973; Lissak, 1973; Smith, 1973; Zimmermann et al., 1973; Broverman et al., 1974).

This chapter cannot examine or review in detail the enormous amount of data in this area, and the reader is referred to the above reviews for details and references omitted here. Although many steroids are secreted by the adrenal gland, and a number of behaviorally important tropic hormones are secreted by the pituitary, we will only deal with a few of the major hormones of the pituitary-adrenal system such as 1) adrenocorticotropic hormone (ACTH) from the adenohypophysis, 2) corticosterone (B), hydroxy-corticosterone (F), and aldosterone (Aldo) from the adrenal cortex, and 3) epinephrine (E) and norepinephrine (NE) from the adrenal medulla. Effects of the catecholamines on the central nervous system (CNS) will also be largely excluded because space limitations preclude adequate coverage of this complex area.

Two basic approaches are available for studying hormone-behavior interactions. One may induce behavioral changes and observe the resulting endocrine responses, or alternatively, one may manipulate the endocrine system and observe the resulting changes in behavior. Problems arise with the use of either approach. When behavioral manipulations result in endocrine changes, the diversity of the training variables that are used often makes it difficult not only to identify which behavioral manipulation consistently produces a specific endocrine change, but also to establish the behavioral significance of that endocrine change. When endocrine manipulations result in behavioral changes, the complex regulatory mechanisms and interrelationships of the different endocrine systems often make it difficult to isolate the behavioral effects of a specific hormone. Furthermore, any apparent behavioral effect of a hormone must be mediated by that hormone's action on the CNS, which, in most instances, is poorly understood.

Hormones of the pituitary-adrenal system exert both "organizing" and "activating" effects on behavior (Levine & Mullins, 1966). Ader (this volume) addresses some important issues regarding the "organizing" effects of the pituitary and adrenal hormones. We will focus on the motivational or "activating" effects of hormones of the pituitary-adrenal system, but in some instances these motivational effects interact with learning phenomena, the subject of another chapter in this volume (Sprott).

A word is perhaps appropriate about the terms motivation and emotion. Both have often been misused when invoked to "explain" poorly understood changes in behavior, and confusion often arises in the use of these terms because variables which exert motivational effects frequently induce changes in emotional behavior, and vice versa. Motivational variables are thought to exert their effects by means of temporary "states" in the organism which result in temporary changes in performance, rather than in relatively permanent changes in performance which presumably reflect learning. Affect, emotion and feeling are all terms that seem best applied to internal, covert events that may activate or arouse the organism (Duffy, 1962; Hebb, 1955), whereas emotional behavior may be viewed as overt expressions of those internal events which may affect the environmental stimuli that elicit the covert emotion of feeling. The possible relationship between the "state" induced by a motivational variable and the covert emotion remains problematic and cannot be addressed in this chapter. Rather, we will focus on the temporary (motivational) changes in performance that may be influenced by the pituitary-adrenal hormones.

We will first briefly summarize the basic regulatory mechanisms of the pituitary-adrenal system and call attention to the physiological consequences of manipulations frequently employed in behavioral studies involving this system. We will then attempt to summarize, in a series of brief statements, the well documented hormone-behavior relationships that have emerged from the rather extensive literature on this topic. Each of these statements will then be examined in view of recent experimental results to determine how they must be qualified, extended or revised. Finally, we will attempt to indicate important directions for future research in this area.

No regulation

REGULATORY DYNAMICS OF THE
PITUITARY-ADRENAL SYSTEM

Fig. 1. is a schematic representation of some interrelationships among various components of the pituitary-adrenal system.
In this diagram, the term stress is used to designate events that
activate this system, but because of varying definitions and class-
ifications of stressors, it cannot be used with great precision
(see Allen et al., 1973 for further details). It is known, however,
that a variety of environmental stimuli (stressors) activate the pituitary-adrenal system, and that these stimuli may represent internal environmental changes, such as hypotension or starvation, as
well as external changes, such as restraint or conditioned and un-
conditioned aversive stimulation. Such stimuli provide afferent
neural input to the hypothalamus or in some cases, though not
designated in the figure, they may act directly on the pituitary.
A component of the hypothalamic response to this input is the release of corticotropin releasing factor (CRF) by neurosecretory
cells of the hypothalamus in the region of the median emminence,
which is located at the base of the hypothalamus above the pituitary. CRF is carried to the anterior pituitary through the hypothalamic-hypophyseal portal veins where it causes rapid release of
stored quantities of ACTH into the systemic circulation and, more
slowly, stimulates synthesis of ACTH in the pituitary (Marks &
Vernikos-Danellis, 1963). Blood-borne ACTH from the pituitary
stimulates cells of the adrenal cortex to synthesize and release
glucocorticoids, predominantly F in man and exclusively B in the
rat.

The adrenal hormones exert feedback effects and thereby regulate release of ACTH from the pituitary. A possible positive feedback effect is illustrated in Fig. 1 and involves E (previously
called adrenaline, and so labelled in the figure). E is released
into the systemic circulation by the adrenal medulla in response
to a variety of stressors which induce activity in the preganglionic
sympathetic (cholinergic) neurons that innervate the medulla. Circulating E may induce ACTH release either by stimulating the hypothalamus and thus inducing CRF release as is suggested by Fig. 1
(Clegg & Clegg, 1969; Allen et al., 1973), or by direct action on
the pituitary. This postulated positive feedback loop is based
on conflicting evidence and is the subject of current debate (Vernikos-Danellis & Marks, 1962; Vernikos-Danellis, 1968; Van Loon,
1973). Fig. 1 also illustrates the negative feedback loop by which
high concentrations of circulating glucocorticoids limit further
ACTH release, either by direct action on the pituitary or by indirect action via the hypothalamus and CRF release, or both. This
negative feedback system will be discussed in greater detail below.

A major function of ACTH is to induce the synthesis and secretion of glucocorticoids (B and/or F), and the rate of release of

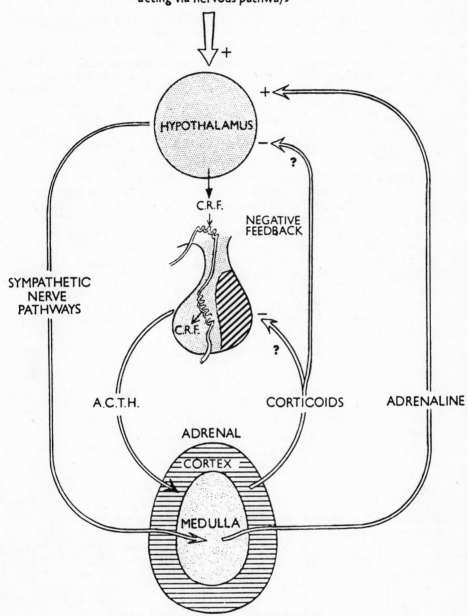

Fig. 1. Schematic diagram of the pituitary-adrenal system. (Fig. 29 from Clegg & Clegg, 1969, with permission.)

these steroids by the adrenal is almost entirely determined by
the amount of ACTH reaching the adrenal cortex in conjunction with
the circulatory dynamics of the adrenal. It is certain that the
hormones of the pituitary-adrenal system play a major role in the
organism's ability to cope with a variety of stressful stimuli,
but at present the way in which increased pituitary-adrenal output
aids survival under stress is not understood. Increased secretion
of adrenal glucocorticoids, elicited either by stress or the anticipation of stress, may facilitate healing processes or reduce the
effects of injury (see Seyle, 1950; Schayer, 1964, 1967 for interesting speculations on this issue).

Figs. 2 and 3 illustrate the typical pattern of pituitary-
adrenocortical responses to stress, in this case surgical stress
in nembutalized rats (Jones et al., 1972). The peak of the pituitary response, as indexed by plasma concentration of ACTH, occurs
around 2.5 min. after stress is applied. Adrenal concentration of
B then increases in response to ACTH and reaches a peak by 10 min.
This is followed by elevation of the plasma concentration of B.
Significant plasma elevations are frequently seen within 5 min.,
but peak concentrations are not usually reached until 20-30 min.
after stress is applied. An ACTH concentration of 3 mU/100 ml of
plasma (see Fig. 2) is usually sufficient to induce a near maximal
adrenocortical response (see Fig. 3), and higher ACTH concentrations result not in a higher but in a more sustained elevation of
plasma B concentrations.

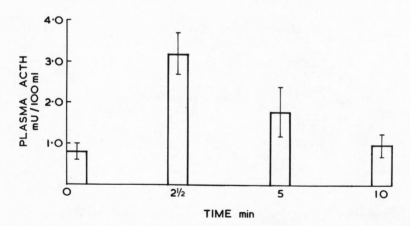

Fig. 2. Plasma concentration of ACTH as a function of time after
surgical stress. Vertical lines indicate 95% confidence limits.
(Fig. 2 from Jones et al., 1972, with permission.)

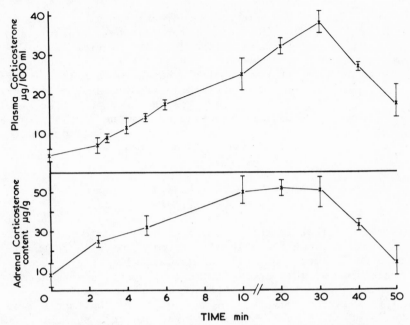

Fig. 3. Plasma (top) and adrenal (bottom) concentrations of B as a function of time after surgical stress. Determinations at 0, 2.5, 5, and 10 min. are from the same experiment and the same animals whose plasma concentrations of ACTH are illustrated in Fig. 2. Vertical lines indicate ± S.E. (Fig. 1 from Jones et al., 1972, with permission.)

It is not surprising that the adrenal medulla, being directly innervated, releases NE and/or E with considerably shorter latency in response to stress than is the case for the adrenocortical response. Furthermore, unlike the adrenal cortex, the medulla stores large amounts of NE and E, the proportions of which vary from one specie to another. Histochemical and electronmicroscopic investigations have determined that there are at least two types of cells in the adrenal medulla, one type selectively storing and secreting NE, and the other E. Different internal and external stimuli can selectively activate one or the other or both cell types with the result that either NE, E, or both may be differentially secreted into the systemic circulation in response to different stressors. The mechanisms governing this selective release are not well understood.

In addition to being sympathetically innervated, the adrenal medulla is also vascularly connected to the adrenal cortex. The importance of this vascular connection is evidenced by the fact that the medullary conversion of NE to E by the enzyme phenylethanolamine N-methyltransferase (PNMT) is dependent on the presence of glucocorticoids. Hypophysectomy, for example, produces

not only a decrease in glucocorticoid concentrations, but also a
decrease in PNMT activity which can be restored by administration
of ACTH or large doses of glucocorticoids. Stimulation of medullary enzyme activity by stress-induced elevations of glucocorticoids can also be seen in intact animals but at a much slower rate
than in hypophysectomized animals (Vernikos-Danellis et al., 1968;
Ciaranello et al., 1969). Given the great dependence of the medulla on the cortex for the synthesis of catecholamines, it is interesting to note that there is no deficiency in the glucocorticoid
response to stress in adrenal demedullated animals.

REGULATION OF ACTH SECRETION BY
ADRENAL GLUCOCORTICOIDS

It is not possible in this chapter to present a complete survey of the literature on the role of corticosteroids in feedback
regulation of ACTH secretion. The focus here will be on steroid
induced inhibition of ACTH secretion in response to stress because
of the potential behavioral significance of this mechanism, and
the reader is referred to Martini & Ganong (1967), Dallman & Yates
(1968), Motta et al. (1969), Smelik (1969), Ganong & Martini (1973),
and Lissak (1973) for extensive reviews of other aspects of ACTH
regulation such as neurochemical control, diurnal and circadian regulation, and "short" feedback regulation.

In the rat there are two temporally distinct periods of inhibition of ACTH secretion in response to stress, which result from
pretreatment with B. These are studied by comparing the magnitude
of the stress response, relative to unstressed controls, at various
times following administration of B. The first, fast feedback inhibition, is of short duration and occurs within the first 20 min.
following administration of a small dose of B (Sayers & Sayers,
1947; Yates et al., 1961; Dallman & Yates, 1969). Fast feedback
has been shown to possess the characteristics of rate sensitivity
and saturation (Jones et al., 1972). Rate sensitivity was demonstrated by complete inhibition of stress-induced ACTH secretion
during an i.p. steroid infusion only when the plasma concentration of B was rising at a rate exceeding 1.3 ug/100 ml/min. Inhibition of ACTH secretion was not related to the absolute plasma
concentration of B. This result is illustrated in Fig. 4. Saturation was shown by the fact that inhibition of the stress response
was abolished when the total amount of infused B was increased
either by increasing the duration of the infusion, or by increasing
the concentration of the infusate (B). Jones et al. (1974) again
illustrate both fast feedback inhibition and saturation of ACTH
secretion in response to ether stress in otherwise unanesthetized
animals following subcutaneous injections of either of two doses
of B. These results are illustrated in Fig. 5. The saturation

effect can be seen 20 min. after injection of the larger of two
doses.

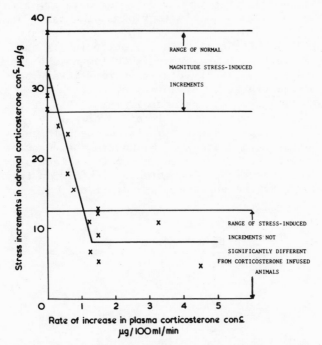

Fig. 4. Relationship between magnitude of stress response and rate
of increase of plasma B concentration induced by i.p. infusion of
B. (Fig. 4 from Jones et al., 1972, with permission.)

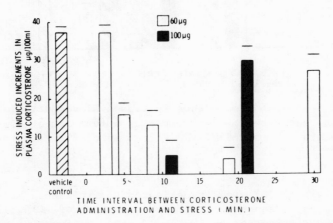

Fig. 5. Fast feedback: Increments in plasma B concentration induced
by 2 min. exposure to ether vapor as a function of time after s.c. injection of 60 or 100 g of B. (Fig. 1 from Jones et al., 1974, with
permission.

The second period of inhibition, slow or delayed feedback, is
of longer duration and refers to the inhibition of ACTH secretion
in response to stress applied from 1 to 24 or more hr. after the
administration of a large, usually supraphysiological, dose of B
(Smelik, 1963; Hodges & Jones, 1964).   This is illustrated in Fig.
6 which shows the inhibition of ACTH secretion in response to either
stress applied at various time intervals following the administration of one of four doses of B.   Plasma steroid levels have returned to normal 1 or more hrs. after an administration of B, so stress
was applied at a time when plasma steroid levels had returned to
normal.   The duration of inhibition is proportional to the dose of
B administered.   Therefore, saturation is not seen in the slow feedback system; whereas larger doses of B shorten the duration of inhibition in the fast feedback system due to the effect of saturation, larger doses increase the duration of inhibition in the slow
feedback system due to the absence of saturation.

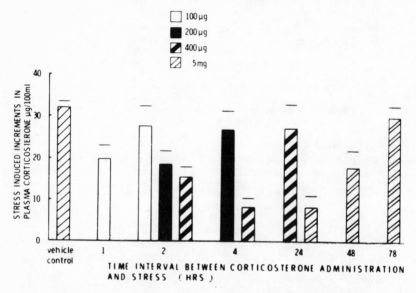

Fig. 6.   Slow feedback: Increments in plasma B concentration induced by 2 min. exposure to ether vapor as a function of time after s.c. injection of 100, 200, 400 g or 5 mg of B.   (Adapted from
Fig. 2 of Jones et al., 1974).

Jones et al. (1974) also investigated the influence of several
steroid molecules on the stress-induced secretion of ACTH.   It was
found that deoxycorticosterone (DOC) and deoxycortisone (S), precursors of corticosterone and cortisol, respectively, interacted
with B differently in fast as opposed to slow feedback.   F, on the

other hand, interacted with B similarly in both fast and slow feedback. Therefore, it can be concluded that not only do the dynamics of the fast and slow feedback systems differ, but also that the
two systems are served by functionally different receptors, which
may or may not be anatomically separated.

Recent evidence indicates that although pretreatment with B
will inhibit ACTH secretion in response to stress, some prior stressors will not (Dallman & Jones, 1973b). When the stress of electric
shock or laparotomy, applied to the animal at time zero, was followed by a second application of the same stress at various intervals up to 24 hr., the endogenous elevation of B in response to
the first stress did not inhibit the pituitary-adrenocortical response to the second stress. It was also found that the stress of
prolonged restraint did not inhibit the response to a minor stress
(sham i.p. injection) given several hours later. However, if the
endogenously produced plasma B levels caused by restraint stress
were mimicked by injections of exogenous B or ACTH, the subsequent
response to injection stress was inhibited. These results indicate
that although exogenous elevations of plasma ACTH and B produce
slow feedback inhibition of ACTH secretion in response to stress,
endogenous elevations of plasma ACTH or B induced by some stressors
do not. Dallman & Jones (1973b) concluded that although B does
inhibit ACTH secretion, stress, per se, may increase the excitability of the pituitary-adrenal system thus rendering it more responsive to a subsequent stress, which in turn would make the inhibition
of that stress response more difficult. However, it is also possible that an adrenal hormone other than B, such as NE or E, which is
also released in response to some stressors, may prevent slow feedback inhibition which would normally result from high circulating
levels of endogenous B induced by those stressors. This hypothesis
is currently being investigated in our laboratory.

Slow feedback inhibition of ACTH secretion has been shown to
depend not only on the dose of steroid administered, but also on
the intensity of the stress to be inhibited. Dallman & Jones (19-
73b) have noted that certain high intensity stressors cannot be
blocked even by high doses of steroids. Furthermore, the response
to one stress may be more easily blocked than the response to
another even when the intensity of the two stressors is held constant at moderate levels. In our laboratory a 2-min. exposure to
ether and a 15-min. exposure to cold produced equal increments in
plasma B concentrations and were therefore judged to be equally
intense stressors. We found that pretreatment with B significantly
inhibited the plasma B response to ether, but not to cold (Froehlich, 1974). One difference between cold and ether stress, which
might account for these results, is that cold induces both ACTH
and TSH (thyroid stimulating hormone) secretion, whereas ether induces ACTH but not TSH release. Therefore, when interpreting the

results of studies on feedback one must consider the possible influence of other hormones which may alter the effectiveness of B
in regulating ACTH secretion in response to certain stressors.

On the basis of this review, we conclude that the fast and
slow feedback inhibition of stress-induced ACTH secretion following
B pretreatment may depend on a number of factors such as: 1) the
dose of steroid administered, 2) the source of B (exogenous or endogenous, 3) the intensity of the stress to be inhibited and 4)
the participation of other hormones in response to a particular
stressor.

The behavioral significance of the feedback mechanisms described above was first suggested by the similarity between the
time scales of slow feedback and the U-shaped retention function
(Kamin Effect) that characterizes many forms of avoidance learning
(see Brush, 1971 for a review of this literature). However, the
rate sensitivity and saturation characteristics of fast feedback
are also potentially significant for behavioral experiments. In
relatively long duration aversive training sessions, it is highly
probable that the aversive stimulation of the first few trials
induces ACTH secretion with subsequent elevation of plasma B at
rates in excess of the critical value (1.3 ug/100 ml/min.). Thus,
ACTH release may be momentarily inhibited, but with the additional
stress of continued training the saturation effect may permit continued ACTH release with no further elevation of plasma B concentration, given that its maximum has been reached. Since behavioral studies have rarely measured plasma concentrations of both ACTH
and B, this is admittedly a speculation. However, Conner et al.
(1971) provide data suggesting that a dissociation between plasma
concentrations of ACTH and B can indeed occur.

Feedback mechanisms may also be important for behavior because of the marked differences in stress duration that occur in
different types of training situations. For example, active avoidance training procedures usually require as many as 100 trials distributed over an hour or more, whereas passive avoidance training
frequently is established in a single trial lasting less than 1 min.
Such gross differences in stress duration will clearly produce
marked differences in ACTH and B secretion during training. Furthermore, long stress durations may induce slow-feedback inhibition
of the response to a later stress, such as a retention test, whereas brief stress durations may not. Indeed, the U-shaped retention
function is routinely found following multi-trial avoidance training but has never been reported following one-trial avoidance
training.

We are postulating that the endogenous rise in plasma B induced by multi-trial avoidance training may induce slow feedback

(and the Kamin Effect), whereas the presumably smaller endogenous elevation of plasma B induced by one-trial avoidance training may not. The finding of Dallman & Jones (1973b) that the plasma B elevations produced endogenously in response to some stressors fail to induce slow feedback may seem damaging to this hypothesis. However, the prodecures used by Dallman & Jones, such as electrical stimulation of nembutalized animals, undoubtedly produced endocrine responses that differ markedly from those produced by protracted avoidance training. Therefore, the finding that some stressors do not induce slow feedback is not incompatible with the hypothesis that protracted avoidance training may be sufficient to do so. In support of our hypothesis, Bowers (1972) found evidence that training procedures sufficient to induce the Kamin Effect also induced slow-feedback inhibition of the plasma B response to mild stress.

SOME PROBLEMS WITH ENDOCRINE MANIPULATIONS FREQUENTLY EMPLOYED IN BEHAVIORAL STUDIES

In an attempt to isolate the behavioral effects of a given hormone many investigators have surgically ablated one or more glands of the pituitary-adrenal system. For example, hypophysectomy is frequently used to produce low levels of ACTH and B. Although this presumably leaves the adrenal medullary response to stress intact, problems arise because it also removes all other tropic hormones, reduces metabolic and growth rates, induces gonadal and adrenal atrophy and alters water and salt metabolism by inducing diabetes insipidus. Selective ablation of the adenohypophysis may seem preferable to total hypophysectomy because diabetes insipidus is avoided, but it is technically difficult to accomplish (De Wied, personal communication), and the functional status of the remaining neurohypophysis may also be questionable. The drastic endocrine changes induced by adeno- or hypophysectomy result in a lethargic, fragile animal which cannot tolerate the food or water deprivation schedules customarily employed in behavioral studies. Such animals also have altered sensory sensitivity, although the evidence is not entirely consistent regarding the roles of ACTH and B in producing these changes (Gispen et al., 1970; Henkin, 1970; Paré & Cullen, 1971; Sakellaris, 1972).

Bilateral adrenalectomy has been frequently used to produce low levels of B and high levels of ACTH which result from the removal of the glucocorticoid feedback signal. In addition, however, adrenalectomy also produces low levels of adrenal catecholamines and aldosterone which alters the metabolism of sodium and other electrolytes. Further complications arise because adrenalectomy not only induces the desired high resting levels of ACTH, but also results in exaggerated stress-induced increments of ACTH release (Dallman & Jones, 1973a). Bilateral adrenalectomy is technically easy, but does not always successfully eliminate the corticosteroids because extra-adrenal steroid-secreting tissue exists in many animals, although this is less of a problem in some rat strains than in others. In the weeks following adrenalectomy, such extra-adrenal steroid-secreting tissue proliferates in response to high levels of ACTH induced by the adrenalectomy. This results in a preparation functionally equivalent to adrenal demedullation. In many experiments using adrenalectomy, the absence of corticosteroids is not assessed by the only adequate test available: the inability to survive longer than ten days without sodium replacement.

Adrenal demedullation is easily accomplished and is reliably used to reduce plasma concentrations of NE and E. However, demedullation results in a temporary deficiency in gluco- and mineralocorticoid secretion with an accompanying elevation of basal ACTH secretion. Experiments by Fortier & De Groot (1959) and Conner & Levine (1969) suggest that adrenocortical regeneration, sufficient to produce a nearly normal response to ACTH, does not occur until approximately 30 days after bilateral adrenal demedullation. However, Buckingham & Hodges (1974) and Buckingham (personal communication) have shown that adrenocortical secretory activity is not completely normal until 64 or more days after bilateral demedullation and that total weight of adrenocortical tissue probably never recovers to the level of unoperated controls. A number of investigators who have failed to find significant behavioral effects of adrenal demedullation have tested their animals only a few days post-operatively. Clearly, a behavioral test at such times must reflect reduced output of cortical as well as medullary hormones.

HORMONE-BEHAVIOR RELATIONSHIPS

The following relatively undisputed hormone-behavior relationships have emerged from a large volume of literature investigating the effects of hormones of pituitary-adrenal system on behavior:

(1) ACTH facilitates extinction performance of active and passive avoidance responses if it is administered during the extinction test. This is a direct behavioral effect of the ACTH molecule and is not mediated by the adrenal steroidogenic response to ACTH since MSH and a number of subfractions of the ACTH molecule, which do not stimulate steroidogenesis, also facilitate extinction performance. The effect is dose dependent and appears in both normal and adenohypophysectomized rats.

(2) Adrenal glucocorticoids such as B or F and nonglucocorticoids such as pregenolone and progesterone inhibit extinction

performance of active and passive avoidance responses. This effect also appears to be dose dependent and direct in action, i.e.,
it is not mediated by steroid-induced suppression of ACTH, since
the effect can also be seen in adenohypophysectomized rats.

(3) Hypophysectomy and adenohypophysectomy interfere with acquisition and performance of both active and passive avoidance
responses. This deficiency can be reversed by both steroidogenic
and nonsteroidogenic fractions of the ACTH molecule in a dose dependent manner.

(4) Adrenalectomy facilitates performance of active and
passive avoidance responses. This facilitation effect can be reversed by B or F in dose dependent manner.

(5) Aversive conditioning or learning paradigms, constituting
a variety of stressful situations stimulate ACTH release and reliably elevate plasma concentrations of B for relatively long
time periods (30 min. to 1 hr. or more).

(6) The relationship between behavior and the adrenal medullary catecholamines is not clear at present. The stress of
avoidance conditioning has been reported to leave plasma concentrations of E at or near basal levels, but has been found to induce marked elevations of plasma NE concentrations, at least for
brief periods of time (under 10 min.). The effects of exogenous
E may be nonlinear such that active and passive avoidance performance may first increase and then decrease as a function of increasing doses of E. Reported effects of bilateral adrenal demedullation are also conflicting, but the data suggest that demedullation interferes with active avoidance responding, an effect
which may be reversed by suitably small doses of exogenous E. We
have not found any reports investigating the effects of exogenous
administration of NE on avoidance performance.

It must be understood that although the above generalizations
are substantiated by a number of investigators, exceptions to each
statement can be found in the literature. Usually these exceptions
appear to result from relatively minor variations in procedure,
the effects of which have yet to be fully explained. In general,
however, the above relationships appear valid and have been the
subject of various attempts of theoretical integration.

One such effort by Levine (1968) led to the hypothesis that
the glucocorticoids act primarily to facilitate the development
of internal inhibition and that the behavioral function of ACTH
is to disinhibit this internal inhibition. This hypothesis is
consistent with a number of the generalizations stated above, and
is compatible with the negative feedback role of the adrenocorti-

cal steroids described above. It is also compatible with the
hypotheses of Lissak & Endroczi (1967), Bohus (1973) and Taylor,
et al. (1971) regarding the action of glucocorticoids and ACTH
in suppressing and activating, respectively, the diencephalic limbic midbrain portion of the reticular activating system. Levine's
hypothesis, however, is difficult to distinguish functionally
from that of Weiss et al. (1969, 1970) who have suggested that
ACTH acts to increase excitability which results in increased generalized fear, whereas corticosterone counteracts this effect of
ACTH by restoring normal levels of excitability. On the one hand,
we have an internal inhibitory process, stimulated by B, which
can be disinhibited by ACTH (Levine); on the other hand we have
excitation, induced by ACTH, which can be inhibited by B (Weiss).
The separation of these two veiws may be tested at the neurophysio-
logical level, but may be difficult to assess at the behavioral
level.

More global efforts at theoretical integration have also
appeared. For example, Di Guisto et al. (1971) note that the
adrenal medullary response to stress is fast relative to that of
the pituitary-adrenocortical system. They postulate, therefore,
that the former is actively involved in early acquisition of aversively motivated behavior, whereas the latter is involved only
later in learning and in performance of previously learned responses.
They also adopt the position of Weiss et al. (1969) that ACTH enhances fear and therefore facilitates avoidance performance. Their
position with respect to the behavioral effects of B, however, appears inconsistent, and recent findings on feedback regulation of
the pituitary-adrenal system require revision of their model.
Broverman et al. (1974) also attempt a major theoretical integration which is based on postulated CNS effects of adrenal cortical
and medullary hormones, but which omits consideration of the well
documented behavioral effects of ACTH. Short-term stress is hypothesized to induce central adrenergic dominance in response to
epinephrine release, thus facilitating performance of overlearned
repetitive tasks and interfering with complex discrimination tasks.
Under conditions of long-term stress, the adrenal corticosteroids
are hypothesized to induce a central cholinergic dominance, by
reducing central monoamine oxidase levels, which is presumed to
exert behavioral effects opposite to those produced by adrenergic
dominance. A perusal of work on brain-pituitary-adrenal interactions cited in the above reviews (especially, De Wied & Weijnen,
1970; Sawyer & Gorski, 1971; and Lissak, 1973) suggests that such
"physiologizing" may be premature. It may be more appropriate to
adopt a cautious empirical approach, such as De Wied's, which has
focused on identifying the neural structures that mediate these
endocrine effects and on specifying the CNS actions of the pituitary-adrenal hormones, before attempting theoretical integration.

RECENT FINDINGS

In this section we will call attention to new findings that may require modification of the hormone-behavior relationships summarized in the preceding section. Each area will be taken up in turn.

Adrenocorticotropin

In spite of the extensive literature documenting the fact that ACTH facilitates extinction performance of avoidance responses, a few significant exceptions have appeared recently. Weijnen & Slangen (1970) used a retractable ledge box to study the effects of $ACTH_{1-10}$ and $ACTH_{4-10}$ on avoidance learning and performance in an automated situation analogous to the manually operated pole-jumping avoidance situation often used by De Wied. De Wied et al., (1972) have repeatedly found that $ACTH_{1-10}$ facilitates extinction performance of the pole-jumping response, but Weijnen and Slangen found that neither $ACTH_{1-10}$ nor $ACTH_{4-10}$ altered performance of the ledge-jumping response. This raises the question of whether consistent behavioral effects of these peptides can be obtained in all avoidance training situations.

Another difficulty is raised by reports showing significant effects of the zinc phosphate vehicle, used in long-acting ACTH preparations, on extinction performance of a two-way shuttle avoidance response. In one experiment, Ley & Corson (1970) used two shock intensities (0.2 and 0.5 mA) and injected their rats with either saline or zinc phosphate vehicle on alternate days throughout acquisition and extinction. The vehicle groups responded significantly more often in extinction than did the saline groups at both shock intensities. In a second report (Ley & Corson, 1971), two groups of rats received either 10 IU/Kg of ACTH or an equal volume of zinc phosphate vehicle on alternate days throughout acquisition and extinction. A saline-injected control group was split in half during extinction, one subgroup continuing on saline the other being shifted to ACTH. When trained with a 0.2-mA shock intensity, the vehicle group responded significantly more often in extinction than did the ACTH group which did not differ from the saline or saline-ACTH control groups. When trained with a 0.5-mA intensity, the vehicle and ACTH groups were not significantly different from each other and both responded more often in extinction than did the saline or saline-ACTH control groups which were not different from each other.

There appears to be no simple explanation of the discrepancy between these results and those of De Wied. However, the significant effect of the zinc phosphate vehicle together with an inter-

action between ACTH and the shock intensity used in training
suggest the need for a careful analysis of effects on performance
which may be due to the interaction of different injection vehi-
cles, dosages, routes of injection and training parameters.

Further concern for such interactions is indicated by the report (Pagano & Lovely, 1972) that ACTH may facilitate extinction
performance of an active avoidance response only during the morning trough of the circadian cycle of plasma B. In contrast, however, Sandman et al. (1971) report that αMSH (ACTH$_{1-13}$) facilitated
extinction performance of a passive avoidance response only during
the evening peak of the circadian cycle. Since both hormonal
treatments and training paradigms differed in these experiments
it is impossible to determine which of these variables is inter-
acting with circadian rhythm. However, holding time of day constant
Guth et al. (1971) and Dempsey et al. (1972) find robust effects
of ACTH and MSH, respectively, on passive avoidance performance.
In each experiment the respective tropic hormone facilitated extinction performance of a passive avoidance response whether it
was injected during approach training, extinction testing, or any
combination thereof.

A number of investigators have found that ACTH and MSH have
significant effects on extinction performance of appetitively
motivated behavior. Using food reward, Sandman et al. (1969)
found that T-maze performance was facilitated by αMSH and Garrud
et al. (1974) reported that straight runway performance was enhanced by ACTH$_{1-39}$, ACTH$_{1-24}$, and ACTH$_{4-10}$ but was retarded by
B. Using water reinforcement for lever-press responding, Guth
et al. (1971) found that extinction performance following continuous reinforcement was enhanced by ACTH. Although these effects
directly parallel those for avoidance behavior, more complex effects of αMSH on reversal learning (Sandman et al., 1972) and extra dimensional shifts in discrimination learning (Sandman et al.,
1974) suggest that peptides like αMSH and ACTH may influence attention, sensory discrimination and memory as well as emotional
arousal and motivation (Bertolini et al., 1969; Sandman et al.,
1971). In any event, it is clear that the effects of hormones
of the pituitary-adrenal system are not limited to stressful a-
versive conditioning situations.

Adrenal Steroids

A significant study by Pappas & Gray (1971) provides the
first report of a state-dependency effect (Overton, 1964) induced
by dexamethasone (Dex) which is a powerful synthetic glucocorticoid. State dependency is evidenced by the inability of an animal to perform a response learned under the influence of a drug

when tested in the absence of that drug (or vice versa), when possible debilitating effects of the drug have been eliminated by
suitable controls. Using a state-dependency design in a passive
avoidance situtation, Pappas and Gray found that animals which
were both trained and tested under the influence of Dex (or its
absence) performed better than those trained under the influence
of Dex and tested in its absence (or vice versa). In accord with
current interpretations of state-dependency, it appears that Dex,
and perhaps endogenous hormones as well, may have stimulus properties which can directly influence behavior.

Hypophysectomy

Few new results have been reported in this area, but one
of interest by Harris (1973) indicates that the avoidance learning and performance decrement, usually seen with hypophysectomy,
can be reversed with a high carbohydrate dietary supplement forti-
fied with sulfamerazine. This result suggests that the performance decrement seen in hypophysectomized rats may not be due to
the absence of ACTH or other hormones. However, the behavioral
effects due to diet and sulfamerazine will have to be separated
before conclusions can be drawn from studies using this procedure.

Adrenalectomy

An important study by Weiss & Gray (1973) implicates Aldo in
mediating the behavioral effects of adrenalectomy. They studied
the effects of pre-exposure to unsignalled shock on asymptotic
free-operant avoidance performance in rats. This pre-exposure
procedure has been shown to stimulate the release of both ACTH
and B (Chalmers et al., 1974) and to facilitate performance in a
passive avoidance situation (Madden et al., 1971) in normal rats.
Weiss and Gray found that hypophysectomy did not alter the preshock effect seen in normal controls, which suggests that ACTH
and B are not involved. However, adrenalectomy abolished the preshock effect, and maintenance doses of DOC of Aldo, but not B,
restored the effect. Furthermore, maintaining normal animals on
high sodium intake (1.5% NaCl in their drinking water) reduced
endogenous production of Aldo and abolished the preshock effect.
Unpublished work by Weiss and his group apparently also indicates
that the facilitation of passive avoidance performance by adrenalectomy (Weiss et al., 1969) is also restored to normal by administration of a long-acting Aldo preparation. These data indicate
that the mineralocorticoids may have significant behavioral effects and force one to question previous interpretations of the
behavioral effects of adrenalectomy in terms of ACTH and the glucocorticoids.

Plasma Elevations of ACTH and B During Conditioning

Some interesting refinements have recently been added to
this area of research. For example, Sandman et al., (1973) reported that foot shocks induce release of both MSH and ACTH,
whereas the conditioned aversive stimuli of the shock-box environment induce release of only MSH. Bassett et al., (1973) examined
the magnitude of the plasma B elevation induced by predictable
vs. unpredictable shock, a parameter of some significance because
of the growing literature of behavioral effects of predictable and
unpredictable aversive events (Seligman et al., 1971). They found
significantly greater plasma B levels when foot shocks were signalled rather than unsignalled, and when the inter-shock intervals
were variable rather than constant. Thus, prediction of shock by
an external signal augments the plasma B response, but prediction
of shock by the passage of time results in a reduced pituitary-
adrenocortical response. Further work in this area is needed to
clarify the hormonal effects of behaviorally significant parameters
such as these.

Significant alterations of the pituitary-adrenocortical response to chronic stress have also been reported. Coover et al.
(1973) found an apparent adaptation of the pituitary-adrenocortical
response to the chronic stress of protracted avoidance training.
Plasma B concentration immediately after daily sessions of shuttlebox avoidance training declined from approximately 62 to 34 ug/100
ml over a period of 20 training days. This decline in plasma B
might be attributed to the decline in shock frequency as avoidance
performance improved were it not for the failure to find signifcant
correlations between plasma B levels and shock frequency in a given
training session.

In a related series of experiments, Sakellaris & Vernikos-
Danellis (1974a and 1974b) find that although the pituitary-adrenocortical system adapts to the stress of chronic water deprivation,
the plasma B response to other stressors such as etherization is
faster after adaptation to deprivation than before. Thus, the possibility exists that the basic time constants of the pituitary-
adrenal regulatory mechanisms may be altered by adaptation to certain forms of chronic stress. This too, is an area of research
that needs further investigation.

Certain manipulations of appetitive learning situations have
also been found to affect pituitary-adrenocortical activity.
Coover et al., (1971a, 1971b) and Goldman et al. (1973) have found
orderly increases and decreases of plasma B concentration as a
result of changes in the schedule of water reinforcement for operant bar pressing. Specifically, decreasing the frequency of reinforcement by changing from continuous reinforcement to extinction

increased the concentration of plasma B above the presession level. Similar shifts from partial schedules (VI-12 sec or FR-20) to extinction as well as shifts of the ratio requirement from FR-20 to FR-40 also elevated plasma B concentration. Conversely, increasing the frequency of reinforcement by shifts from VI-12 sec. or FR-20 to continuous reinforcement reliably reduced the plasma B concentration below the presession level. Also a brief period of water consumption in the home cage reduced the plasma B concentration 20 minutes later relative to the level immediately prior to the drinking session. The authors interpret these results in terms of a "frustration effect" from downward shifts and an "elation effect" from upward shifts in reinforcement frequency. Regardless of one's interpretation, however, it is clear from these and the previously cited results that manipulations of appetitive as well as aversive learning situations can affect the pituitary-adrenocortical system.

No

Behavior and Adrenal Medullary Catecholamines

Relatively little research has been reported which clarifies the confusion regarding the behavioral effects of NE and E. Recent studies of learning have reported that passive avoidance acquisition is retarded by injections of 6 hydroxydopamine (6 OHDA) which decreases systemic NE of neural origin (Di Giusto, 1972). Decreasing systemic NE and E by adrenal demedullation had no effect on passive avoidance acquisition when tested 20 days (Leshner et al., 1971) or 30 days post operatively (Di Giusto, 1972). Treatment with 6 OHDA has also been reported to retard acquisition in difficult, but not easy, active avoidance learning paradigms (Di Giusto & King, 1972). Clear cut motivational effects of NE or E have not been reported. However, Hucklebridge & Nowell (1974) found that exposure of mice to repeated bouts of fighting with a trained fighter induced significant plasma elevations of E but had no effect on plasma NE concentration. There was no change in plasma concentration of either NE or E in response to the conditioned stimuli of the fighting situation. The hormone-behavior interrelationships involving NE and E remain unclear, but theorizing continues (Di Giusto & King, 1972).

CONCLUDING REMARKS

It is apparent from the foregoing review that although consistent hormone-behavior relationships can be derived from the extensive research on this topic, new findings require constant revision of our understanding of those relationships. Any hormone-behavior relationship involving the pituitary-adrenal system is likely to be the product of interactions among many variables, and further deliniation of those interactions is needed. Appre-

ciation of the complexity of the problem will hopefully foster
more detailed and careful research.

Particular attention needs to be paid to pituitary-adrenal
responses induced by behavioral manipulations, but more precise
measurement of those endocrine responses is also needed. For
example plasma B concentration is routinely used to index pituitary-adrenocortical activity, but that measure reflects the integrated effects of many mechanisms: synthesis, release, binding,
feedback and metabolic degeneration of various hormones. It seems
to us to be highly desirable to determine ACTH output more directly and to use the most reliable, specific and sensitive techniques
available (see Chayen et al., 1972).

Conversely, more careful analysis of the specific behavioral
effects induced by the pituitary-adrenal hormones is needed. Recent findings suggest that important behavioral effects of some
hormones have been overlooked (Aldo) and that further refinement
and variation of behavioral testing situations will help to de-
lineate the range of psychological functions that are controlled
by these hormones.

Recent advances in our understanding of the positive and negative feedback mechanisms of the pituitary-adrenal system have suggested that fast and slow feedback regulation of the pituitary response to stress may have direct behavioral significance. Furthermore, adaptation to chronic stress may alter those regulatory mechanisms and thereby have important implications for behavior.

Finally, the search for CNS sites and modes of action of
the pituitary-adrenal hormones is crucial for further advances
in this area. It is hoped that neurobiochemical and electrophysiological analyses will be used in combination with behavioral
manipulations in an attempt to provide an integrated understanding of hormone-behavior relationships.

REFERENCES

ALLEN. J. P., ALLEN, C. F., GREER, M. A., & JACOBS, J. J., 1973, Stress-induced secretion of ACTH, in "Brain-Pituitary-Adrenal Interrelationships," (A. Brodish, & E. S. Redgate, eds.), pp. 99-127, S. Karger, New York.

BASSETT, J. R., CAIRNCROSS, K. D., & KING, M. G., 1973, Parameters of novelty, shock predictability and response contingency in corticosterone release in the rat, Physiol. Behav. 10:901.

BERTOLINI, A., VERGONI, W., GESSA, G., & FERRARI, W., 1969, Induction of sexual excitement by the action of adrenocorticotropic hormone in brain, Nature 221:667.

BOHUS, B. 1973, Pituitary-adrenal influences on avoidance and approach behavior of the rat, in "Drug Effects on Neuroendocrine Regulation, Progress in Brain Research," (E. Zimmerman, W. H. Gispen, B. H. Marks, & D. De Wied, eds.) 39:407, Elsevier, Amsterdam.

BOWERS, J. M., 1972, The role of shock and plasma corticosterone levels in retention of an avoidance response (unpublished Ph.D. thesis) University of Oregon Medical School.

BRODISH, A., & REDGATE, E. S. (eds.) 1973, "Brain-Pituitary-Adrenal Interrelationships," International Symposium on Brain-Pituitary-Adrenal Interrelationships, S. Karger, New York.

BROVERMAN, D. M., KLAIBER, E. L., & VOGEL, W., 1974, Short-term versus long-term effects of adrenal hormones on behaviors, Psychol. Bull. 81:672.

BRUSH, F. R., 1971, Retention of aversively motivated behavior in "Aversive Conditioning and Learning," (F. R. Brush, ed.), pp. 401-460, Academic Press, New York.

BUCKINGHAM, J. C., & HODGES, J. R., 1974, The redox bioassay technique for the direct assessment of pituitary adrenocorticotrophic activity in the rat, Clin. Endocrin. 3:347.

CHALMERS, D. V., HOHF, J. C., & LEVINE, S., 1974, The effects of prior aversive stimulation on the behavioral and physiological responses to intense acoustic stimuli in the rat, Physiol. Behav. 12:711.

CHAYEN, J., LOVERIDGE, N., & DALY, J. R., 1972, A sensitive bioassay for adrenocorticotrophic hormone in human plasma, Clin. Endocrin. 3:219.

CIARANELLO, R. D., BARCHAS, J. D., & VERNIKOS-DANELLIS, J., 1969, Compensatory hypertrophy and phenylethanolamine N-methyl transferase (PNMT) activity in the rat adrenal, Life Sci. 8:401, part 1.

CLEGG, P. C., & CLEGG, A. G., 1969, "Hormones, Cells and Organisms, the Role of Hormones in Mammals," Stanford University Press, Stanford.

CONNER, R. L., & LEVINE, S., 1969, The effect of adrenal hormones on the acquisition of signalled avoidance behavior, Horm. Behav. 1:73.

CONNER, R. L., VERNIKOS-DANELLIS, J., & LEVINE, S., 1971, Stress, fighting and neuroendocrine function, Nature 234:564.

COOVER, G. D., GOLDMAN, D. L., & LEVINE, S., 1971a, Plasma corticosterone levels during extinction of a lever-press response in hippocampectomized rat, Physiol. Behav. 7:727.

COOVER, G., GOLDMAN, D. L., & LEVINE, S., 1971b, Plasma corticosterone increases produced by extinction of operant behavior in rats, Physiol. Behav. 6:261.

COOVER, G. D., URSIN, H., & LEVINE, S., 1973, Plasma corticosterone levels during active-avoidance learning in rats, J. Comp. Physiol. Psychol. 82:170.

DALLMAN, M. F., & JONES, M. T., 1973a, Corticosteroid feedback control of stress-induced ACTH secretion, in Brain-Pituitary-Adrenal Interrelationships," (A. Brodish & E. S. Redgate, eds.), pp. 176-196, S. Karger, New York.

DALLMAN, M. F., & JONES, M. T., 1973b, Corticosteroid feedback control of ACTH secretion: Effect of stress-induced corticosterone secretion on subsequent stress responses in the rat, Endocrinology 92:1367.

DALLMAN, M. F., & YATES, F. E., 1968, Anatomical and functional mapping of central neural input and feedback pathways of the adrenocortical system, in "The Investigation of Hypothalamic-Pituitary-Adrenal Function," (V. H. T. James & J. Landon, eds.), pp. 39-72, Cambridge University Press, Cambridge.

DALLMAN, M. F., & YATES, F. E., 1969, Dynamic asymmetries in the corticosteroid feedback path and distribution-metabolism-binding elements of the adrenocortical system, Ann. N. Y. Acad. Sci. 156:696.

DEMPSEY, G. L., KASTIN, A. J., & SCHALLY, A. V., 1972, The effects
    of MSH on a restricted passive avoidance response, Horm.
    Behav. 3:333.

DE WIED, D., VAN DELFT, A. M. L., GISPEN, W. H., WEIJNEN, J. A.
    W. M. & VAN WIMERSMA GREIDANUS, Tj. B., 1972, The role of
    pituitary-adrenal system hormones in active avoidance condi-
    tioning, in "Active Avoidance Conditioning," (S. Levine, ed.),
    pp. Academic Press, New York.

DE WIED, D., & WEIJNEN, J. A. W. M. (eds.), 1970, "Pituitary,
    Adrenal and the Brain, Progress in Brain Research," v. 32,
    Elsevier, Amsterdam.

DI GIUSTO, E. L., 1972, Adrenaline or peripheral noradrenaline de-
    pletion and passive avoidance in the rat, Physiol. Behav.
    8:1059.

DI GIUSTO, E. L., CAIRNCROSS, K., & KING, M. G., 1971, Hormonal
    influences on fear-motivated responses, Psychol. Bull. 75:
    432-442.

DI GIUSTO, E. L., KING, M. G., 1972, Chemical sympathectomy and
    avoidance learning in the rat, J. Comp. Physiol. Psychol.
    81:491-500.

DUFFY, E., 1962, "Activation and Behavior," Wiley, New York.

FORTIER, C., & DEGROOT, J., 1959, Adenohypophyseal corticotrophin
    and plasma free corticosteroids during regeneration of the
    enucleated rat adrenal gland, Amer. J. Physiol. 196:589.

FROEHLICH, J. C., 1974, The effect of injected corticosterone on
    the adrenal response in rats exposed to ether and cold stress,
    (Unpublished M. S. Thesis), Syracuse University.

GANONG, W. F., & MARTINI, L. (eds.), "Frontiers in Neuroendocrin-
    ology," 1969, Oxford, New York.

GANONG, W. F., & MARTINI, L. (eds.), 1973, "Frontiers in Neuro-
    endocrinology," Oxford, New York.

GARRUD, P., GRAY, J. A., & DE WIED, D., 1974, Pituitary-adrenal
    hormones and extinction of rewarded behaviour in the rat,
    Physiol. Behav. 12:109.

GISPEN, W. H., VAN WIMERSMA GREIDANUS, TJ. B., & DE WIED, D.,
    1970, Effects of hypophysectomy and $ACTH_{1-10}$ on responsive-
    ness to electric shock in rats, Physiol. Behav. 5:143.

GOLDMAN, L., COOVER, G. D., LEVINE, S., 1973, Bidirectional effects of reinforcement shifts on pituitary adrenal activity, Physiol. Behav. 10:209.

GUTH, S., LEVINE, S., & SEWARD, J. P., 1971, Appetetive acquisition and extinction effects with exogenous ACTH, Physiol. Behav. 7:195.

GUTH, S., SEWARD, J. P., & LEVINE, S., 1971, Differential manipulation of passive avoidance by exogenous ACTH, Horm. Behav. 2:127.

HARRIS, R. K., 1973, Acquisition of conditioned avoidance response by hypophysectomized rats, J. Comp. Physiol. Psychol. 82:254.

HEBB, D. O., 1955, Drives and the C. N. S. (conceptual nervous system), Psychol. Rev. 62:243.

HENKIN, R. I., 1970, The effects of corticosteroids and ACTH on sensory systems, in "Pituitary, Adrenal and the Brain, Progress in Brain Research," (D. De Wied & J. A. W. M. Weijnen, eds.), 32:270-294, Elsevier, Amsterdam.

HODGES, J. R., & JONES, M. T., 1964, Changes in pituitary corticotropic function in adrenalectomized rat, J. Physiol. 173: 190.

HUCKLEBRIDGE, F. H., & NOWELL, N. W., 1974, Plasma catecholomine response to physical and psychological aspects of fighting in mice, Physiol. Behav. 13:35.

JAMES, V. H. T., & LANDON, J. (eds.), 1968, "The Investigation of Hypothalamic-Pituitary-Adrenal Function," Cambridge University Press, Cambridge.

JONES, M. T., BRUSH, F. R., & NEAME, R. L. B., 1972, Characteristics of fast feedback control of corticotrophin release by corticosteroids, J. Endocrin. 55:489.

JONES, M. F., TIPTAFT, E. M., BRUSH, F. R., FERGUSSON, D. A. N., & NEAME, R. L. B., 1974, Evidence for dual corticosteroid receptor mechanisms in the feedback control of adrenocorticotrophin secretion, J. Endocrin. 60:223.

LESHNER, A. I., BROOKSHIRE, K. H., & STEWART, C. N., 1971, The effects of adrenal demedullation on conditioned fear, Horm. Behav. 2:43.

LEVINE, S., 1968, Hormones and conditioning, in "Nebraska Symposium on Motivation," (W. J. Arnold, ed.), pp. 85-101,

University of Nebraska Press, Lincoln.

LEVINE, S. (ed.), 1972, "Hormones and Behavior," Academic Press, New York.

LEVINE, S., & MULLINS, R. F., JR., 1966, Hormonal influences on brain organization in infant rats, Science 152:1585.

LEY, K. F., & CORSON, J. A., 1970, Effects of ACTH and zinc phosphate vehicle on shuttlebox CAR, Psychon. Sci. 20:307-309.

LEY, K. F., & CORSON, J. A., 1971, ACTH and zinc phosphate vehicle interact with UCS parameters to influence shuttlebox CAR, Horm. Behav. 2:149.

LISSAK, R. (ed.), 1973, "Hormones and Brain Function," Plenum Press, New York.

LISSAK, R., & ENDROCZI, E., 1967, Involvement of limbic structures in conditioning, motivation, and recent memory, in "Structure and Function of the Limbic System. Progress in Brain Research," (W. R. Adey & T. Tokizane, eds.) 22:246-253, Elsevier, Amsterdam.

MADDEN, J., ROLLINS, J., ANDERSON, D. C., CONNER, R. L., & LEVINE, S., 1971, Preshock-produced intensification of passive avoidance responding and of elevation in corticosteroid level, Physiol. Behav. 7:733.

MARKS, B. H., & VERNIKOS-DANELLIS, J., 1963, Effects of acute stress on the pituitary gland: Action of ethionine on stress-induced ACTH release, Endocrinology 72:582.

MARTINI, L., & GANONG, W. F. (eds.), 1967, "Neuroendocrinology," Academic Press, New York.

MOTTA, M., FRASCHINI, F., & MARTINI, L., 1969, "Short" feedback mechanisms in the control of anterior pituitary function in "Frontiers in Neuroendocrinology," (W. F. Ganong & L. Martini, eds.) pp. 211-254, Oxford, New York.

OVERTON, D. A., 1964, State dependent or "dissociated" learning produced with pentobarbital, J. Comp. Physiol. Psychol. 57:3.

PAGANO, R. R., & LOVELY, R. H., 1972, Diurnal cycle and ACTH facilitation of shuttlebox avoidance, Physiol. Behav. 8:721.

PAPPAS, B. A., & GRAY, P., 1971, Cue value of dexamethasone for fear-motivated behavior, Physiol. Behav. 6:127.

PARE, W. P., & CULLEN, J. W., 1971, Adrenal influences on the
aversive threshold and CER acquisition, Horm. Behav. 2:139.

SAKELLARIS, P. C., 1972, Olfactory thresholds in normal and adrenalectomized rats, Physiol. Behav. 9:495.

SAKELLARIS, P. C., & VERNIKOS-DANELLIS, J., 1974a, Alteration of
pituitary-adrenal dynamics induced by a water deprivation
regimen, Physiol. Behav. 12:1067.

SAKELLARIS, P. C. & VERNIKOS-DANELLIS, J., 1974b, Hyper-reactivity
of the pituitary-adrenal system in rats adapted to chronic
stress, Endocrinology (in press).

SANDMAN, C. A., BECKWITH, B. E., GITTIS, M. M., & KASTIN, A. J.,
1974, Melanocyte-stimulating hormones (MSH) and overtraining
affects on extradimensional shift (EDS) learning, Physiol.
Behav. 13:162.

SANDMAN, C. A., DENMAN, P. M., MILLER, L. H., KNOTT, J. R., SCHALLY,
A. V., & KASTIN, A. J., 1971, Electroencephalographic measures
of melanocyte-stimulating hormone activity, J. Comp. Physiol.
Psychol. 76:103.

SANDMAN, C. A., KASTIN, A. J., & SCHALLY, A. V., 1969, Melanocyte-
stimulating hormone and learned appetitive behavior, Experientia 25:1001.

SANDMAN, C. A., KASTIN, A. J., & SCHALLY, A. V., 1971, Behavioral
inhibition as modified by melanocyte-stimulating hormone (MSH)
and light-dark conditions, Physiol. Behav. 6:45.

SANDMAN, C. A., KASTIN, A. J., SCHALLY, A. V., KENDALL, J. W.,
MILLER, L. H., 1973, Neuroendocrine responses to physical and
psychological stress, J. Comp. Physiol. Psychol. 84:386.

SANDMAN, C. A., MILLER, L. H., KASTIN, A. J., & SCHALLY, A. V.,
1972, A neuroendocrine influence on attention and memory,
J. Comp. Physiol. Psychol. 80:54.

SAWYER, C. H., & GORSKI, R. A. (eds.), 1971, "Steroid Hormones and
Brain Function, UCLA Forum in Medical Sciences, Number 15,"
University of California Press, Berkeley.

SAYERS, G., & SAYERS, M. A., 1947, Regulation of pituitary adrenocorticotrophic activity during the response of the rat to acute
stress, Endocrinology 40:265.

SCHAYER, R. W., 1964, A unified theory of glucocorticoid action, Perspect. Biol. Med. 8:71.

SCHAYER, R. W., 1967, A unified theory of glucocorticoid action, II, on a circulatory basis for the metabolic effects of glucocorticoids, Perspect. Biol. Med. 10:409.

SELIGMAN, M. E. P., MAIER, S. F., & SOLOMON, R. L., 1971, Unpredictable and uncontrollable aversive events, in "Aversive Conditioning and Learning," (F. R. Brush, ed.) pp. 347-401.

SELYE, H., 1950, "Stress," ACTA, Montreal.

SMELIK, P. G., 1963, Relation between blood levels of corticoids and their inhibiting effects on the hypophyseal stress response, Proc. Soc. Exp. Biol. Med. 113:616.

SMELIK, P. L., 1969, The regulation of ACTH secretion, Acta Physiol. Pharm. 15:123-135, Netherlands.

SMITH, G. P., 1973, Adrenal Hormones and Emotional Behavior, in "Progress in Physiological Psychology," (E. Stellar & J. M. Sprague, eds.), pp. 291-351, Academic Press, New York.

TAYLOR, A. N., MATHESON, G. K., & DAFNY, N., 1971, Modification of the responsiveness of components of the limbic-midbrain circuit by corticosteroids and ACTH, in "Steroid Hormones and Brain Function, UCLA Forum in Medical Sciences, Number 15," (C. H. Sawyer & R. A. Gorski, eds.), pp. 67-68, University of California Press, Berkeley.

VAN LOON, G. R., 1973, Brain catecholamines and ACTH secretion, in "Frontiers in Neuroendocrinology," (W. F. Ganong & L. Martini, eds.), pp. 209-247, Oxford Press, New York.

VERNIKES-DANELLIS, J., 1968, The pharmacological approach to the study of the mechanisms regulating ACTH secretion, in "Pharmacology of Hormonal Polypeptides and Proteins," (N. Back, L. Martini, and R. Paoletti, eds.), pp. 175-189, Plenum Press, New York.

VERNIKOS-DANELLIS, J., CIARANELLO, R. D., & BARCHAS, J. D., 1968, Adrenal epinephrine and phenylethanolainine N-methyl transferase (PNMT) activity in the rat having a transplantable pituitary tumor, Endocrinology 83:1357.

VERNIKOS-DANELLIS, J., & MARKS, B. H., 1962, Epinephrine-induced release of ACTH in normal human subjects: A test of pituitary function, Endocrinology 70:525.

WEIJNEN, J. A. W. M., & SLANGEN, J. L., 1970, Effects of ACTH
    analogues on extinctions of conditioned behavior, in "Pitui-
    tary, Adrenal and the Brain, Progress in Brain Research,"
    (D. De Wied & J. A. W. M. Weijnen, eds.), 32:221-235,
    Elsevier, Amsterdam.

WEISS, J. M., & GRAY, P., 1973, Hormones and avoidance behavior:
    A different approach points to a role for mineralocorticoids,
    in "Drug Effects on Neuroendocrine Regulation, Progress in
    Brain Research," (D. De Wied & J. A. W. M. Weijnen, (eds.)
    39:471-480, Elsevier, Amsterdam.

WEISS, J. M., MCEWEN, B. S., SILVA, M. T., & KALKNUT, M. F., 1970,
    Pituitary-adrenal alterations and fear responding, Amer.
    J. Physiol. 218:864.

WEISS, J. M., MCEWEN, B. S., TERESA, M., SILVA, A., & KALKUT, M. F.,
    1969, Pituitary-adrenal influences on fear responding, Science
    163:197.

YATES, F. E., LEEMAN, S. E., GLENISTER, D. W., & DALLMAN, M. F.,
    1961, Interaction between plasma corticosterone concentration
    and adrenocorticotrophin-releasing stimuli in the rat: evi-
    dence for the reset of an endocrine feedback control, Endo-
    crinology 69:67.

ZIMMERMANN, E., GISPEN, W. H., MARKS, B. H., & DE WIED, D. (eds.)
    "Drug Effects on Neuroendocrine Regulation, Progress in Brain
    Research, Volume 39," Elsevier, Amsterdam.

SUBJECT INDEX

Pages 1-439 will be found in Volume 1, pages 441-806 in Volume 2